# Applications of Counseling in Speech-Language Pathology and Audiology

# Applications of Counseling in Speech-Language Pathology and Audiology

EDITOR

## THOMAS A. CROWE, Ph.D.

Chair and Professor
Department of Communicative Disorders
Director, Center for Speech and Hearing Research
The University of Mississippi
University, Mississippi

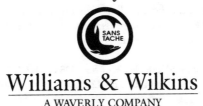

## Williams & Wilkins
### A WAVERLY COMPANY

BALTIMORE • PHILADELPHIA • LONDON • PARIS • BANGKOK
BUENOS AIRES • HONG KONG • MUNICH • SYDNEY • TOKYO • WROCLAW

*Editor:* John P. Butler
*Managing Editor:* Linda S. Napora
*Production Coordinator:* Anne Stewart-Seitz
*Copy Editor:* Joann Nash
*Designer:* Dan Pfisterer
*Typesetter:* Peirce Graphic Services, Inc., Stuart, Florida
*Printer:* Vicks Lithograph & Printing, Yorkville, New York

Copyright © 1997 Williams & Wilkins

351 West Camden Street
Baltimore, Maryland 21201–2436 USA

Rose Tree Corporate Center
1400 North Providence Road
Building II, Suite 5025
Media, Pennsylvania 19063–2043 USA

*Printed in the United States of America*

**Library of Congress Cataloging-in-Publication Data**

Applications of counseling in speech-language pathology and audiology
/ editor, Thomas A. Crowe
p.      cm.
Includes bibliographical references and index.
ISBN 0–683-02216-4 (alk. paper)
1. Communicative disorders—Patients—counseling of. I. Crowe, Thomas Ashley,
1947—.
[DNLM: 1. Speech Disorders—therapy.   2. Language Disorders—therapy.   3. Counseling—methods. 3.   4. Hearing Disorders—therapy.
WM 474 A652 1997]
RC423.A656 1997
616.85′506—dc20
DNLM/DLC
for Library of Congress                                                                96–9331
                                                                                                           CIP

*The publishers have made every effort to trace the copyright holders for borrowed material. If they have inadvertently overlooked any, they will be pleased to make the necessary arrangements at the first opportunity.*

To purchase additional copies of this book, call our customer service department at **(800) 638–0672** or fax orders to **(800) 447–8438.** For other book services, including chapter reprints and large quantity sales, ask for the Special Sales department.

Canadian customers should call **(800) 268–4178,** or fax **(905) 470–6780.** For all other calls originating outside of the United States, please call **(410) 528–4223** or fax us at **(410) 528–8550.**

**Visit Williams & Wilkins on the Internet:** **http://www.wwilkins.com** or contact our customer service department at **custserv@wwilkins.com.** Williams & Wilkins customer service representatives are available from 8:30 am to 6:00 pm, EST, Monday through Friday, for telephone access.

96 97 98 99 00
1 2 3 4 5 6 7 8 9 10

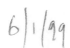
6/1/99

To Sandra, Mark, and Brad
—my life-counselors—

steadfast, true, sustaining

# Foreword

I share with the editor and authors of *Applications of Counseling in Speech-Language Pathology and Audiology* the hope that training in counseling will expand from inclusion in a few programs to become an integral part of the training of speech-language pathologists and audiologists. We are aware that, although many teachers and supervisors in training programs agree on the importance of counseling skills, there is very little room for such training in their programs. There probably are a number of reasons for this lack, two of which come quickly to mind.

First, the certifying arm of ASHA emphasizes knowledge of individual disorders, their differences, and the different treatments deemed appropriate for each. This medical model has resulted in neat categories for certification, but has left little room for work in additional areas. Thus, we have produced numbers of professionals who are extremely knowledgeable about disorders, but quite unaware of the other factors that affect therapy. Furthermore, because so many of the teachers and supervisors have been trained in this model, they cannot be faulted for reluctance to argue for including this new task for which they have little background.

The second reason for lack of emphasis on counseling is today's marvelous technology. It is so easy to put a program into the computer and have it produce a total plan for clients of a given age group with a certain type of disability. Unfortunately, no computer program can deal successfully with all the various contingencies that can arise during a therapy session. This is where the professional's skill in counseling is needed.

However, it has not always been the case that counseling has been de-emphasized. For a period of time during and after World War II, a small number of professionals engaged in speech-language therapy and audiology; most worked in schools. Few of us had many ideas about what to do for a new population disabled by war. This was the toddlerhood of our professions; there was so much to learn in a very short time. We learned from each other and from others who understood disabilities and human behavior: school therapists and teachers, psychologists, nurses, social workers, and others. People in our professions learned from all of them and dared to try new approaches. This reminiscence is *not* to imply that those were the "good old days." Rather, it is to point out that the necessity of learning what to do with an unknown group of clients fostered communication and led to new ideas. Dr. Crowe and his contributors know about counseling and practice it; they discuss counseling as a therapeutic process and they also encourage readers to communicate about the subject and keep on learning.

The book is arranged, as are most texts, with each chapter highlighting a different disorder category. This arrangement is for convenience. These authors understand that, although each person is unique, all share a universe of similar needs, concerns, and emotions. They may also show similar coping behaviors. As you read, think of your own situation and try to apply suggestions to your own population, whatever their disorders may be. I think you can enjoy and learn from this exercise.

As you consider your case load, please do not overlook parents, family members, and other caretakers. You know that a disability has serious ramifications for those people closest to the identified client; they also should be viewed as clients in need of all that counseling entails.

Here you may begin to think anxiously about stumbling blocks to your success in counseling. First, you have not had the same experiences as any client. Of course not; each person builds his or her unique world of experience, never to be duplicated by another. This is not a deterrent to successful practice because it is not on the basis of shared experience that we truly relate to people. Rather, we grow to understand each other better at the level of emotions, values, and attitudes. Anyone old enough to read this book probably has experienced the whole universe of emotions: love, joy, hurt, anger, loss, disappointment, satisfaction. Clients, of course, will not experience these emotions as you did, but if you can remember how you felt, you can imagine something of what a client may be feeling and voice your compassion, thus relating on a more meaningful basis than just the experiential level.

Another stumbling block for many people is lack of time. There probably will never be enough time for all you would like to do, but I think of what I remember Carl Rogers saying at a convention long ago, "If you only have fifteen minutes with a client, you can make it the best fifteen minutes you have to give." This book should prove helpful and enjoyable as well.

Elizabeth J. (Betty) Webster, Ph.D.

*Professor Emeritus, University of Memphis*
*Deerfield Beach, Florida*

# Preface

The question of whether counseling should be essential to the clinical practice of speech-language pathology and audiology is rhetorical. Counseling, in fact, does occur in almost every therapy encounter, whether it is intentionally employed by clinicians to achieve specific therapy goals, or whether it happens spontaneously and unguided toward any purpose. Intentional, informed counseling involves clinicians' use of their personal theory of counseling and counseling and psychotherapy techniques to (a) gain insight into the interpersonal and intrapersonal ramifications of clients' speech, language, and hearing disorder (e.g., by taking case histories in an interrogatory manner and clinical atmosphere that encourages clients to reflect on and fully articulate their concerns, rather than only permitting clients to give limited response to sets of standard questions); (b) impart information to clients that does not increase their anxiety (e.g., interpreting diagnostic test results in a didactic way that leads to goal-setting and positive action by clients); and (c) help clients and their significant others positively adjust to the realities of communicative disorders and to the new behaviors and concept of self that emerge in therapy so as to have maximally productive and contented lives. Unintentional counseling happens, for instance, when clients read meaning into clinicians' inadvertent facial expressions, gestures, voice tone, or comments and modify their attitudes or behaviors because of those impressions. Uninformed counseling occurs when clinicians attempt to influence clients' attitudes or behaviors without having adequate training in counseling, knowledge of and practice with helping skills, and a personal theory of counseling.

Although many speech-language pathologists and audiologists agree that counseling is an elemental and essential aspect of therapy, they disagree on what constitutes counseling, the extent to which counseling should be emphasized in therapy, the balance clinicians should maintain in therapy between counseling and programmatic and technology-based strategies, and whether or not graduate training programs should require coursework and clinical practicum training in counseling. The questions raised include: To what ends should counseling be employed? What approaches to counseling are most applicable to speech-language pathology and audiology? How directive and prescriptive should counseling be? What training in counseling should speech-language pathologists and audiologists receive? How does one build a personal theory of counseling? What particular counseling issues are potentially associated with various communicative disorders?

The purpose of this book is to consider these questions through discussion of general counseling issues and applications and from the perspective of counseling needs and uses specific to speech-language pathology and audiology. The book is organized in two sections.

In Section I (Chapters 1 to 5), counseling is defined generally and then is compared to and distinguished from psychotherapy. A synoptic history of the practice of counseling is provided as well as a rationale for the use of counseling in speech-language pathology and audiology. The influence of emotional variables on the status and treatment of communicative disorders is discussed and an argument for holistic treatment of persons with communicative disorders is presented. Construction of a personal theory of counseling is considered relative to theories of personality development and approaches to counseling. The importance of culturally based factors to the nature of the counseling relationship and the process of the counseling experience is discussed.

Section II (Chapters 6 to 15) concerns counseling within the context of specific disorders of speech, language, and hearing. Although the basic counseling needs for individuals in distress are essentially the same, regardless of what is perceived by them to be the precipitating event of their distress, each individual's unique circumstances present unique challenges that might need to be addressed in counseling. This is true for individuals with speech, language, and hearing disorders. These individuals, their parents, and their significant others share many similar feelings and experiences irrespective of the nature of each individual's disorder type. But each type of communicative disorder carries with it potentially unique crises and challenges for clients and their supporting others, although the status of those crises and challenges is largely dependent on highly individualized client characteristics. In this second section of the book, counseling is discussed relative to general, rather than individualized, disorder features and client characteristics.

It is hoped that speech-language pathologists and audiologists' recently renewed interest in counseling as a therapeutic process continues to grow so that their clients, not just their clients' communicative facility, will benefit maximally from therapy. In an indictment of the fundamental problem in Western culture, Carl Jung posited, well before our current computer culture existed, that through technology humankind had mastered the world at the cost of its soul. That thought is a bit extreme perhaps, but it should serve as a caution to speech-language pathologists and audiologists that they should interact with the client as well as with the machine and should help the person as well as the disorder.

Thomas A. Crowe

*Oxford, Mississippi*

# Acknowledgments

I am especially indebted to my wife, Sandra C. Crowe, for her expert and exacting technical assistance with preparation of the manuscript and for her unflagging enthusiasm for and encouragement of the project; she should by rights be designated co-editor.

My sincere appreciation is extended to my research assistants at the University of Mississippi, Anthony DiLollo and Bradley T. Crowe, who spared me much of the library servitude attendant to such an undertaking, helped me prepare the references for Chapters 1 through 4, and inspired me to maintain my excitement for the project by their constant and genuine expression of interest in it.

Special thanks to Mark A. Crowe who researched articles for me in the Lister Hill Library at the University of Alabama School of Medicine.

I am grateful to Dean H. Dale Abadie for facilitating my sabbatical leave to complete this book; without that respite from the demands and distractions of chairing an academic department the project would have been unduly protracted.

My thanks also are extended to my departmental colleagues and staff who covered for me in my absence for the better part of a year and cheered me down the interminable homestretch. I should like to thank one colleague in particular, Sue T. Hale, who assumed the duties of department chair while I was on sabbatical leave; that really was above and beyond behavior and I am most grateful to her for it. My secretary, Maribel Sullivan-Gonzalez, played a major role in managing logistic aspects of the project and I appreciate her conscientious work. I am grateful as well to my many other colleagues in speech-language pathology, audiology, and psychology who advised and assisted me in the conception and production of the book.

I am sincerely appreciative of the good work by all of the contributing authors; working with them was an eminently pleasurable as well as an intellectually profitable experience.

John P. Butler and Linda S. Napora at Williams & Wilkins made my editorial tasks appreciably less onerous with their patient guidance throughout the process; I am grateful for their positive instruction.

# Contributors

Jerome G. Alpiner, Ph.D.
*Department of Veterans Affairs Medical Center*
*Coordinator of Audiology*
*Audiology and Speech Pathology Services*
*Denver, Colorado*

Kenn Apel, Ph.D.
*Associate Professor*
*Department of Speech Pathology and Audiology*
*Western Washington University*
*Bellingham, Washington*

Dolores E. Battle, Ph.D.
*Professor*
*Department of Speech-Language Pathology*
*State University College at Buffalo*
*Buffalo, New York*

Eugene B. Cooper, Ed.D.
*Professor and Chair Emeritus*
*Department of Communicative Disorders*
*The University of Alabama*
*Tuscaloosa, Alabama*

Thomas A. Crowe, Ph.D.
*Chair and Professor*
*Department of Communicative Disorders*
*Director, Center for Speech and Hearing Research*
*University, Mississippi*

Stuart I. Gilmore, Ph.D.
*Visiting Professor*
*Department of Communicative Disorders*
*The University of Mississippi*
*University, Mississippi*

Mary Blake Huer, Ph.D.
*Professor*
*Department of Speech Communication*
*Program in Communicative Disorders*
*California State University-Fullerton*
*Fullerton, California*

Julie J. Masterson, Ph.D.
*Professor*
*Department of Communication Sciences and Disorders*
*Southwest Missouri State University*
*Springfield, Missouri*

Betty Jane McWilliams
*Professor*
*Communication and Dental Medicine*
*Director Emeritus*
*Cleft Palate Craniofacial Center*
*University of Pittsburgh*
*Pittsburgh, Pennsylvania*

Lisa Lucks Mendel, Ph.D.
*Associate Professor*
*Coordinator of Audiology*
*Department of Communicative Disorders*
*Assistant Director*
*Center for Speech and Hearing Research*
*University of Mississippi*
*University, Mississippi*

Paul R. Rao, Ph.D.
*Executive Director of Clinical Services*
*National Rehabilitation Hospital*
*Adjunct Professor*
*Audiology and Speech Pathology*
*Gallaudet University*
*Washington, D.C.*
*Department of Speech Pathology, Loyola College*
*Baltimore, Maryland*

R. E. (Ed) Stone, Jr., Ph.D.
*Director, Speaking Arts & Sciences Associate Professor*
*The Vanderbilt Voice Center*
*Nashville, Tennessee*

# Contents

Section 1.

# Theoretic Foundations
# of Counseling

# 1. Counseling: Definition, History, Rationale

Thomas A. Crowe

The general nature of counseling is considered in this chapter. Although a consensus definition of counseling is difficult to elucidate (Tyler, 1969), general statements can be made about what it is and what it is not. The evolution of counseling as a clinical process is summarized in this chapter and the relationship of current day counseling practices to the guidance movement is discussed. After defining counseling in terms of its aspects and origins, a rationale is presented for the application of counseling to clinical practice in speech-language pathology and audiology.

## COUNSELING DEFINED

Counseling is a scholarly discipline, a social science, and a clinical or helping process, which makes it an applied science. The process of counseling is an art that derives from theoretic foundations within the science. The discipline of counseling is grounded in various other disciplines including philosophy, religion, psychology, education, anthropology, and sociology. Glanz (1974) noted that economics is also a foundation discipline in counseling in that the study of economics includes research and intervention with interpersonal relationships in the workplace.

The art-science nature of counseling and its multidisciplinary character make it difficult to define counseling concisely and inclusively. Difficulty arises also from various lay and professional opinions of the degree of synonymy among counseling, interviewing, guidance, and psychotherapy. In particular, confusion about the demarcation between the clinical provinces of counseling and psychotherapy are troublesome to clinicians not schooled in psychotherapy technique. Therefore, rather than risk their counseling efforts becoming or being construed as psychotherapy, some clinicians avoid counseling altogether as part of their practice.

In the following discussion counseling is considered as an art and as a science, as a process applicable to numerous disciplines, and as a clinical endeavor distinguishable from, although overlapping with, psychotherapy.

### Counseling as an Art and as a Science

THE ART OF COUNSELING

As an art, counseling involves both the personal attributes of clinicians that are important to their general effectiveness as counselors and the helping skills that ensure the efficacy

3

of the client-clinician relationship. The art of counseling also involves the degree to which clinicians can appropriately use their personal attributes and helping skills to assist clients of various ages, sexes, and cultures; clients with different belief systems; and clients with problems varying in type and severity. Nystul (1993) describes the art of counseling as the clinician's flexibility and creativity in therapy.

The personal attributes and interpersonal skills that successful clinicians bring to the art of counseling determine the nature of the client-clinician relationship and the clinician's congruency in that relationship. The American Psychological Association (1947) identified the following characteristics as personal attributes of persons suited to be counselors and psychotherapists: resourcefulness, versatility, curiosity, respect for the integrity of other individuals, awareness of own personality traits, humor, tolerance, ability to relate warmly to others, industry, responsibility, integrity, stability, and ethics. Rogers (1959) suggests that for clinicians to be successful in counseling they must be capable of being congruent in the counseling relationship, have unconditional positive regard for their clients, and display empathic understanding of their clients' internal frame of reference. Truax and Mitchell (1971) concur that effective counselors are genuine and authentic, and show nonpossessive warmth for their clients. Concrete expression of feelings and experiences, by both clinician and client, is also considered to be a primary facilitating characteristic of successful counseling relationships (Carkhuff & Berenson, 1967).

Desirable helping skills for counselors to possess include verbal and nonverbal skills they can use to help clients identify and modify maladaptive behaviors and recognize and resolve emotions that are barriers to therapy progress (Egan, 1982; Kanfer & Goldstein, 1980; Okun, 1987). Hackney and Cormier (1988) identify three general types of skills counselors should possess: *interpersonal skills, discrimination or conceptualization skills,* and *intervention skills.* These skills are used in counseling to help clients develop an understanding of themselves and others, to comfort clients and help them manage crises, and to help them take action that results in positive changes in their behavior (Brammer, 1973).

Clinicians can promote clients' *self-understanding* by using the skills of *listening, indirect and direct leading, reflecting, summarizing, confronting, interpreting,* and *informing.* Listening skills, in particular, are important to counselors, especially as used in nondirective counseling (Moursund, 1990). If clients perceive that a clinician is assiduously *attending* to their verbalizations about themselves and their problems, then the clients will be more inclined to attend to the thoughts and feelings represented in those verbalizations. Attending to and reflecting on their own verbalizations helps clients *clarify* and understand their *thoughts, feelings,* and *behaviors*—the three interactive dimensions of the client-clinician relationship. This in turn establishes the conditions for change to occur in a client's thoughts and feelings and consequently in behavior or, conversely, for changes to occur in behavior that result in changes in thoughts and feelings.

In addition to attending, listening skills include the use of *paraphrasing, perception checking, summaries,* and *I statements. Paraphrasing* (e.g., "You're saying that you think your father is responsible for your having developed stuttering and you are angry with him for that") and *perception checking,* (e.g., "I take it, from what you've said, that you think that therapy is not going to help you improve your speech. Is that accurate?") are both used by clinicians to clarify a client's comments and to determine the accuracy of the clinician's understanding of them. *Summaries* are used to open or close discussion of an issue, to assess the progress of counseling, to focus a client's thoughts and feelings so that he or she can more fully examine issues at hand, and to reinforce progress in therapy. *I statements* convey a clinician's thoughts and feelings to clients, thereby establishing a congruent counseling relationship and promoting a client's self-understanding (e.g., "I think you, rather than I, should determine your goals in therapy" and "It is not clear to me why you think your hearing loss has caused others to lose their positive regard for you").

Helping skills used to *comfort during crises* include *reassuring support* of clients, *crisis intervention* through consolation and hope building, *centering strategies* used to help clients identify their strengths and remember positive past experiences, and *referral* to other services at critical instances in the counseling process. Skill with referral is especially important. Although on the surface referral might not appear to be a counseling skill, it does require an acute perception of the client's verbal and nonverbal behaviors that signal the need for referral and an understanding of those behaviors to make appropriate and timely referrals.

Clinicians can also use *silence* to demonstrate support and caring for clients during crises and to facilitate progress in therapy. Through silence, which may be induced by the counselor or by the client, a counselor can express a number of therapeutic messages to a client, from disagreement with a client's behavior to empathic understanding of any concerns. Clinicians can use silence to help clients reflect on their comments and defensive emotions and to discover for themselves strategies to resolve their crises (Hackney & Cormier, 1988).

Brammer (1973) notes that clients can be helped to take *positive action* toward changing behaviors by learning to solve problems and make decisions. To facilitate the acquisition of *problem-solving* and *decision-making* skills by the client, counselors can help them identity and analyze their problems, explore possible solutions to the problems, select plans of action, view their problems in terms of goals and, once the present problems are resolved, generalize the effective strategies used to resolve them to new problems that might arise. Numerous models of problem-solving can be found in the literature (e.g., Dixon & Glover, 1984; Stewart, Winborn, Johnson, Burks, & Engelkes, 1978).

*Contract building* is a technique clinicians can use to help clients develop problem-solving and decision-making skills. Contracting for behavioral change can help a client learn to identify maladaptive behaviors, establish priorities among the behaviors targeted for change, develop sequences of intermediate goals and end-goals of therapy, establish strategies to achieve the behavior change goals, set time limits for change to occur, and form a partnership with the clinician that is defined in terms of the expected roles and commitments of both. A discussion of contract building is found in Moursund, 1990; Steiner, 1974; Webster, 1977.

THE SCIENCE OF COUNSELING

Counseling, as a science, involves applying standard scientific process to the helping relationship. The scientific process is composed of observing, stating presuppositions, drawing inferences, forming hypotheses, testing hypotheses, and establishing theories. The theories then form the bases for clinicians on how to approach counseling practice, and how to apply their personal attributes, helping skills, and counseling adaptability and ingenuity. Not everyone, however, accepts the premise that science is a descriptor that can be applied to counseling or that scientific process and counseling practice are mutually dependent activities.

Can counseling be science and application or is it application only? Can its underlying theories be tested? The answers are yes and no. Certainly, the efficacy of clinical intervention through counseling can be stated by gathering empirical data through systematic observation of therapy and presenting those data as individual case studies or as longitudinal group findings. Personality development theories can be tested through observation of the temporal manifestations of behaviors assumed to mark epigenetic stages. Thus, one could argue that Freud's psychosexual developmental stages, or aspects thereof (e.g., the

Oedipus complex) or Erickson's eight ages of man have been scientifically validated by decades of careful empirical testing and thereby have moved from inference to theory. But this argument can be carried only so far in defending counseling as a science. It becomes difficult to satisfy fully a definition of counseling in terms of scientific process in a practice that deals with elements of being and change that to a large extent are hidden from the eye of empirical observation, whether one regards those elements as unconscious or merely unspoken.

Pepinsky and Pepinsky (1954) suggest that the relationship between the science and the practice of counseling is a symbiotic one and present a model to illustrate this mutually dependent interrelationship. The scientist-as-counselor or counselor-as-scientist model serves to increase the accountability of counseling services to the client's benefit. Through research, the counselor-as-scientist continually tests his or her personal approaches to therapy and the theories on which they are based. That testing, in turn, leads clinicians to make continuing adjustments both to their personal theories and to their clinical technique. The relevance of theory to the practice of counseling and the importance of constructing personal theories of personality and counseling are discussed more fully in Chapter 3.

## The Multidisciplinary Nature of Counseling

Because of its multidisciplinary base, counseling is difficult to define inclusively, as one's conceptualization of counseling as an art or as a science is unavoidably determined to a large extent by the discipline to which it is applied. Counseling might have quite different specific denotations, although not so many different general connotations, to a minister than to a psychologist or to a cultural anthropologist than to a speech-language pathologist or audiologist. Professionals from diverse disciplines explore different questions when counseling. They are exposed to varying aspects of counseling during their professional education, address different problems in the practice of counseling, and expect different outcomes of counseling practice. An economist might have counseling questions chiefly about workplace dynamics, whereas a philosopher's questions might center on less prosaic concerns, such as questions about human behavior relative to the meaning of existence. There is far less exposure to clinical counseling theory and practice in the study of economics and philosophy than in the study of clinical psychology and ministerial religion; counseling training in speech-language pathology and audiology falls somewhere in the middle with the type and amount of training varying appreciably among training programs.

It might be said that the basic focus of counseling from any professional vantage is on stress, anxiety, guilt, and depression, and on the roles emotions play in personality formation and human behavior, particularly when out of both conscious control and typical proportion. The assumed causes of states of feeling becoming unhealthy are different when viewed from the various foundation disciplines of counseling—for instance, sociologists look to urban malaise; ministers look to spiritual vacuity or vacillation; speech-language pathologists and audiologists look to communicative disorders. Regardless of one's discipline, it might be said that the universal aim of counseling inquiry and intervention is a society composed of self-actualizing, reality oriented citizens who can cope, although one's discipline does to an extent dictate desired outcome of counseling. Successful counseling outcome to an economist might be measured not only by degree of positive changes in the attitudes of employees toward their jobs and co-workers, but also by the degree of change in product enhancement or production volume as a result of changes in workers' attitudes. A speech-language pathologist or an audiologist might measure the success of counseling by the extent to which they are able to help clients or the parents of clients become or re-main fully functioning and self-actualizing individuals despite having to encounter life with speech, language, or hearing problems. They might also judge the success of coun-seling by how effective it is in improving the prognosis for successful therapy with a client's communicative disorder or by how effectively counseling can be used to treat certain com-municative disorders.

A consensus definition for counseling is elusive also within the contexts of individual disciplines because numerous theoretic bases for counseling study and practice exist within each of its foundation disciplines. Although all of the foundation disciplines of counseling share a general base of counseling theories, professionals within each discipline operate from differing composite personal theories of normal and abnormal personality develop-ment, behavior, and behavioral intervention. The theories to which individuals within each discipline ascribe determine, in large measure, their definition of counseling, regardless of their discipline. Add to this these facts: that the field of counseling is relatively new; it is growing rapidly; new theories and approaches to practice are frequently being introduced; thus, the problem with defining counseling becomes a difficult one (Hansen, Stevic, & Warner, Jr., 1982). Shertzer and Stone (1971) note that the different uses by various authors of the term "guidance" to convey their personal opinions and biases ultimately made that term meaningless. To an extent, the same is true for the term counseling.

## Counseling and Psychotherapy

As discussed in more detail later in this chapter, modern counseling practices originated to a considerable degree in the guidance movement of the 1930s through the 1960s. Early in the movement, during the first half of the 20th century, the counseling emphasis in schools was on vocational and educational guidance only. Personal adjustment counseling, rarely recommended for students, was left to professionals other than school counselors. As the guidance movement progressed, school counselors were expected to acquire the psy-chotherapy skills necessary to help students resolve emotional and self-concept barriers to achieving their vocational and educational goals and to becoming fully functioning indi-viduals. This created a dilemma that still exists, both for school counselors and for all pro-fessionals who employ counseling to achieve the desired outcomes respective to their pro-fessions. Namely, the dilemma was and is: Is counseling necessarily psychotherapy and, if not, how is one distinguishable from the other? Is there a definable demarcation between the two? How far can psychotherapy skills be taken by clinicians in counseling students or clients before the counseling is more accurately termed "psychotherapy?"

These questions were important in the 1960s, both to school counselors and to those who practiced in the specialized areas of counseling that had emerged or were gaining more attention in the 1970s; for example, marriage counselors, family mediators, drug and alcohol counselors, pastoral counselors, community mental health counselors, psychiatric social workers, and counselors of the disabled. A legitimate fear was that clinicians might inadvertently extend beyond their ethical practice by not knowing the answers to those questions, which is perhaps the single most important reason that speech-language pathologists and audiologists often avoid counseling with clients altogether. To dispel any notions that they use psychotherapy to any degree in clinical intervention with speech, lan-guage, and hearing disordered persons, they conceptualize counseling to be interviewing, case history taking, information giving in a didactic sense, and discussing fees for services. Counseling as a clinical technique or process is, however, not only these activities. By some definitions it is psychotherapy, but distinctions between the terms counseling and psychotherapy can be drawn.

In terms of clinical process, counseling and psychotherapy have been viewed as being synonymous (Albert, 1966; Ard 1966; Balinsky & Blum, 1951; Curran, 1968). Although not identical clinical processes, counseling and psychotherapy share therapy techniques so that each one constitutes, in part, the other. Hinsie and Campbell (1970) define counseling as:

> A type of psychotherapy of the supportive or re-educative variety; often the term is applied to behavioral problems not strictly classifiable as mental illnesses, such as vocational or school or marriage problems. (p. 166)

And psychotherapy as:

> Any form of treatment for mental illnesses, behavioral maladaptions, and/or other problems that are assumed to be of an emotional nature . . . for the purpose of removing, modifying, or retarding existing symptoms, of attenuating or reversing disturbed patterns of behavior, and of promoting positive personality growth and development.
>     There are numerous forms of psychotherapy—ranging from guidance, counseling, persuasion, and hypnosis to re-education and psychoanalytic reconstructive therapy. . . . (p. 631)

In the above definitions, counseling is described as a type of psychotherapy and psychotherapy as a type of counseling. This would not appear at first glance to help significantly distinguish between the two terms, but several differences are suggested in these definitions. First, one can infer from them that counseling is used to treat less severe problems and disorders than are treated with other types of psychotherapy. Second, indicated in these definitions is that counseling addresses behavioral problems that are consequential to external events, roles, role identities, decisions, and life circumstances. For instance, problems within families and marriages or difficulty in choosing a vocation or educational direction, can result in thought, emotional, and behavioral problems that are not conducive to an individual experiencing positive growth and productive self-insight; these problems are treated by counseling. Although not external to the individual in the same sense as are role problems or problems of vocational-educational choices, communicative disorders might be perceived by individuals who are communicatively disordered to be the cause of the secondary maladaptive reactions experienced by them (e.g., they might perceive, accurately or inaccurately, that their communicative disorder is causing a vocational problem). Psychotherapy is defined not as much in terms of related contexts as is counseling, but more in terms of the client's maladaptive symptoms relative to basic problems in personality development and personal adjustment. Third, if, as the definitions above instruct, counseling typically concerns an individual's problems relative to a role or to a dynamic phenomenal field psychotherapy essentially concern individuals with mental illness, then it can be said that counseling is applicable more to interpersonal problems and psychotherapy to intrapersonal problems. Fourth, Hinsie and Campbell (1970) indicate that counseling is a supportive and re-educative type of psychotherapy, which is in reference to Wolberg's (1988) classification of psychotherapy into three basic approaches: supportive, re-educative, and reconstructive.

The *supportive approach* to psychotherapy is used when a client's abilities can be enhanced to attain an optimal state of self-control. Techniques used in supportive therapy include environment control, catharsis, persuasion, reassurance, and desensitization. These techniques are not altogether unfamiliar to most speech-language pathologists and audiologists and at times can occur clinically, spontaneously, and undirected; they have a positive effect in counseling when used by clinicians in a deliberate, controlled manner. *Re-educative therapy* involves helping a client understand the nature of conscious conflicts being experienced and resolve those conflicts by using personal assets. The psychotherapy techniques of relationship therapy, attitude therapy, and reconditioning are used in re-educative therapy. Group therapy is used in both the supportive and re-educative approaches to psychotherapy; in supportive therapy it is inspirationally oriented, and it is insight-oriented in re-educative therapy. In the *reconstructive approach,* importance is placed on recognition and resolution of unconscious conflicts and general reconstruction of the personality using psychoanalytic techniques and psychotherapy procedures. Wolberg (1988) suggests that the supportive and re-educative approaches to psychotherapy are appropriate for counselors to practice and that the reconstructive approach is appropriate for psychotherapists only.

Another indication of the overlap between counseling and psychotherapy is in the desired outcomes of both processes. Although the subgoals of therapy and the strategies used to achieve them might differ, counseling and psychotherapy both are designed to help individuals become fully functioning, adaptive, flexible, socialized beings who are in charge of their lives and who make full use of their potentialities for their own and society's benefit. On the goals of psychotherapy, Wolman (1989) states:

> Through interaction with the clinician and experimentation outside the therapeutic situation, the patient acquires more adaptive skills in interpersonal relations. Consequently, psychotherapy is not a form of treatment for a disease (formerly called neurosis), but it represents a more or less systematic attempt to help a patient achieve maturity, autonomy, responsibility, and skill in adult living. (p.276)

These goals of psychotherapy are not inconsistent with those of counseling.

The techniques and goals shared between counseling and psychotherapy are appreciable and make it difficult to separate them neatly into two distinct clinical activities. Patterson (1980) states that not only are counseling and psychotherapy indistinguishable to the nature of the client-clinician relationship, therapy process, and clinical techniques used in the therapy process, but the array of theories that support both also overlap. A view seemingly in converse exception to the position taken by Patterson is expressed by Belkin (1975): "Counseling is built upon an underlying philosophical foundation, while psychotherapy is built upon an underlying psychopathology, theory of personality, and corpus of specific techniques." (p. 29)

Such disagreement about the identifying essences of counseling and psychotherapy have led some scholars to take a middle-of-the-road approach to the issue. In this view, counseling and psychotherapy are seen as positions on opposite ends of a continuum (Hansen, Stevic, & Warner, 1982; Vance & Volsky, 1962; Wolberg, 1988). Thus, counseling and psychotherapy are seen as related processes, with each one capable at times of approximating the other to some extent depending on the degree of assimilation or sharing of characteristics that define their respective positions on the continuum. Some of these characteristics were discussed earlier in this section.

One of the most frequently mentioned continuum factors that separates counseling and psychotherapy is the severity of the client's problem. Counseling is described as being effective with the "normal" individual; with persons who (*a*) can take responsibility for their growth; (*b*) function adequately; (*c*) have role problems; (*d*) have normal problems; (*e*) have interpersonal problems; or (*f*) have problems of living; and with neurotic persons (Aubrey, 1967; Blocher, 1974; Bordin, 1968; McDaniel & Shaftel, 1956; Mowrer, 1950). Psychotherapy is considered to be appropriate in treating persons suffering from mental illness; those who have conflicts deep within the personality structure; "sick," "seriously disturbed," "neurotic," "pathological," persons; persons with intrapersonal problems; and psychotic persons.

The differences in seriousness of the problems encountered in counseling and psychotherapy indicate that the objectives of therapy might be different for the two activities.

Counseling is designed to help clients examine their personality and behavior relative to specific roles in their lives and to resolve role problems by developing a better under- standing of themselves through that examination (Hansen, Stevic, & Warner, 1982). Psy- chotherapy seeks to reorganize personality in order to bring the client into a state of con- scious control and productive reality. Owing to psychotherapy's focus on deep, complex processes and structures, it is usually more intense, less direct, and lasts longer than coun- seling (Belkin, 1975; Perry, 1955). Nystul (1993) estimates that counseling typically re- quires 3 to 12 weeks for resolution of role-related short-term goals, whereas psychother- apy typically requires 3 to 6 months, or longer, to achieve long-term goals related to severe mental disorders.

Viewed from the perspective of the continuum model, however, two types of problems (role problems and intrapersonal disturbances) can be related and treatment approaches can therefore overlap. For instance, psychotherapy can shift into counseling in treating role problems that have precipitated, exacerbated, or maintained an intrapersonal problem. Once these problems are resolved, short-term therapy is shifted back along the continuum toward psychotherapy for long-term treatment of the intrapersonal problem. On the con- tinuum model, the counselor might use some psychotherapy skills in treating role prob- lems and even mild intrapersonal problems, but at no time would practice completely at the psychotherapy end. Psychotherapists, on the other hand, can ethically perform both the short-term counseling at one end of the continuum and the intensive psychotherapy at the other end.

The continuum model illustrates the relationship between counseling and psy- chotherapy relative to the type and severity of clients' problems. Role problems are repre- sented as responding well to direct guidance and counseling, which become less effective as problems tend to be of a more intrapersonal nature. Problem intensity also determines whether counseling or psychotherapy is the proper treatment, with more intense problems toward the psychotherapy end of the continuum. But it should be noted that a person might have problems at either end of the continuum that vary in degree from mild to se- vere. Although generally speaking intrapersonal problems are more severe than are typi- cal role problems, role problems can at times be very serious, even without the co- existence of an intrapersonal problem. If an intrapersonal problem is present with severe role problems, the intensity level of the intrapersonal problem determines if psychother- apy is advisable and indicates how easily the role problems might respond to counseling.

Brammer and Shostrom (1977) note that counseling involves problems of which the client is consciously aware, use of problem-solving and decision-making skills to resolve those problems, and specific situational contexts in which the client's problems are signif- icant. Psychotherapy is characterized by treatment of unconscious emotional problems, an emphasis on deep probing, and analysis of the client's personality and behavior.

Psychotherapy often takes place in private practice and medical settings; it is practiced chiefly by psychiatrists, clinical psychologists, and psychiatric nurses; all states in the United States require licensure for practice. Counseling occurs in a variety of settings in- cluding schools, health professions clinics, marriage counseling clinics, vocational bureaus, and churches. Whereas psychotherapists practice both counseling and psychotherapy, counseling is practiced by an array of professionals and lay persons who are not qualified to practice psychotherapy and who are not necessarily required to be licensed as coun- selors.

Blocher (1966) suggests that there is also a difference in the client-clinician relation- ships of counseling and psychotherapy. He points out that in psychotherapy the person being helped is regarded as a patient and, as such, does not participate in establishing the goals of therapy. In counseling, the person being helped is called a client. Being regarded as a client serves to create a teacher/student relationship between the counselor and coun-selee wherein they act as partners in determining therapy goals. Counseling is a three-way relationship, with the counselor and client directly interacting with each other and with a role problem. In psychotherapy, the clinician relationship is a direct, two-way one between psychotherapist and client (Hansen, Stevic, & Warner, 1972).

It has been noted in this section that overlap between counseling and psychotherapy does exist in that counselors use psychotherapy skills in counseling. These skills include general personal attributes and helping skills behaviors, but also involve techniques, philosophies, and approaches to counseling that are associated with various schools of psychotherapy. Belkin (1975) considers the various schools of psychotherapy in actuality to be counseling theories and contends that each school has some degree of applicability to both counseling and psychotherapy. In Belkin's view, schools that are grounded to a greater extent on philosophy have more applicability to counseling. Schools that are based on a theory of personality focus on psychopathology and use psychoanalytic techniques have more relevance to psychotherapy.

There are several reasonable inferences that might be drawn from the foregoing de-scriptions of counseling and psychotherapy to attempt to differentiate one from the other. One inference is that counseling asks the question "How?" in regard to how the client's role problems can be resolved; how the client can learn new more effective response pat-terns for decision-making and problem-solving with support from the counselor; and how the client can reduce mild neurotic symptoms (anxiety, depression, stress, guilt) with help from a counselor who uses psychotherapy skills in direct, short-term therapy. Another in-ference is that psychotherapy asks the question "Why?" as well as "How?" Psychotherapy asks how best to help the client using psychotherapy skills applied in intense, long-term therapy; how to reconstruct the client's personality to resolve severe mental disorders (neuroses and psychoses); and how the client's intrapersonal problems are affecting his or her interpersonal relationships. Psychotherapy also asks why the client's personality is dis-ordered, why the client is resistant to change, and why the client has repressed unresolved conflicts and impulses from conscious awareness. Lastly, it can be inferred that counseling and psychotherapy are different processes and are used to treat different types of and de-grees of problems. Overlap of the two does exist, however, and it is not always easy to de-termine when a clinician is practicing one as opposed to the other. One safeguard speech-language pathologists and audiologists can use in identifying the boundaries of counseling is to develop a mindset predicated on the widely accepted descriptors for counseling and psychotherapy.

## Definition of Counseling

Counseling, then, is an applied social science that may be defined as either an art or a sci-ence. The art of counseling concerns its clinical practice and the talents and skills the clini-cian brings to it. The science of counseling concerns the theories that support the art of prac-tice; the formation of those theories through scientific process; and the testing, revision, and validation of theories through ongoing research. The art and the science of counseling are mutually dependent, mutually enhancing dimensions. Because of its multidisciplinary base, the definition of counseling varies among disciplines. Because individual professionals within specific disciplines tend to form their own personal composite theoretic frameworks for counseling research and practice, the definition of counseling also varies within disci-plines. Counseling and psychotherapy are different, although overlapping, activities. Dif-ferent types and degrees of problems are treated in counseling than in psychotherapy, al-though some of the techniques used to treat problems are shared between the two clinical endeavors. In speech-language pathology and audiology, counseling is a helping process that occurs in dyads and in groups. The success of counseling with clients depends to great extent on clinicians' personal attributes and how effectively they use their helping skills. Counseling involves interviewing, guidance, and some measure of psychotherapy, yet is not wholly synonymous with any of those three activities. The purposes of counseling in speech-language pathology and audiology are to:

- gather and convey information
- prevent communicative disorders from developing or from becoming more severe and involved
- help clients adjust emotionally to their disorders and to resist developing defensive behaviors in reaction to their disorders
- help and be supportive of families and significant others in coping with a client's disorder
- help clients correct their communicative disorders by learning decision-making and problem-solving skills and maintaining high motivation levels for therapy
- provide a clinical setting for clients that is optimal for changes to occur in their thinking, feeling, and behaving
- help clients develop the self-reinforcement behaviors and coping strategies that are critical to successful carryover and generalization of therapy results

## HISTORICAL PERSPECTIVE OF COUNSELING

In this section, the development of counseling as a clinical process is cursorily reviewed. This review is intended as a perspective on the historical influences that led to the modern philosophy of intervening in a person's life through counseling. There are basically four periods germane to a discussion of the development of counseling: early origins, up to the 18th century; the Victorian Period; the modern era—namely, the early part of the 20th century; and the 1930s through the 1960s, during which time the guidance movement occurred.

### Early Origins

Discussion of human personality and behavior, and of the need to intervene with maladaptive behavior, can be found in very early scholarly texts. Hippocrates (circa 460–377 B.C.), for example, described abnormal personality in his writings and classified mental illnesses as states resulting from natural causes. Plato (427–347 B.C.) believed, as did the other great thinkers in early Greek society, that by recognizing and directing the internal resources for achievement each person possesses, individuals will prosper and society as a whole will benefit. Plato developed a systematic theory of psychological states and wrote of the influence of those states on human behavior. Through dialogues in works such as *Meno* and *Republic,* Plato questioned the role of human psychology in education, morality, and theology.

Aristotle (384–322 B.C.), a student of Plato, also made appreciable, important contributions to the future professions of counseling and psychology, most particularly in his study of the dynamics of individuals' interactions among themselves and with their general environment. Other notable early influences on counseling thought and practice include the traditions and literature of early religious societies and leaders within those societies, such as St. Augustine (354–430 B.C.) who instructed emotional control through what now might be termed self-analysis.

The Middle Ages saw little progress toward the shaping of what was to become the modern practice of counseling. This was in part owing to the fact that youth guidance was basically within the province of the church during the Middle Ages and therefore consisted largely of spiritual instruction. Gibson and Higgins (1966) point out, however, that occasional attempts at establishing the practice of vocational counseling of youth did occur as kingdoms in Europe expanded their colonial empires.

After the Middle Ages, during the 16th and 17th centuries, philosophers and educators began to recommend guidance of youths into occupations according to their personality traits and individual talents. At this time, books began to appear throughout Europe that contained detailed descriptions of various occupations, the education required for those occupations, recommended schools, and sources of available funding for professional education. From this time into the mid-20th century, the term counseling was used synonymously with vocational guidance or placement.

## The Victorian Period

In the 19th century there was appreciable momentum toward the emergence of modern counseling practice. It also was the time during which the emerging professions of psychiatry, psychology, and counseling became interrelated in their development. In the 19th century the medical specialty of psychiatry began to come into its own. This was accomplished through the works of physicians such as Philippe Pinel (1745–1826), a Parisian psychiatrist whose descriptions of neuroses and psychoses helped to systematize the study of mental disorders and who was influential in abolishing some of the barbaric methods used to treat persons with mental disorders. The work of Jean-Martin Charcot (1825–1893) and his studies of hypnosis to treat hysteria can also be regarded as the springboard to the practice of counseling and psychotherapy (or earlier, to Franz Anton Mesmer, 1733–1815, who was the first to demonstrate hypnotism, in Vienna in 1775). Charcot, a French neurologist, was the first physician to use psychotherapy techniques to treat emotional disorders on an individual case basis. The Viennese physiologist Josef Breuer (1841–1925) abandoned hypnosis in treating hysteria and favored a "talking or cathartic method," which might also be considered as critical to giving rise to the modern practices of counseling and psychotherapy. Breuer's first use of talking as treatment was in 1880 with his famous case known as Anna O., which is viewed as the case that led to the founding of psychoanalysis (Gay, 1988). Sigmund Freud (1856–1939), who studied under both Charcot and Breuer, stated on several occasions that Breuer, rather than himself, should be regarded as the founder of psychoanalysis. One does tend, however, to regard Freud as the father of psychoanalysis and the seminal work of psychoanalysis to be *Studies on Hysteria,* published by Freud, in 1895, with Breuer as first author; Freud's psychoanalytic theory is discussed in Chapter 3. Whichever figure or work is considered to be the key factor in the advent of psychoanalysis as a technique to treat mental disorders and the emotional problems associated with physical disorders, the work of these 19th century French and Austrian physicians has had lasting influence on the practice of counseling and psychotherapy.

At the close of the 19th century, the drama involving Freud's personality theory, the acceptance of psychiatry by the medical community, and the practice of psychoanalysis and other forms of psychotherapy by Freud and his disciples, such as Carl Jung (1875–1961) and Alfred Adler (1870–1937), set the stage for the development in the 20th century of new theories of personality, behavior, and counseling. It also ensured the professional security of psychiatry and contributed to development of the disciplines of psychology and counseling. Within a 30-year span, from 1880 to 1910, Emil Kraepelin (1856–1926) identified mental disease entities and systematized mental disorder classification by differentiating various types of psychoses; the first experimental psychology laboratory was founded at the University of Leipzig in 1879 by Wilhelm Wundt (1832–1920), known as the father of modern psychology; William James (1842–1910), published his theories of emotions and states of consciousness in *Principles of Psychology;* Ivan Pavlov (1849–1936) described the experimental procedure known today as classical conditioning; Eugen Bleuler (1857–1939) published what remains today the definitive text on schizophrenia, and recommended using the term schizophrenia to describe the condition; and Freud systematized psychotherapy and published, amid much fanfare, *Interpretation of Dreams.*

The years between 1880 and 1910 were a signal period of growth and acceptance of psychiatry and psychology; the American psychologist and educator, G. Stanley Hall (1844–1924) established the first counseling center for children and was the first educator to apply the findings of child psychology research to classroom instruction. As with Hall, the French psychologist Alfred Binet (1857–1911) was interested in child psychology and during the same period published, along with his colleague Theodore Simon, the first intelligence tests for children, enabling teachers and clinicians to determine a child's intelligence quotient and thereby the child's mental age (Gazzaniga, 1973; Gleitman, 1986). One particularly noteworthy event that occurred during this period was the 1908 publication of the book, *A Mind That Found Itself* (1962)by Clifford Beers (1876–1943). Beers, a former mental institution patient who had been treated for schizophrenia, founded what is now the National Association for Mental Health. He is credited with being an influential leader of the mental hygiene movement which ultimately led to humanitarian reforms in the treatment of persons with mental disorders, increased research into mental illnesses, the establishment of counseling agencies and counseling programs in institutions, recognition of the need for therapy with the less severe forms of maladjustments, and greater awareness of the need to recognize and intervene with the adjustment problems of youths (Gibson & Mitchell, 1986; Shertzer & Stone, 1971).

## Modern Era

The establishment of the Vocational Bureau in Boston in 1908 by Frank Parsons is viewed as the beginning of the modern era in counseling. Parsons is considered the father of the guidance and counseling movement in education in the United States and the architect of the guidance counselor profession (Traxler & North, 1957). There are also others whose work ranks prominent in the advent of modern counseling as a professional practice. Jesse B. Davis, for example, incorporated vocational counseling into the curriculum of a Michigan high school the year before Parsons established his bureau. These and other events that occurred during the first decade of the 20th century not only launched the modern practice of counseling but also heightened the efforts to (*a*) develop training programs for counselors, (*b*) describe human personality and behavior through scientific research, and (*c*) use empirical data on normal and abnormal personality and behavior to develop accountable theories of counseling and psychotherapy.

The major influences on the work of American pioneers such as Parsons and Davis and on the continued development into the 20th century of the guidance and counseling movement are detailed by Shertzer and Stone (1971) and Traxler (1957). A brief discussion of those and other influences follows.

HUMANITARIAN MOVEMENTS

The influx of immigrants into the United States in the early part of the 20th century created societal problems on a mass scale, particularly in major urban areas. These problems included squalid living conditions, poverty, poor education, inadequate health services, crime, and child and sweatshop labor practices. Driven by the practical good sense of maximizing human resources to enhance the overall prosperity of society or, in some cases, by utopian ideals carried over from the previous century, philanthropists provided the financial resources for vocational guidance agencies, such as Parsons' bureau, and for counseling programs in educational settings.

## RELIGION

Since the Middle Ages, the church has sought to counsel youth in the importance, both to themselves and to humankind, of leading moral lives. The religious emphasis on the need for early moral guidance of children influenced schools to provide such moral guidance. For example, Davis' first public school guidance program included both moral and vocational counseling. However, the role of religion in the general educational guidance process for young children has been and continues to be one of serious debate.

## THE MENTAL HYGIENE MOVEMENT

As discussed, the 1908 publication of Beers' book led to sweeping reforms in the institutional living conditions of persons with mental disorders and in the general availability of treatment services to those persons. The mental hygiene movement effected new laws to protect persons with mental disorders; funding for research on the causes and treatment of mental disorders; and establishment in 1909 of the National Committee for Mental Health (later renamed the National Association for Mental Health).

## SOCIAL REFORM

School enrollments increased rapidly because of a number of factors including the fast-growing national population, unemployment brought on by this growth and by economic depression, a demand for technicians and skilled workers in the quickly expanding technological labor force, compulsory education, and the passage of child labor laws. The enlarged school enrollments, in turn, signaled the need for increased educational and vocational counseling services to help students plan curricula and choose professions suited to their individual attitudes and abilities.

## WAR

At the end of World Wars I and II, many ex-service personnel returned to school on government benefit programs provided through the Veteran's Administration vocational rehabilitation programs. Federal legislation passed after World War I established the Veteran's bureau and provided, as part of the Bureau's services, vocational counseling services to veterans. Gibson and Mitchell (1986) note that interest increased in the development and standardization of group psychological tests as a result of World War I. Also, the residual psychological impact of war on individuals focused concern on the personal adjustment of veterans. Adjustment problems exhibited by Korean War and Vietnam War veterans resulted in the creation of counseling subspecialties to treat those problems.

## INTELLIGENCE MEASUREMENT

The term mental test was coined in 1890 by James McKeen Cattell. As noted, it was 1905 before Binet and Simon published the first standardized intelligence scale; the Stanford-Binet revision of the Binet-Simon scale was published in 1916. Interest in both individual and group intelligence testing continued to increase thereafter. The Army Alpha Test (1917) was the first group intelligence test to be used with a large population and its development contributed to the gathering momentum of the testing movement between the two world wars; it was later replaced in World War II by the Army General Classification Test. The Army testing program helped facilitate more effective group counseling practices. The movement in intelligence testing served to increase awareness of differences among individuals and of the need to collect reliable information about those differences to provide effective, individualized counseling services.

## STUDENTS AS INDIVIDUALS

The testing movement led to objective classification of students as individuals. This, in turn, impelled schools to know and counsel students according to each one's unique intellectual and personality profile. Testing afforded schools the means to systematize individual descriptions of students, which resulted in more reliable guidance services.

## EMERGING NEW PROFESSIONS

The same influences that drove the guidance counseling movement created an impetus in the 1920s for the emergence of other new helping professions. The basic credo of the guidance movement, "each person has worth and each person's worth should be recognized, respected, and facilitated," engendered a climate of concern for the complete well-being of the individual so everyone could lead a productive and contented life. New specialties rapidly developed in medicine, health- related professions, social work, and counseling at a rate that has yet to abate. The founding during that period of what today are the professions of speech-language pathology and audiology are examples new specialties established to serve the disadvantaged and disabled. In part, the guidance movement reinforced the need for counseling to be a part of the standard services provided by personnel within each emerging new profession.

## FEDERAL LEGISLATION

The evolution of counseling was sustained from the 1920s to midcentury by federal government support to establish counseling agencies and train counselors. Several critical legislations were enacted. The Civilian Vocational Rehabilitation Act (1920) after World War I established the Veteran's Bureau. The National Mental Health Act (1946) created the National Institute of Mental Health. The National Defense Education Act (1958) provided generous funding to operate university-based counselor training programs and to support school- based counseling services. Its primary goal was to counsel students to enter science professions so the United States could keep pace technologically with the Soviet Union's burgeoning space program and military-industrial might.

## NONDIRECTIVE THERAPY

One of the major and relatively recent positive influences on the development of the practice of counseling was the work of Carl R. Rogers. Rogers developed his nondirective approach to counseling in the 1940s, first known as client-centered therapy and later renamed person-centered therapy. Rogers' approach to counseling recognizes the individual capacity for change and for enhancement of the self through self-discovery and insight rather than through rigid direction from counselors who treat every person and every problem with a set protocol. Person-centered therapy is a holistic approach to counseling in that it is used to treat the functioning of the whole person instead of only a disorder or a disability. It lends itself well for use in group therapy and can be used by a variety of helping and health care professionals who might have limited training in counseling and psychotherapy. Rogers' theory of personality development is discussed in Chapter 3 and person-centered therapy is discussed in Chapter 4.

## Guidance Movement

Miller (1961) describes the two major emphases of guidance that had been established by the 1930s. Chronologically, the first is *vocational guidance*. Parsons is credited with originating this form of counseling and with coining the term "vocational guidance." Vocational guidance based on the Parsonian model involves a process of matching individuals to occupations based on a fit between the personal traits of individuals and the characteristics of an occupation. This approach to guidance fell in step with the testing movement, which was occurring simultaneously with Parsons' work. To effect optimal matches between persons and vocations, detailed objective data were needed on each. Shertzer and Stone (1971) note that the assessment of an individual's traits and abilities prior to vocational matching was a unique step in counseling. But there have been views expressed that counseling was not altogether served by the early vocational guidance movement. Namely, it is held by some that the vocational guidance models conveyed the impression that counseling is a short-term, formulary process used for vocational concerns only. The use of the term *guidance,* or rather its use interchangeably and redundantly with counseling (i.e., guidance counseling), also led to confusion in attempts to define counseling. Although guidance was the accepted term for counseling until the 1960s, particularly in regard to vocational and educational counseling, its use is now viewed as outdated (Gibson & Mitchell, 1986).

The development of a second major type of counseling practice, *educational guidance,* is often credited to John M. Brewer and the publication of his book *Education as Guidance* (1932). The term educational guidance was used as early as 1914, however, and the concept of education as being synonymous with guidance had earlier been presented by various educators. Also, as has been mentioned, the actions of Davis in establishing moral and vocational counseling as part of the educational process were significant in placing the responsibility for a child's complete well-being and development within the purview of schools. Educational guidance advocates stressed the importance of identifying each child's individuality and fitting their educational experiences to that individuality. They also stated the importance of letting each child recognize and exercise his or her individuality, under the educational guidance of counselors and teachers. During the 1920s and 1930s the concept of guidance as identical with education grew in popularity among educators in both primary and, later, secondary schools, leading to the opinion by some that every teacher should be considered a guidance counselor (Shane, Shane, Gibson, & Munger, 1971). This very conceptualization of education and counseling as being identical processes has been suggested to have had a negative influence on modern counseling. Counseling in an educational guidance context tends to be didactic and impersonal, particularly when counseling occurs in formal group or class settings.

Other approaches to counseling developed from the 1930s through the 1960s as models within the vocational-educational framework. Although these models may not seem relative to counseling in health care professions, in fact they are. It was through these models, developed mainly for the practice of educational guidance, that various counseling issues were played out—the professionalization of counseling, the scope of counselors' practices, direct versus indirect counseling, the role of science in counseling, the responsibilities of the counselor versus those of the client, what is counseling versus what is psychotherapy, treatment of the person versus treatment of the problem, and so forth. The techniques of and approaches to counseling that comprise each model are, to varying degrees, generally viable counseling practice today.

Counseling as *distribution and adjustment* is one such model. Although Proctor (1925) is credited with initiating this approach to counseling, the influence of the mental hygiene movement should also be noted. The distributive aspect of Proctor's approach pertains to the counselor helping students identify life goals, personal as well as vocational, relative to environment and self-concept. The adjustment function concerns crisis management counseling when a student's goals are in conflict with either environment or self-concept. This approach is noteworthy for emphasizing that personal adjustment to vocational and avocational goals is as important as attainment of those goals. This approach also stresses the value of making choices based on a knowledge of self and one's environment. But implicit to this approach is the unfortunate suggestion that counseling occurs at crisis points only.

In the late 1930s, Paterson (1938) and Williamson (1939) introduced models of counseling based on *clinical process.* This approach was founded on work in the testing movement started by Binet and Simon in France and introduced in the United States by Cattell. Group mental testing during World War I also influenced the development of this approach to counseling. The emphasis of this model is on guiding an individual's educational and vocational decisions by organizing the data necessary in making choices. If an individual is having difficulty making choices, the data organized by the counselor should clarify what interpersonal problems are inhibiting action or causing the individual not to make the best long-term choices for him- or herself. Psychological testing is used extensively in this approach to reveal adjustment problems and skills deficits that are barriers to an individual's progress through school and career. The clinical process approach to counseling is directive and objective, owing to its reliance on problem-solving through the scientific method and to its emphasis on research and analytic diagnostic techniques. It is felt to be an efficient approach to counseling that permits the counselor to work with a larger number of students in a given time than does other approaches. This approach is criticized, on the other hand, for making the counselor too responsible for diagnosing the individual's problems and for relying too much on external testing for diagnosis. It involves discrete analysis of an individual's characteristics with limited consideration of the significance in the interrelationships of his or her problems. Development of this approach, however, did influence counselors becoming true professionals with formal training in scientific method and clinical psychology.

In the 1940s, another emphasis on counseling appeared, *decision-making.* This approach, credited to Jones (1970) and Myers (1941), stresses the importance of students being able to make growth- sustaining decisions at critical periods in their lives. It also emphasizes the importance of self-direction in problem-solving and decision-making. The role of the counselor oriented to this approach is to guide students through early crisis periods, helping them make optimal choices for themselves by teaching them to use independently a decision-making model. This enables students to exercise a degree of autonomy in making life choices and gives them decision-making skills to use during critical periods throughout life. A disadvantage of this counseling model, as with the distribution and adjustment model, is it suggests that counseling need occur only during life crises.

During the 1950s the *developmental counseling* approach was introduced, partly in response to the emphasis of the distribution and adjustment model and of the clinical process model on counseling intervention occurring only during crisis periods in an individual's life. The general concept of the developmental approach to counseling was presented by Little and Chapman (1955) and later expanded by others. At the time this counseling approach was introduced, concurrent focus in psychology on human skills development strengthened its viability. An individual's personal growth and educational and vocational skills development are seen in developmental counseling as overlapping, cumulative, unending processes tied to ego functions. This means that students require continuing, consistent guidance to ensure that they develop to their maximal potential. Developmental counseling addresses the student's emerging self-concept as it relates to life growth in general, rather than only to educational and vocational choices as did earlier counseling models. The developmental approach to counseling also stresses the importance of a team approach to student growth that involves school administration, teachers, and other school professionals, and counselors in the guidance process. The team concept of developmental counseling is one of the most difficult aspects of its premise to effect because, questions of cooperation aside, not all administrators and teachers are qualified through training or experience to participate in the counseling process. There was renewed interest in the developmental approach to counseling in the 1970s and it remains a viable approach to counseling today.

In the 1960s other approaches to counseling were developed, including the *eclectic systems approach*, which disparaged the single position or theory approach to counseling as too limiting and recommended that counselors should equip themselves with opinions and techniques from a variety of interdisciplinary theories. Original authorship of this approach is not attributed to any one scholar, but rather to opinions expressed by a number of writers (e.g., Ennis, 1960; Strang, 1964; Traxler & North, 1957; Wilkins & Perlmutter, 1960). Diagnosis is emphasized in this approach in order that the counselor might know each student as an individual. But in diagnosis and in the subsequent counseling based on diagnostic findings, the counselor is free to use parts of any theories or methods of counseling to provide the best individually tailored services. This approach has been criticized for encouraging counselors not to adhere to a specific philosophic position. It is argued that in not doing so, the counselor, in essence, becomes a "jack-of-all-trades and master of none." Practically speaking, it is difficult for counselors to receive sufficient training to be proficient in more than one method, so the attempt to practice several approaches to counseling might result in less than accountable services. It has also been noted that with the eclectic systems approach it is difficult to establish standards for counseling practice.

One of the most lasting and widely used models of counseling was also introduced in the early 1960s by Hoyt (1962), who developed the *constellation of services* model in reaction to changes that were then being proposed for the practice of counseling. Development of Hoyt's model coincided with the National Defense Education Act (1958) and the ample funds it provided for counselor training. With the funds came suggested reforms for counseling practice and Hoyt objected to most of them. It was suggested that detailed job descriptions be established for counselors, expanded practical training specific to counseling should be developed and required, and counselors should not have to follow the same educational track as classroom teachers. Also, sentiment was increasing against the use of the term guidance, as it was thought to connote a directive process rather than one of choice; Hoyt argued that use of the term should not abandoned. Hoyt saw the school counselor as the liaison between professional services, within and available to the school, and the classroom teachers. And although he felt that students' well-being was the responsibility of all professionals within the school, the interdisciplinary team concept is not configured in his model. The roles of other specialists—school psychologists, social workers, psychometrists, nutritionists, speech-language pathologists, and audiologists, are thus seen as adjunctive only, rather than as fundamental to the health and performance of students as are the roles of administrators, teachers, and school counselors. The constellation of services counseling model classifies these other professionals as "consultants" and tends thereby to relegate them to lower status in the school personnel hierarchy. For decades, this satellite services concept proved to be the bane of speech-language pathologists and audiologists employed in schools.

The *science of purposeful action* model of counseling, developed by Tiedeman and Field (1963), conceptualizes counseling as a science of action toward specific purposes, framed within the educational context. It places the responsibility of choosing goals largely with students rather than with counselors. With their model, Tiedeman and Field sought to elevate the status of counselors above that of technicians to promote counseling to a fully organized profession. Their model emphasizes choice over prescription, openness over bias, and freedom over control. Students therefore realize through this approach that it is their responsibility to develop to full potential and to make the appropriate choices in their lives. The role of the counselor is to help students learn the process of taking purposeful action in making life choices. One key criticism of this approach is that there is no theoretic base that accounts for both behavioral change and individual independence in the process of change.

Shoben (1962) presented a model of counseling as *social reconstruction* based on his opinion that schools unintentionally direct students to aspire to specific life styles, prescribe life goals for students, and encourage them to accept societal values that originate with the school or with a segment of society rather than within themselves. Shoben's approach to counseling promotes expression of individuality through introspection, attempts to offset the impersonal character of modern education, and aims to reconstruct the role of schools and society in shaping the individual. Students should be exposed to a variety of potential role models, according to Shoben, and should be permitted to examine themselves relative to those models. What emerges then is a composite self-concept, unique in itself, composed of both intrinsic personality characteristics and the assimilated characteristics of others. Counselors using this approach should encourage students to examine continually their self-concept relative to life goals and should serve primarily as a source of feedback in a student's self-examination and goal setting. Shoben holds that this approach might promote more successful counseling owing to an increased sense of trust between counselor and student. A criticism of this approach is the high level of training and experience counselors would need to facilitate the self-actualization process in students. Also, the magnitude of the task in reconstructing education's and society's influence on the development or inhibition of student individuality is daunting.

Students' overall *personal development* as being as central a responsibility of schools as is their intellectual development was proposed by Kehas (1970). This model comes almost full circle from the concept of Brewer that education and counseling are synonymous. Kehas suggests that rather than defining education as basically a function of teachers, with auxiliary support from counselors only when vocational and higher education decisions are involved, education should be defined as "involvement with learning." This definition of education makes counselors equal partners with teachers in student learning. Learning in this sense means growth in all personal and interpersonal aspects of being as well as in intellectual processes. The outcome of this approach ideally is students in control of their personal development with a positive sense of being and with realistic goals set by themselves. Kehas opines that teachers are not the only nor the primary professionals responsible for the development of students. He argues instead that all the professional school personnel have equal responsibility for the students, although the type of responsibility differs among them. For example, the teacher has primary responsibility for a student's intellectual development and the counselor has primary responsibility for a student's personal development. This compartmentalization of professional responsibilities is one criticism of Kehas' model. There is significance in this model for the roles assumed by speech-language pathologists and audiologists in schools. They and other professionals in schools are often considered auxiliary to teachers, Kehas argues, and they receive referrals only when aspects of a student's behavior are considered by teachers to be possible barriers to academic success and intellectual growth. This attitude prohibits equal involvement with teachers by speech-language pathologists, audiologists, and other professionals in identifying and intervening with problems of students. Although the problems might not influence the students' intellectual development, they might influence the life and career goals they set, their self-concept, and the degree to which they become socialized, fully functioning individuals.

By the 1970s, some of the counseling issues philosophically debated throughout the guidance movement had been more or less resolved. Students were treated more as individuals with potential to be self-directing. Their overall development—personal, interpersonal, and intellectual, was of concern to schools, and counseling was considered to be integral to facilitating students' development. Counseling became less prescriptive and was designed more to help students understand themselves, in terms of personality traits and capabilities, and become self-actualizing individuals. Professionals in schools, other than teachers, increasingly were viewed as being equal in status and importance to teachers. Vocational and educational guidance were no longer the only or main counseling emphasis in the school setting; emphasis only on information giving was augmented with an emphasis on introspection. Counseling had evolved toward recognition as a profession and had made significant progress toward establishing professional counseling practice and certification guidelines; certification for counselors was begun in 1982 with establishment of the National Board for Certified Counselors by the American Personnel and Guidance Association (later to become the American Counseling Association). Counseling had essentially replaced guidance in professional parlance; the American Psychological Association in 1951 renamed its counseling and guidance division, counseling psychology. Another reason for the disuse of the term guidance was the growing awareness that guidance personnel needed some measure of psychotherapy skills to counsel with students, not just about their setting vocational and educational goals and determining methods of reaching those goals, but also about emotional and personal problems that might prevent them from achieving their goals and from becoming self-actualizing adults.

## RATIONALE FOR COUNSELING IN SPEECH-LANGUAGE PATHOLOGY AND AUDIOLOGY

Having considered what counseling is and what its origins are, the logical next question is whether counseling is applicable to clinical practice in speech-language pathology and audiology. Although counseling is indicated as being not only appropriate but necessary by the American Speech-Language-Hearing Association (1993) and by scholars who represent the breadth of specialty areas of communicative disorders (Backus, 1960; Clark & Martin, 1994; Luterman, 1991; Scheuerle, 1992; Shipley, 1992; Webster, 1977), there appears to be a somewhat general reluctance among speech-language pathologists and audiologists to practice purposeful counseling (Clark, 1994; Rollin, 1982). This reluctance might be due in part to clinician trepidation about committing inadvertent ethical violation of psychotherapy's purview. Or it might be due to clinicians' personal feelings of educational and practical inadequacy to employ counseling as a helping process that is more than interviewing clients for case histories and interpreting diagnostic findings and therapy goals to them. But whatever the reason for speech-language pathologists and audiologists' uncertainty about and avoidance of counseling, it needs to be resolved so that clients can receive maximally accountable services that include both adjustment and informative counseling.

Clinicians should apply their counseling skills to:

- give information to and receive information from clients
- advise clients how to develop and use decision-making and problem-solving skills both in modifying their communicative disorders and in living life as persons with communicative disorders

- help clients resolve life problems resulting directly or indirectly from their communicative disorder

- help clients develop or regain positive self-concepts and become self-actualizing, fully functioning individuals, even in cases where the prognosis for successful therapy is guarded

- help parents, spouses, and significant others develop realistic, supportive acceptance of their child's or partner's communicative disorder

It is an arguable point that these objectives might be accomplished indirectly by the clinician and client working together toward correction of or compensation for the client's communicative problem. In other words, if a client's communicative disorder is the primary causal and maintaining factor in his or her personality maladjustment and general maladaptive behavior, improvement or elimination of the communicative problem might remove perforce its attributive personality, adjustment, and role problems. This argument becomes specious, however, if one presupposes that behavioral correction of a communicative disorder does not necessarily eliminate all of its cognitive and emotional sequelae. Also, not all communicative disorders can be modified appreciably in therapy; communicative disorders that typically do not respond well to therapy are more likely not to do so if the client is not fully functioning. Any change in a client's communicative behavior, even toward normative standards, might create a new set of adjustment and role problems for the client. In this view, the potential need for counseling in the treatment of communicative disorders is never obviated, even with clients for whom therapy is highly successful.

The following indications and contraindications of the need for counseling are presented as a clear rationale that counseling with clients and their families should be practiced by speech-language pathologists and audiologists, although their practice of counseling carries with it certain caveats.

## Indications of the Need for Counseling

### TOTAL REHABILITATION OF THE CLIENT

Total rehabilitation involves treating clients in a holistic sense, regarding them in Gestalt terms of their whole persons, rather than only as a communicative problem to be fixed. Their thoughts and emotions about their speech, language, and hearing and about themselves as communicators are as important to their sense of well-being as is their actual communicative behavior. The holistic approach to therapy is discussed further in Chapter 2.

### TREATMENT OF COMMUNICATIVE DISORDERS

Counseling is at times the primary technique used in treating communicative disorders, particularly voice and fluency disorders. Some communicative disorders in fact have psychogenic causes that might at times be appropriately and successfully resolved through counseling.

### STABILIZATION AND CARRYOVER OF THERAPY RESULTS

Clients less likely to maintain the new behaviors attained in therapy are those who have become too dependent on the client-clinician relationship, who are still struggling with disabling emotions engendered by their concept of self as persons with communicative disorders, and who do not possess the ego strength necessary to maintain coping behaviors in lieu of defensive ones. For example, perhaps the issue of greatest irony in therapy for stuttering is that clients can master the clinical strategies to achieve fluent speech and can in fact achieve asymptotic behavior in therapy, yet remain persons who stutter outside of the clinic, particularly after therapy terminates. In such cases, a client's ego functions might be in defensive rather than coping control, possibly owing to therapy not having addressed the cognitive and affective components of the client's self-concept as a person who stutters.

## CLIENT'S PERCEIVED NEED FOR THERAPY IN ABSENCE OF A DISORDER

In addition to demonstrating didactically to such clients that their speech, language, or hearing does not require clinical intervention, clinicians should counsel with them to be certain that all of the client's fears and concerns have been dispelled and that the client's belief that a disorder does exist is not a manifestation of psychological disturbances that might call for referral to a psychologist or psychiatrist. Clinicians should not dismiss such clients' concerns too quickly; in counseling with them it is important to keep in mind that their perceived disorders are very real to them.

## INTERPERSONAL NATURE OF COMMUNICATION

Communication is the defining behavior of the socialization process. Functional speech, language, and hearing and effective communication are two different considerations. Clients might at times require counseling to help them learn to use effectively new communicative skills in interpersonal communication. Speech, language, and hearing are completely functional only if their use helps individuals to meet their emotional as well as physical needs, and if their use of communication serves to enhance and reinforce their self-concepts and self-actualizing behaviors. These objectives are achieved through effective interpersonal communication, not simply by being able to communicate. Attitudes toward interpersonal communication govern its effectiveness and these attitudes are responsive to counseling. If the intent of speech-language pathologists and audiologists is to help their clients become maximally effective communicators, clients' attitudes toward the interpersonal process of communication must be measured and addressed. Clients' attitudes about themselves as communicators, rather than their actual ability or potential to communicate often chiefly determine the degree of success they will have with interpersonal relationships. Barbara (1958) notes that persons with communicative disorders, especially those who also are neurotic, often place premiums on unrealistic ideals of communication skills, believing their attainment of those skills to be the only requisite necessary for self-actualization and successful relationships.

## CLIENT'S SELF-CONCEPT

Self-concept is represented in communicative behaviors. Self concept, personality, and communicative behavior are inextricably linked one to the other (Barbara, 1954, 1958). A change in one might produce changes, not necessarily desired or positive changes, in the others. This issue is further addressed in Chapter 2.

## RESIDUAL SEQUELAE

The disordered communication of a client might be changed but reactions to it remain a problem. Counseling is indicated for clients and their parents or significant others if communicative disorders cause them to experience disabling emotions or maladaptive behaviors that remain after the communicative disorders have been successfully treated.

## PARENTS' SHATTERED DREAMS

The shattered dreams of parents represent one of the most critical counseling occasions in speech-language pathology and audiology (Moses, 1985). Counseling with parents might be required to involve them fully and productively in their child's therapy, particularly if the parents exhibit defensive behaviors that deny and distort the reality of their child's condition.

## CULTURAL BARRIERS

Counseling might be used to address cultural barriers to therapy that inhibit full participation by all parties in the therapy experience. If these barriers are ignored therapy might not be maximally effective or may even be futile (Robinson & Crowe, 1994). Cultural barriers and related strategies for counseling are discussed in Chapter 5.

## CLINICIAN EMPATHY

Oftentimes, accurately or not, clients perceive that their speech-language pathologist or audiologist is the only person who understands their travail and is the only person in whom they can confide their fears and concerns about living life as persons with communicative disorders. If clinicians counsel with their clients about these concerns, mainly by being empathic listeners, their clients might not only resolve their fears but in the process also take responsibility and find direction to correct their communicative disorders.

## CLIENT-AS-CLINICIAN

Optimal therapy situations are those in which clients want to share responsibility with the clinician to modify their speech, language, or hearing disorder. As indicated, creating such a counseling environment with clients helps to facilitate their taking charge of their lives.

## GUARDED PROGNOSIS

The reality of communicative disorders is that some of them have a guarded prognosis of being responsive to therapy or have a prognosis that indicates that therapy will be long and arduous. In such cases, counseling is used to help clients, their parents, and significant others adjust to problems that are not going to go away, at least not in the short-term and without hard work.

## INACCURATE PERCEPTIONS AND NONPRODUCTIVE ATTITUDES

If clients' perceptions of themselves, their environments, and their disorders do not match external reality, they may have difficulty setting realistic goals in therapy and in assessing their progress toward these goals. Clients who have nonproductive attitudes toward therapy and life in general are less likely to be motivated and self-reinforcing in therapy.

## MOTIVATION

Counseling can be used by clinicians to help clients maintain focus on the objectives of therapy. At times a client's attention tends to become diffused and is focused on secondary manifestations of the problems, such as the negative effects of anxiety and the defenses that the client has constructed against anxiety (Wolberg, 1988).

## DIFFICULT CLIENTS

Some clients are not congruent to the client-clinician relationship and may be openly aggressive toward their clinicians, although they might have volitionally enrolled in therapy. Shipley (1992) identifies difficult clients as those who are angry, overprotective, overtalkative, insatiable, hostile, paranoid, and grieving; and those who feel entitled and tend to intellectualize. McFarlane, Fujiki, and Brinton (1984) note that reluctant clients are challenges for the clinician: the tardy/absent client, the yes-but client, the pleaser client, and the semi-successful client. Counseling might be used with difficult clients to improve the client-clinician relationship and enhance the prognosis for successful therapy.

## ROLE PROBLEMS

As discussed, one of the primary applications of counseling is to address role problems. Communicative disorders can create role problems for clients that might need to be resolved before clients can move forward in therapy or that need to be addressed directly, regardless of the progress of therapy. Success in therapy also can create role problems for clients who have improved, controlled, or eliminated their communicative disorders; these clients might suddenly find new demands placed on them and new, challenging roles assigned to them that create new anxieties associated with communication.

## CATASTROPHIC, CHRONIC, AND GLOBALLY INVOLVING ILLNESSES AND CONDITIONS

Clients presenting with communicative disorders related to catastrophic illnesses, (e.g., cancer, amyotrophic lateral sclerosis); chronic illnesses (e.g., Parkinson's disease); chronic conditions (e.g., papillomatosis); and potentially globally involving conditions and events (e.g., cerebral palsy, stroke, traumatic brain injury), might have counseling needs that speech-language pathologists and audiologists find challenging, if not beyond their scope of practice. These client's anxieties may go well beyond concerns about coping with a communicative disorder, although if they can develop effective communication, other anxieties about daily living might be somewhat allayed. Clinicians should attempt counseling in such cases, being careful to keep it within the context of a client's communicative disorders. If the clients' emotions are atypically labile or intense; if their anxieties about their conditions, their living or their imminent death are immobilizing; or if their health conditions have created interpersonal problems, such as marital difficulties, then clinicians should make appropriate referrals to other counseling specialists. They should be carefully circumspect in making referrals. These clients may already be seeing a host of health care professionals; referral to additional ones might possibly add logistic complications to their daily routines, increase their financial concerns, and emphasize to them that they have even more problems that have to be treated.

## PREVENTION

Counseling to prevent communicative disorders is typically thought of as preventing-by-informing but it might also involve adjustment counseling with at risk clients or their parents. Crowe (1995) suggests that the syndrome of stuttering might be prevented in at-risk disfluent children by counseling their parents on how to ensure healthy ego development for their children in the preschool years. Whereas counseling can be used effectively for primary prevention of communicative disorders, it is most effective when used for secondary and tertiary prevention.

## SCOPE OF PRACTICE

The American Speech-Language-Hearing Association includes counseling in the scope of practice of speech-language pathologists and audiologists and in its preferred practice patterns (American Speech-Language-Hearing Association, 1993). Even so, clinicians should be careful not to exceed their professional boundaries in counseling with clients nor attempt to employ helping skills that they do not fully comprehend how and when to use.

DIFFERENCE VERSUS DISORDER VERSUS HANDICAP

The type and severity of a client's speech, language, and hearing concerns largely determine whether they are communicative differences, disorders, or handicaps. But in some cases, clients' reactions to their speech, language, or hearing problems might cause them to perceive their problems as disorders or handicaps, which they in fact are only because of the clients' cognitive and affective reactions to them. Counseling can help such clients match their perceptions with external reality and view their speech, language, or hearing problems as disorders that can be helped in therapy rather than as hopeless handicaps causing tension, anxiety, loss of self-esteem, and a lowered quality of life. Similarly, clients who perceive themselves as disordered but present with nonproblematic speech, language, or hearing differences can be assisted through counseling, as discussed.

## Contraindications of the Need for Counseling

PRIMARY PROBLEMS

If the emotional problems of clients are judged to eclipse severely their problems with communication, then referral is indicated. Also, at times clients present with mental disorders that are unrelated to their communication disorders. Treatment for their speech, language, or hearing problems would be considered secondary to psychotherapy or medical treatment for their mental disorders.

PROFESSIONAL BOUNDARIES

If a need is indicated for specialized counseling, even if it is related to a client's communicative disorder, then referral is appropriate. For instance, if a client is experiencing sexual or relationship problems due to a communicative disorder (e.g., aphasia, laryngectomy, and so forth) the clinician can go only so far in counseling with the client and the client's spouse before the communicative disorder is no longer the focus of the counseling. Speech-language pathologists and audiologists should at all times keep their counseling within the context of their clients' communicative disorder.

INADEQUATE TRAINING

Simply put, if clinicians are not trained to counsel with clients they should not attempt it. Speech-language pathologists and audiologists often are at a loss as to where and how to obtain the training, credentials, and identity that will enable them to provide accountable counseling and feel comfortable in doing so.

One source of training in counseling is college course work. Speech-language pathologists and audiologists in training should avail themselves of any courses on counseling offered in their academic departments. If their departments do not have courses on counseling, or if they simply wish to take additional courses, they might take counseling or psychotherapy courses in psychology and counseling psychology departments. Unfortunately, presently it is easier said than done for speech-language pathologists and audiologists to obtain course work in counseling. Culpepper, Lucks Mendel, and McCarthy (1994) reported the results of a survey they conducted of the counseling experience and training offered by graduate programs accredited by the Educational Standards Board of the American Speech-Language-Hearing Association. Among their findings was that only 43% of the responding programs (121 returned of 193 programs surveyed for a return rate of 63%) offered course work in counseling within their departments. Only 51% of the responding programs indicated that counseling courses were available to their students through other departments. It is hoped that this situation will improve. In addition to course work in counseling, clinicians ideally should have course work in general human growth and de-velopment, normal personality development, abnormal psychology, fundamentals of learning, and principles and processes of behavior change as background preparation for counseling with clients. Clinicians already practicing without having had this academic preparation can take credit or noncredit courses at night. Guided practice in counseling should be provided in clinical practicum as a follow-up to course work.

Counseling training can also be obtained by other formal or informal means. Formal means include special workshops, seminars, and programs on counseling other than tra-ditional college courses. Private institutes established to provide training and credential-ing in specific approaches to counseling and psychotherapy regularly sponsor workshops and seminars. Information on these programs are available through university academic departments and professional societies for counseling and psychology. Informal means of counseling training include self-study and informal mentoring experiences, although mentoring can also be a formal arrangement.

## REFERENCES

Albert, G. (1966). If counseling is psychotherapy—what then? *Personnel Guidance Journal, 45,* 124–129.

American Psychological Association. (1947). Recommended graduate training program in clinical psychology: Report of the committee on training in clinical psychology. *American Psychologist, 2,* 539–558.

American Speech-Language-Hearing Association. (1993). Preferred practice patterns for the professions of speech-language pathology and audiology. *ASHA, 35* (3), Supplement, 1–102.

Ard, B. N. (Ed.). (1966). *Counseling and psychotherapy.* New York: Science and Behavior Books.

Aubrey, R. (1967). The legitimacy of elementary school counseling: Some unresolved issues and conflicts. *Personnel Guidance Journal, 46,* 355–359.

Backus, O. (1960). The study of psychological processes in speech therapists. In D. A. Barbara (Ed.). *Psychological and psychiatric aspects of speech and hearing.* Springfield, IL: Charles C. Thomas.

Balinsky, B. N., & Blum, M. L. (1951). *Counseling and psychology.* Englewood Cliffs, NJ: Prentice-Hall.

Barbara, D. A. (1954). *Stuttering: A psychodynamic approach to its understanding and treatment.* New York: Julian Press.

Barbara, D. A. (1958). *Your speech reveals your personality.* Springfield, IL: Charles C. Thomas.

Beers, C. W. (1962). *A mind that found itself.* New York: Longmans, Green, & Company; reprinted by Doubleday & Company.

Belkin, G. (1975). *Practical counseling in the schools.* Dubuque, IA: William C. Brown.

Blocher, D. (1966). Wanted: A science of human effectiveness. *Personnel Guidance Journal, 44,* 824–839.

Blocher, D. H. (1974). *Developmental counseling* (2nd ed.). New York: Ronald Press.

Bordin, E. S. (1968). *Psychological counseling.* New York: Appleton-Century-Crofts.

Brammer, L. (1973). *The helping relationship: Process and skills.* Englewood Cliffs, NJ: Prentice-Hall.

Brammer, L., & Shostrum, E. (1977). *Therapeutic psychology: fundamentals of counseling and psychotherapy* (3rd ed.). Englewood Cliffs, NJ: Prentice-Hall.

Breuer, J., & Freud, S. (1955). *Studies on hysteria. Standard Edition, 2,* 1–305. London: Hogarth Press. (Originally published 1895).

Brewer, J. M. (1932). *Education as guidance.* New York: Macmillan.

Carkhuff, R., & Berenson, B. (1967). *Beyond counseling and therapy.* New York: Holt, Rinehart, and Winston.

Clark, J. G. (1994). Audiologists' counseling purview. In J. G. Clark, & F. N. Martin (Eds.), *Effective counseling in audiology: Perspectives and practice.* Englewood Cliffs, NJ: Prentice-Hall.

Clark, J. G., & Martin, F. N. (1994). *Effective counseling in audiology: Perspectives and practice.* Englewood Cliffs, NJ: Prentice-Hall (1994).

Crowe, T. A. (1995). Preventive counseling with parents at risk. In C. W. Starkweather, & H. M. F. Peters (Eds.), *Proceedings of the First World Congress on Fluency Disorders.* Nijmegen, Netherlands: University Press.

Culpepper, B., Lucks Mendel, L., & McCarthy, P. A. (1994). Counseling experience and training offered by ESB-accredited programs. *ASHA, 36,* 55–58.

Curran, C. A. (1968). *Counseling and psychotherapy.* New York: Sheed & Ward.

Dixon, D. N., & Glover, J. A. (1984). *Counseling: A problem solving approach.* New York: John Wiley & Sons.

Egan, G. (1982). *The skilled helper: Model, skills, and methods for effective helping* (2nd ed.). Monterey, CA: Brooks/Cole.

Ennis, M. (1960–61). The need for a philosophy of guidance still haunts us. *Vocational Guidance Quarterly, 9,* 138–140.

Freud, S. (1955). *Interpretation of dreams.* London: Hogarth Press. (Original work published 1900)

Gay, P. (1988). *Freud: A life for our time.* New York: WW Norton.

Gazzaniga, M. (1973). *Fundamentals of psychology: An introduction.* New York: Academic Press.

Gibson, R., & Mitchell, M. (1986). *Introduction to counseling and guidance* (2nd ed.). New York: Macmillan.

Gibson, R., & Higgins, R. (1966). *Techniques of guidance: An approach to pupil analysis.* Chicago, IL: Science Research Associates.

Glanz, E. G. (1974). *Guidance foundations, principles, and techniques* (2nd ed.). Newton, MA: Allyn and Bacon.

Gleitman, H. (1986). *Psychology* (2nd ed.). New York: WW Norton.

Hackney, H., & Cormier, L. S. (1988). *Counseling strategies and intervention* (3rd ed.). Englewood Cliffs, NJ: Prentice-Hall.

Hansen, J., Stevic, R., & Warner, R., Jr. (1972). *Counseling: Theory and process.* Newton, MA: Allyn and Bacon.

Hansen, J., Stevic, R., & Warner, R., Jr. (1982). *Counseling: Theory and process* (3rd ed.). Newton, MA: Allyn and Bacon.

Hinsie, L. E., & Campbell, R. J. (1970). *Psychiatric dictionary* (4th ed.). New York: Oxford University Press.

Hoyt, K. (1962). Guidance: A constellation of services. *Personnel Guidance Journal, 40,* 690–697.

James, W. (1890). *Principles of psychology.* New York: Henry Holt.

Jones, A. J. (1970). *Principles of guidance* (6th ed.). Revised by B. Stefflre & N. Stewart. New York: McGraw-Hill.

Kanfer, F. H., & Goldstein, A. P. (1980). *Helping people change: A textbook of methods* (2nd ed.). Elmsford, NY: Pergamon Press.

Kehas, C. (1970). Education and personal development. In *Introduction to guidance: selected readings.* Boston, MA: Houghton Mifflin.

Little, W., & Chapman, A. (1955). *Developmental guidance in the secondary school.* New York: McGraw-Hill.

Luterman, D. M. (1991). *Counseling the communicatively disordered and their families* (2nd ed.). Austin, TX: Pro-Ed.

McDaniel, H. B., & Shaftel, G. A. (1956). *Guidance in the modern school.* New York: Holt, Rinehart & Winston.

McFarlane, S. C., Fujiki, M., & Brinton, B. (1984). *Coping with communicative handicaps: Resources for the practicing clinician.* San Diego, CA: College Hill Press.

Miller, C. (1961). *Foundations of guidance.* New York: Harper and Brothers.

Miller, F. W. (1968). *Guidance: Principles and services* (2nd ed.). Columbus, OH: Charles E. Merrill.

Moursund, J. (1990). *The process of counseling and therapy.* Englewood Cliffs, NJ: Prentice-Hall.

Moses, K. L. (1985). Dynamic intervention with families. In E. Cherow (Ed.), *Hearing impaired children and youth with disabilities.* Washington, DC: Gallaudet College Press.

Mowrer, O. (1950). *Learning theory and personality dynamics.* New York: Ronald Press.

Myers, G. (1941). *Principles and techniques of vocational guidance.* New York: McGraw-Hill.

Nystul, M. S. (1993). *The art and science of counseling and psychotherapy.* New York: Merrill.

Okun, B. F. (1987). *Effective helping, interviewing, and counseling techniques* (3rd ed.). Monterey, CA: Brooks/Cole.

Paterson, D. G. (1938). The genesis of modern guidance. *The Educational Record, 16,* 36–46.

Patterson. C. (1980). *Theories of counseling and psychotherapy* (3rd ed.). New York: Harper & Row.

Pepinsky, H., & Pepinsky, P. (1954). *Counseling: Theory and practice.* New York: Ronald Press.

Perry, W. G. (1955). The finding of the commission on counseling and guidance on the relation of psychotherapy and counseling. *Annals of the New York Academy of Science, 63,* 396–407.

Plato. (1989). Hamilton, E., & Cairns, H. (Eds.). *The Collected Dialogues of Plato.* Princeton, NJ: Princeton University Press.

Proctor, W. M. (1925). *Educational and vocational guidance.* Boston, MA: Houghton Mifflin.

Robinson T. L., Jr., & Crowe, T. A. (1994). *Speech fluency in multicultural populations: Issues in assessment and treatment.* Paper presented at the American Speech-Language-Hearing Association Convention, New Orleans, LA.

Rogers, C. R. (1959). A theory of therapy, personality, and interpersonal relationships as developed in the client-centered framework. In S. Koch (Ed.), *Psychology—A study of a science* (Vol. 3). New York: McGraw-Hill.

Rollin, W. J. (1982). *The psychology of communication disorders in individuals and their families.* Englewood Cliffs, NJ: Prentice-Hall.

Scheuerle, J. (1992). *Counseling in speech-language pathology and audiology.* New York: Merrill.

Shane, J., Shane, H., Gibson, R., & Munger, P. (1971). *Guiding human development: The counselor and the teacher in the elementary school.* Worthington, OH: Charles A. Jones.

Shertzer, B., & Stone, S. (1971). *Fundamentals of guidance* (2nd ed.). Boston, MA: Houghton Mifflin.

Shipley, K. G. (1992). *Interviewing and counseling in communicative disorders: Principles and procedures.* New York: Merrill.

Shoben, E., Jr. (1962). Guidance: Remedial functions or social reconstruction? *Harvard Education Review, 32,* 430–443.

Steiner, C. (1974). *Scripts people live: Transactional analysis of life scripts.* New York: Grove Press.

Stewart, N., Winborn, B., Johnson, R., Burks, H., & Engelkes, J. (1978). *Systematic counseling.* Englewood Cliffs, NJ: Prentice-Hall.

Strang, R. (1964). *Counseling techniques in college and secondary schools.* New York: Harper and Brothers.

Tiedeman, D., & Field, F. (1963). Guidance: The science of purposeful action applied through education. *Harvard Education Review, 32,* 483–501.

Traxler, A. E., & North, R. D. (1957). *Techniques of guidance* (3rd ed.). New York: Harper & Row.

Truax, C. B., & Mitchell, K. M. (1971). Research on certain therapist interpersonal skills in relation to process and outcome. In A. E. Bergin, & S. L. Garfield (Eds.), *Handbook of psychotherapy and behavior change.* New York: John Wiley & Sons.

Tyler, L. (1969). *The work of the counselor* (3rd ed.). New York: Appleton-Century-Crofts.

Vance, F. L., & Volsky, T. C., Jr. (1962). Counseling and psychotherapy: Split personalities or Siamese twins. *American Psychologist, 17,* 565–570.

Webster, E. J. (1977). *Counseling with parents of handicapped children: Guidelines for improving communication.* New York: Grune & Stratton.

Wilkens, W., & Perlmutter, B. (1960). The philosophical foundations of guidance and personnel work. *Review of Education. Research, 30,* 97–104.

Williamson, E. (1939). *How to counsel students: A manual of techniques for clinical counselors.* New York: McGraw-Hill.

Wolberg, L. (1988). *The technique of psychotherapy* (4th ed.). New York: Grune & Stratton.

Wolman, B. B. (1989). *Dictionary of behavioral science.* New York: Academic Press.

## 2. Emotional Aspects of Communicative Disorders

Thomas A. Crowe

---

| Emotional Responses to Communicative Disorders | Self-Concept and Communicative Behavior |
|---|---|
| Grieving Process | |
| Other Clinically Relevant Emotions | Holistic Approach to Counseling |

---

Disorders of communication can cause persons who have them to develop strong reactive emotions (Barbara, 1958; Luterman, 1991; Rollin, 1987). When these emotional reactions are present, which is not with every client, they are at times more debilitating to persons with communicative disorders than are their speech, language, or hearing problems. Parents, spouses, and significant others of communicatively disordered persons also often experience distracting, unpleasant, and potentially problematic emotions as a direct result of their loved one's congenital or acquired communication problems. One reason individuals have high emotional involvement with their speech, language, and hearing might be that self-concept is displayed to the world through communication. Luterman (1991) notes that communicative disorders distort a basic defining characteristic of an individual's humanness. If individuals feel that they cannot accurately portray their self-concepts or if they are frustrated in efforts to develop a positive self-concept, emotional responses may occur. The emotional responses to communicative disorders are identified in this chapter and discussed relative to their effects on the client and the clinical process. Following that discussion, brief consideration is given to the clinical relevance of clients' self-concepts and to the rationale for holistic treatment of communicative disorders.

### EMOTIONAL RESPONSES TO COMMUNICATIVE DISORDERS

Emotions have been discussed both as reactions to communicative disorders caused by physical, physiological, or learning circumstances and as possible causative variables in the onset of speech, language, and hearing disorders. For example, Van Riper (1982), in his equational description of the onset of stuttering, attributes prominent causal roles to penalty, frustration, anxiety, guilt, hostility, fear, and stress. West (1931) views stress and emotional disturbances as possible precipitating agents in the breakdown of speech fluency; Johnson and Knott (1936) speak of stuttering as a struggle behavior caused by fearful anticipation of a struggle. Sheehan (1953) characterizes stuttering as an approach-avoidance behavior that results from internalized conflicts between the desire to speak and the fear of doing so. Bloodstein (1987), in describing the influence of communicative pressure on fluency failure, states:

> the likelihood cannot be ignored that there are certain personality traits (e.g., the tendency to be unusually sensitive, fearful, dependent, perfectionistic, easily frustrated, or too anxious for approval) that render a child more vulnerable to the provocations and pressures that may lead to anticipatory struggle behavior. (p. 64)

And, there are the psychoanalytic interpretations that stuttering is behavior symbolic of unconsciously repressed emotional or sexual needs or that it is consciously or unconsciously developed behavior by individuals for epinosic gains (e.g., Barbara 1954; Brill, 1923; Coriat, 1928; Fenichel, 1945; Gemelli, 1982a, 1982b; Glauber, 1958).

Emotions as causal factors are associated with other disorders of fluency, voice, articulation, language, and hearing, in particular communicative disorders that manifest as conversion symptoms. It is, however, the emotional responses of clients and their families to communicative disorders that most often are of clinical concern to speech-language pathologists and audiologists. Intense emotions associated with communicative disorders can lead to a client's experiencing neurotic states of being that in turn can effectively block any chance of maximal or lasting success in therapy. Emotional reactions to communicative disorders also can cause clients to (*a*) set unrealistic goals for themselves, (*b*) have difficulty setting any goals at all, (*c*) actualize only part of their creative potential, (*d*) be noncongruent to their phenomenal fields and to the therapy experience, (*e*) avoid experiences and relationships, and (*f*) place negative valuations on themselves because of these behaviors. Strong reactive emotions can have a substantively greater impact than actual disorders on individuals leading "lives of quiet desperation," in which the daily quality of living is diminished by distracting emotions attendant to illness, injury, and disability. Whether clients and their supporting others' emotional states are ones of distraction or disturbance, acute or chronic, or whether their emotions should be addressed in counseling or psychotherapy, emotional responses to communicative disorders should be recognized and assessed. If emotions constitute a problem, they should be resolved to enhance a client's psychological, somatic, and social well-being, and thereby improve the prognosis for successful outcomes of therapy, outcomes in which success is not measured solely by objective improvement in speech, language, and hearing. Arnold (1960), in his revision of the James-Lange theory of emotions, which held that physiological reactions to environmental stimuli precede and therefore motivate emotions, suggested instead that emotions, as determined by individuals' perceptions and interpretations of themselves and their experiences, form the core of the motivational process and serve to direct their behavior.

## Grieving Process

What are the emotions speech-language pathologists and audiologists might find clinically relevant in that they might adversely influence clients' motivational states and erode their confidence in themselves and in therapy? The emotional-perceptual stages of grief is a good place to start because parents and significant others of communicatively disordered children and adults and the clients themselves often encounter grief due to the onset of speech, language, and hearing problems (Tanner, 1980). A client and supporting others must work their way through grief if the client is to achieve wellness in a holistic sense (Bristor, 1984; Moses, 1985).

Grieving is a natural process. If experienced normally, grief is a beneficial process wherein individuals work their way through various emotions to positive acceptance of distressing circumstances. It is usually thought of as a process associated with dying or death. Grieving, however, can be activated by a loss of any type (e.g., a failed marriage, a lost job, a financial crisis, and so forth) that causes grief for what was but is now lost or for what might have been.

In an existential sense, speech, language, and hearing problems can be viewed as boundary situations, which are situations that force individuals to confront existential issues such as being and nonbeing. Confronting death is the most significant boundary situation individuals experience; death confrontation can be real or symbolic. Perceptions of symbolic death or nonbeing might be present, for example, in:

- the unrealized dreams for a physically perfect child of parents of a cleft palate child
- the feelings a person with aphasia has of being suddenly marooned in a parallel universe, dead to his or her former existence for lack of communication with it
- the isolation persons with hearing impairment feel when ignored because of the difficulty others have in communicating with them
- the dejection a person who stutters feels when apprehensions of fluency failure are painfully confirmed

Grief is very real for persons who confront communicative disorders. It can become despair, supplant a client's goal-directed behaviors with stasis, and generally lower the quality of life. With death, terminal dying, or a one-time loss with short-term restitution of that which was lost, the grieving process typically is limited in respect to the time required for an individual to resolve grief and re-enter emotional wellness. This is not necessarily so with persons who have communicative disorders. Their sense of loss might be reprised and reinforced daily, thereby interminably protracting their grieving process. They can enter therapy discouraged and despondent to the point of inactivity, although they might say the things the clinician wants to hear. It should be considered a clinical imperative for clinicians to use counseling techniques, to explore the characteristics of grieving displayed by clients and their families, to determine how related their states of grief are to therapy outcomes, and to help them work their way through the grieving stages from symbolic death to holistic wellness.

This is not to say that boundary situations, involving death encounters, whether real or symbolic, are without value. They can strengthen one's inner resolve to accomplish goals while there is still time to do so, bring avoided important issues to the fore, enhance one's acceptance of self, and increase one's appreciation and awareness of living. Grief does not have to injure the psyche of those experiencing it and grief is not a condition to be avoided whenever possible. Instead, grief is a coping process wherein an individual hurtfully mourns, but also wherein there can be self-examination and evaluation of present circumstances relative to future growth. Grief serves to help an individual accept the shock of sudden, unwanted, new realities. Speech-language pathologists and audiologists should not attempt to negate their clients' grieving; instead, they should help them maintain a normal grieving state and avoid a morbid one, which manifests as melancholia or depression.

Although various models of the grieving process have been proposed (e.g., Bowlby, 1969, 1973, 1980; Engel, 1964), the one presented by Kubler-Ross (1969, 1975) perhaps has had the most widely interdisciplinary application. Kubler-Ross explains the grieving process as consisting of five stages: (a) denial, (b) anger, (c) bargaining, (d) depression, and (e) acceptance. These stages can be recognized in parents, significant others, and clients who are working their way toward acceptance of a communicative disorder. Although these stages are not immutable in terms of their presence, intensity, or progression for all grieving persons, they do tend to appear to varying degrees in most persons who must confront loss. Clinicians should note that most models of the grieving process suggest that the grieving process is linear. In fact, clients often progress through grief in a cyclical fashion; emotions are experienced and resolved only to be re-experienced in response to unpredicted stimuli or due to clinical setbacks.

## DENIAL

*Denial,* the first stage in the grieving process, is a primitive defense used to reject the existence of a painful or frightening reality. Persons with communicative disorders can present in states of total or varying degrees of denial. Clients in total denial might disavow the existence of their communicative disorders, whereas a client in a lesser state of denial might admit to the presence of a communicative disorder but deny that the disorder is of concern. As with the grieving process in general, denial is a normal reaction to an unpleasant circumstance beyond one's control. It serves as a buffering state that buys time for an individual to ease into new reality and begin to move through the grieving process toward ultimate acceptance of the illness or disability (Kubler-Ross, 1969). Although temporary denial may be normal and may serve helpful protective functions, it prevents clients from modifying their communicative disorders to the fullest extent. If a client fixates in the denial stage of the grieving process, the prognosis for improvement in speech, language, or hearing remains guarded and he or she will not move toward resolution of grief. Although clients might return to any stage of grief, including denial, when physical or psychological setbacks occur with progressive or recurring illness and disability, they must move beyond initial denial in order to begin the processes of resolution of grief and amelioration of their communicative disorder.

Kubler-Ross (1969) identified three factors that might influence the existence and recalcitrance of denial in grieving. First, the accuracy and completeness of information about the illness or disorder determine if and for how long an individual will experience denial. If accurate and full insight emerge only after considerable time, denial might also extend over time and acceptance be delayed. Second, the time an individual needs to resolve grief might affect duration and intensity. This is a somewhat equivocal factor in that an individual who has only a short time to work through the stages of grief (e.g., imminent death) might do so expeditiously because he or she feels the pressure of time and wants to come to terms with fate before ultimately confronting it. Others might view the imminence and irreversibility of fate with such dread that they fixate in denial or in a subsequent emotional stage of grief. The unpredictability of a client's reaction to the time factor in grieving is also seen in individuals who face long-term illnesses or disabilities. They may feel in no hurry to come out of denial owing to the absence of critical time pressure to do so. On the other hand, individuals who quickly decide that their illnesses or disabilities are real and are not going away and that they can have long, productive lives despite those factors, might be anxious to work through their grief and get on with therapy. Clinicians can explore and favorably influence how clients view this time factor relative to denial. Third, an individual's premorbid tendency to rely on denial as a defense against life's pressures increases the probability and intensity of its presence with illness or disability. Individuals with a long-standing proclivity to use denial as defensive reaction to unpleasant circumstances are more likely to use it as a buffer to news that they or their children have communicative disorders. Denial might in fact be the most prominent stage of the grieving process for them—one to which they revert with each new revelation about their disorder or disappointment in therapy.

As with the grieving process in general, denial is a natural reaction to disturbing news and clinicians should not indicate to clients that it is otherwise. Clinicians should be concerned, however, if a client remains in denial long after having been counseled to the nature and prognosis of the disorder and to the course of therapy. A client's grieving might continue for some time into therapy, but denial should soon show signs of weakening and give way to other defenses that do not impede therapy. If clients' denial of the realities of their communicative disorders shows little or no sign of remission after appreciable time in therapy, they may have needed more time at the outset to voice opinions, ask questions, or adjust to new realities before therapy commenced. It might mean that the clinician presented diagnostic results as an efficient technician rather than as an empathic counselor or that counseling was approached in too direct and prescriptive ways, as in the early models of guidance. Perhaps the clinician did not know how to recognize subtle or covert denial or may not have felt competent to address denial or chose to ignore it, thinking that modification of speech, language, and hearing was the only goal and that denial would probably take care of itself. Or, rather than helping a client work through denial by listening to expressions of denial and responding in ways that encourage introspection (e.g., clarifying diagnostic and prognostic data and demonstrating understanding of a client's reactions to those data), the clinician instead might have attempted to repudiate the client's denial by arguing the irrationality of its existence in the face of objective evidence. Moses and Van Hecke-Wulatin (1981) suggest that dialogue structured to help clinicians understand clients' perceptions is more effective in resolving denial than is argument. Argument with clients about denial might, in fact, serve only to make it more impervious to change.

Denial is most effective as a defense mechanism for persons who are in weakened ego states. In the ego psychology paradigm of personality and behavior, persons in denial are viewed as having diminished strength in their controlling functions—the functions of the ego that enable one to focus on tasks and goals without being distracted by emotions (Kroeber, 1964). In this paradigm, denial is represented as the defense mechanism in opposition to concentration—the coping behavior; the stronger the state of denial, the weaker the ability to concentrate. Clients should be helped to substitute concentration for denial to come to terms with their communicative disorder. If clients are unable to concentrate on tasks, therapy does not progress well, if at all. Clinicians should be sensitive to client denial and consider helping resolve it a potential first goal of therapy.

ANGER

*Anger* is the second stage of Kubler-Ross's (1969) grieving process model. For communicatively disordered persons and their supporting others, this is the point at which the realities of their speech, language, or hearing problems have entered conscious awareness. It is the stage where clients ask, literally and rhetorically, "Why?" "Why me?" and "What did I do to deserve this?" Their fundamental belief systems may have been shaken in a very basic sense. The philosophies or religions on which their self-concepts were partially grounded and which were based on the keystone tenet that rewards accrue to lives lived truly and productively might now seem sophistic to them. Their natural, spontaneous anger over developing or having children born with communicative disorders might not easily be resolved if their catechismal processes for accepting unwanted fate can no longer be trusted.

A client's degree of anger cannot be predicted. Some clients will react with intense anger when confronting mild, easily correctable disorders, whereas others with severe disorders and dismal prognoses often react with equanimity. The degree of a client's anger can be surmised, however, as can the intensity of denial, bargaining, and depression experienced. Although not true for all clients, the degree of anger and other emotions clients experience when first confronted with a communicative disorder might depend to an extent on the disabling potentiality of the disorder and on its prognosis. More intense emotional responses might be anticipated to potentially debilitating disorders that have guarded prognoses than to those that are essentially cosmetic problems with favorable prognoses. The degree of anger might be related in an oxymoronic sense to a client's perception of the disorder's normalcy. Clients who perceive their speech, language, or hearing to be *different* rather than *disordered* and do not perceive that others do regard it as disordered are less likely to experience anger when confronted with the realities of their disorders than those who perceive otherwise. Another possible predictor of the degree of anger a communicatively disordered person might experience is the relation of the disorder to the status of their general health. Clients with organic communicative disorders are more likely also to be confronting chronic or catastrophic illness. Communicative disorders due to organic causes often are more severe and disabling; they carry more guarded prognoses than do nonorganically based communicative disorders. Organic communicative disorders also often involve secondary related crises for clients, such as financial concerns and role problems.

Many other factors may figure into the degree of anger experienced by clients in the grieving process, concerns that predated or are independent of the communicative disorder, or are perceived by clients to be due to their disorders (e.g., marital or relationship problems, job-related conflicts, unrelated physical problems, mental health problems, and self-concept crises). Caution should be observed in considering any possible predictor of degree of anger valid across clients and disorders; predictors of degree of anger should serve only to alert clinicians to the fact that anger is more likely to be a counseling issue for certain communicative disorders and certain clients.

The rate of dissipation is another aspect of anger in the grieving process that is just as difficult to predict as is its relative degree. The duration of anger as a defensive behavior varies from client to client. For some, anger may be nonexistent, whereas others may carry it well into the therapy process as a conscious or unconscious defense and never completely resolve it. The rising and diminishing rates of anger vary widely from case to case and may, in part, be determined by the chronicity and severity of the disorders and by the rate and degree of success in therapy. Some clients' anger rises and resolves in relatively smooth gradients, whereas other clients' anger recurs and is mercurial, spiking and dissipating in sharp gradients. In some cases in which it does not quickly subside, anger gives way to a less intense emotional state that might be called resentment. This feeling of resentment, of having been treated wrongly and unjustly, sometimes proves to be a persistent residue of anger. In cases of enduring or residual anger, clinicians should be sensitive both to the effect that anger has on clients and to its consequences for family members, employers or employees, friends, and others with whom it is important for the client to maintain positive, productive interpersonal relationships. If a client is displacing anger onto significant others with no signs of the displacement defense abating after counseling, clinicians might productively redirect the psychic energy of a client's anger to therapy. Clinicians should move such clients into therapy in an intensive way, with a structured plan that places high demands and expectations on the client. A client might be helped to use sublimation to supplant displacement behaviors as a defensive reaction to anger. This might be accomplished by the clinician's (a) strong, consistent reinforcement in a nonjudgmental clinical atmosphere of the client's attempts to accomplish tasks and goals and (b) continued counseling encouragement of the client to examine and express anger and channel it in productive directions. Sublimation as a response to anger then permits the client to direct the psychic energy expended on anger toward setting and accomplishing therapy goals.

Because a client might hide anger, clinicians often have difficulty determining whether it even exists, much less how quickly it is diminishing. Subtle signs of anger that might be observed in clients who do not verbally express it include (a) little enthusiasm for therapy; (b) vocal and nonvocal displacement behaviors directed toward clinicians or family members; (c) inattention; (d) subdued or atypically controlled affect; and (e) a high level of frustration.

Generally speaking, the rate at which a client's anger dissipates might be related to the factors suggested above as possibly influencing the degree of anger experienced. Clients who are more likely to sustain their anger are those with disorders that are:

- potentially seriously disabling
- perceived by themselves and others in their environments to be disorders by virtue of the type, rather than degree, of the problem
- organically based communicative disorders that possibly involve general health concerns
- communicative disorders not likely to be resolved in the short-term or ever

Clients who present with disorders that fit an opposite profile might resolve their anger relatively quickly, keeping in mind, however, as with degree of anger, such predictions can only be surmised because tendencies for emotional reaction to external or internal stimuli are highly individualized.

Several factors might help clients accelerate resolution of their anger. Three, in particular, are critical to helping clients work through their anger in relatively quick fashion. First, strong support from family and significant others, both for the client and for therapy, extends the security and comfort of therapy to a client's home, school, social settings, and work environments. They have both the clinician and a network of sympathetic individuals for anger transference and ultimately catharsis of their anger. Second, the dissipation rate of a client's anger is in part determined by the skill of clinicians as counselors. Clinicians who can recognize anger in their clients and who create a clinical atmosphere that encourages externalization of anger (i.e., an atmosphere that promotes expression and introspection by clients rather than rumination) are more effective in factoring anger out of the therapy equation. Third, the degree of success early in therapy determines if a client's anger will be long-lived. A client who sees quick, appreciable progress in therapy is more inclined to supplant anger with pride of accomplishment and hope for continued improvement.

Anger is a normal, expected reaction to news that one's well-being is threatened or injured, a reaction that helps an individual accept bad news. But anger clouds the therapy process, making it difficult for a client to see the purpose and course of therapy. Anger also can make it difficult to establish a relationship in which the client and clinician interact with the congruency necessary for optimal therapy progress. The anger clients with communicative disorders experience might be directed toward their families, their physicians, God, themselves, or their speech-language pathologists and audiologists; they might also experience a frustrating, directionless feeling of anger. Clinicians should be aware that a client's anger may be directed toward them and they should not react defensively to these expressions of anger. By using the suggestions for hypothesizing potential degree and dissipation rate of anger in clients as subjective predictors, clinicians might build strategies to assess and counsel anger into their prediagnostic interviews, diagnostic protocols, and treatment plans. Anger exhibited by clients has specific causes and it is the clinician's responsibility to determine what they are and help clients resolve them, either by counseling or by referral. When clients experience anger about their communicative disorder, they may perceive an external locus of control to be responsible for the existence of their disorder and, more importantly, for whether or not their disorder can be modified. Clients might have this perception, in some cases, owing to life problems that existed before the onset of their communicative disorder or to problems that occurred after (e.g., marital, academic, or vocational problems). In some instances, clients perceive their disorder to be under the influence of an external locus of control they cannot define or can define in metaphysical terms only. Speech-language pathologists and audiologists should counsel such perceptions only within the context of the client's communicative disorder and refer clients to other professionals for concerns that have achieved problem status independent of or only tangentially related to communicative disorders.

## BARGAINING

*Bargaining* is the third stage in Kubler-Ross's (1969) grieving model. Individuals are inculcated from childhood with the belief that bargaining is the behavior with which one obtains material possessions and spiritual goals. Bargaining can be secular or religious, open or tacit, self- or other-directed, realistic or unrealistic. It is used by individuals in attempts to delay acceptance of illness or disability, to revert from the present to the past, to barter for less severe involvement of an illnesses or disability and to have a more favorable prognosis of therapy.

Bargaining is a universal and life-sustaining behavior. It helps individuals set and achieve goals by bargaining with themselves through self-reinforcement. Bargaining helps individuals live moral, responsible lives because of their belief in present- and after-life rewards for doing so; maintain relationships by negotiating middle-ground when interpersonal disputes occur; and gradually absorb the shock of illness and disability.

Persons with communicative disorders and their family members might attempt to bargain with themselves, God, or their clinicians that they will behave in some exemplary manner if their speech, language, or hearing problem is corrected or improved. Parents may promise to be attentive and loving to their communicatively disordered children, to bring them to every therapy session, to do all at home that the clinicians suggest; in return, they expect complete or significant improvement of their children's problems. The same likelihood of bargaining is true for adult clients and can continue throughout the period of therapy, especially if it is reinforced in any way.

This is a point in the grieving process where the stage can be set for therapy success or failure. Clients who believe in their bargaining potency are eager to initiate therapy and negotiate therapy contracts with their clinicians. The bargaining stage is a hopeful one, although often somewhat desperately so, and remains hopeful when a client receives the expected returns. This is a cautious time for clinicians; they should take precautions, through counseling, to avoid the implication that a bargain has been struck to the effect that if the client enters and regularly attends therapy and is compliant to all of the clinician's instructions, the communicative disorder will be cured. This is a good time to negotiate clinical contracts with clients, but clinicians need to design them with realistic goals and make sure they have not inadvertently bargained with their clients for unrealistic outcomes. Clinicians should carefully explain all diagnostic findings, prognostic indicators, and therapy strategies to clients, and probe to determine the accuracy of a client's comprehension of those explanations. Clinicians should explore clients' expectations regarding returns throughout the course of therapy and, when found to be unrealistic, counsel to realign them with reality.

## DEPRESSION

If clients' perceive attempts at bargaining to have been futile, and if they feel impotent to negotiate for help from any source, they may next experience *depression*, Kubler-Ross's (1969) fourth stage of grieving. Depression occurs when a client realizes that denial, anger, and bargaining were to no avail and that he or she is left with no course other than to accept the facts of an illness or disability. This acceptance is, of course, the desired outcome of the grieving process, but it often comes only after the precursory state of depression. In this regard, depression is almost welcomed, as it is the emotional harbinger of acceptance. Depression, however, does not always readily give way to acceptance; it can become self-perpetuating and one of the foremost barriers to progress in therapy. Tanner (1980) states: "Depression should not be considered abnormal or pathological" (p. 922). This is true, insofar as depression is a typical stage in the grieving process. If, however, depression is to be distinguished as an emotional state different than dejection, which English and English (1958) suggest is a better term to describe "normal" depression, and other synonymic lay terms for only the mood aspect of depression, depression must be viewed, if not as an abnormal state, at least as one that is undesirable. Nacht and Racamier (1960) define depression as a pathological emotional state in which individuals consciously experience guilt and psychic suffering. Wolman (1989) notes that depression is differentiated from terms such as sadness, unhappiness, and sorrow because depression, unlike those emotions, involves feelings of helplessness and a personal sense of guilt for being helpless. Perhaps what is typically observed in persons with communicative disorders is a feeling state less related to clinical depression than it is to other emotions; the matter is somewhat a semantic one as well as a question of degree. It is important, however, for clinicians not to view a client's depression as necessarily a normal feeling state that will give way in time to more pleasant emotions. A client who is experiencing depression tends to give up on therapy and abandon hope for improvement. A depressed client's self-blame can lead to loss of self-esteem which, in turn, makes the individual more susceptible to guilt feelings which, in turn, deepens depression, creating a downward emotional spiral. Depression is a diminished state of mental and psychomotor activity; while clients are experiencing depression, progress toward clinical modification of their communicative disorder is minimal.

Depression, in a way, is the reverse feeling state of anger—one of its preceding states. Whereas individuals experiencing anger in the grieving process are inclined to rail against their fate and become aggressive toward all perceived *particeps criminis* associated with it, depressed persons tend to give up and become passive, although anxiety can increase during depression and obsessive thoughts and behaviors develop. Depression, as with anger or any emotion, occurs in varying degrees and lasts for varying periods of time across clients. The variables suggested above as possible factors in an equational prediction of degree and duration of the anger experienced by persons grieving their loss of communicative function—the actual disabling potential of the loss; clients' perceptions of difference versus disorder versus handicap; organic versus functional loss, especially regarding general health concerns; prognosis for correction or compensation of the loss—might also be possible predictors of degree and duration of a client's depression. As with anger, the degree and duration of depression are determined by the highly individualized affective and cognitive make-ups of clients, which largely determine how they react to loss of speech, language, or hearing function.

There also might exist external realities apart from but directly attributable to clients' communicative disorders that cause concern or frustration but which they feel powerless to control. For example, as a result of a communicative disorder or concomitant health or physical problems, a client frequently incurs large medical bills or has to deal with disfigurement. Sometimes a client has to alter or restrict social life and give up vocations and avocations. These clients can become alienated from their families and develop marital problems, triggered by their or others' emotional reactions to their communicative disorders. These circumstances can induce reactive or exogenous depression, which is depression in reaction to an external event; if the event is positively terminated or altered, the contingent depression might spontaneously remit. Speech-language pathologists and audiologists can help clients resolve reactive depression through counseling, being careful to keep counseling within the context of a client's communicative disorder. Clinicians should refer to other professionals if the event producing a client's reactive depression indicates the need for specialized counseling (e.g., financial or marital counseling) or if a client's emotional reactions to external events produced by a communicative disorder or by its causes transcend the limits of what might be judged to be nonpathological reactions.

It is natural for a client to experience depression or milder feeling states recognized as depression. In fact, almost everyone experiences a sense of depression from time to time; therefore, it could be considered a normal emotion. Perhaps questions of degree, duration, or control of depression determine whether it is a normal or pathological emotional state. Perhaps whether a period of depression is spent in introspection or rumination determines its normalcy. Whether normal or pathological, the general problem with a client's depression, as with denial and anger, is it reduces or prevents forward progress in therapy. It is important for a client to work through depression so that it does not linger and interfere with concentration on therapy goals. Although depression can recur throughout therapy, its resolution, through counseling, reduces the likelihood that the external events effecting a client's depression will continue to do so.

If clients' depression is directly related to the communicative disorder, corrective or compensatory changes in speech, language, or hearing effected in therapy can prove to be the best means of resolving their depression. This is a Catch-22 situation, however, as progress in therapy serves to reduce depression but depression hinders progress in therapy. If depression persists for clients with communicative disorders and if no related external events are determined responsible for its persistence, therapy might not be working in some respect—unrealistic client expectations, the client is not trying or concentrating, the clinician is ineffective in delivery of therapy or is incongruent in the counseling relationship, or the client's communicative disorder is less responsive to therapy than was predicted by evaluation and indicated in prognosis. Of course it could also mean that the client's depression is endogenous or internally generated, perhaps precipitated by onset of a communicative disorder but now self-feeding. In such cases, referral to a clinical psychologist or psychiatrist is appropriate.

ACCEPTANCE

Kubler-Ross's (1969) last stage of grieving is *acceptance*. This is the last stage if a client has had the time, inner resources, and helping support to resolve the preceding stages successfully. Although it is the final stage in the linear design of the Kubler-Ross grieving process model, a client might revert at any time during therapy to earlier stages of grief, which means that grieving does not necessarily cease completely once the acceptance stage is reached. Acceptance symbolizes a client's conscious awareness of the reality that he or she is and may always be a person with a communicative disorder until an earnest attempt is made to do something about it. Acceptance implies that denial, anger, and bargaining have lost value as defensive reactions to the client's losses and the fog of depression has lifted. A client who is in the acceptance stage should be appreciably better able than earlier in the grieving process to concentrate on therapy and to make goal-directed decisions.

It should be noted that acceptance, as spoken of in this stage, should not be construed to mean resignation (Tanner, 1980). Resignation conveys acceptance of fate by virtue of one's being helpless to do anything about the future. Acceptance, on the other hand, acknowledges only the realities of one's fate. Clinicians should observe clients' vocal and nonvocal behaviors carefully to ascertain whether their clients are displaying acceptance of their communicative disorders rather than resignation, which in actuality might be depression masked as acceptance.

Clients work their way at different rates through the grieving process. How soon they arrive at the acceptance stage depends on numerous variables, including the characteristics of their disorders, the degree and quality of family support, individual personalities, and their clinician's counseling skills. Some clients are already in the acceptance stage of grief when they report for therapy. Kubler-Ross (1969) suggests that grief, in particular grief attendant to the death of a loved one, typically lasts up to a year after the loss, as evidenced in long-standing cultural traditions in which a wife must symbolically mourn the death of her husband for one year. Regardless of how quickly and easily clients arrive at the acceptance stage of grief, clinicians can do two things to help them remain in acceptance and to make maximal clinical use of it. First, although they may have done so earlier, clinicians should explain to clients, carefully and in detail, evaluation results, prognoses, and therapy procedures and rationales. A client's accurate awareness of a disorder must precede acceptance of its realities and the responsibility for addressing those realities in therapy. If entering the acceptance stage of grief with faulty knowledge about the disorder or with an inaccurate perception of what can be accomplished in therapy, the client is more likely to regress to earlier stages of grief than if given complete and accurate information. Second, although acceptance does not imply passivity on the part of clients (Bristor, 1984), neither does it ensure action by them. Clinicians should remain vigilant to their clients' levels of motivation and not assume that acceptance prompts motivation. Acceptance is a feeling state in which motivation can be generated and sustained, although not necessarily spontaneously. A client who is quickly motivated is likely also to achieve therapy goals quickly; each success in therapy decreases the probability that a client will revert to earlier stages of grief.

Speech-language pathologists and audiologists should be knowledgeable about and sensitive to the feelings of loss experienced by their clients. They should help their clients through the grieving process by:

- creating an accepting, nonjudgmental clinical setting
- being empathic listeners
- using nondirective counseling techniques
- allowing clients to remain in control of their progress through grief

It is a clinical imperative that clinicians help communicatively disordered clients accept their loss as well as modify their disorders, which serves to enhance clients' general well-being and clinicians' clinical accountability.

## Other Clinically Relevant Emotions

In the admixture of a communicatively disordered client's emotions are several other clinically relevant emotions in addition to those constituting the grieving process discussed above. Three emotions in particular—anxiety, guilt, and feelings of isolation—are experienced often by persons who have communicative disorders and by their parents and significant others. These emotions, which can exist concurrently with the emotions typically associated with grief, can play equally important roles in clients' and parents' experiencing loss.

### ANXIETY

Hartbauer (1978) notes that *anxiety* often observed in clients during the initial clinical interview stems from client worries about therapy prognosis, clinician competency, and how they will be perceived by the clinician. It is reasonable to expect clients to feel some level of anxiety on entering an unfamiliar setting to begin an evaluation and treatment process with no prior informed expectations. Anxiety about therapy might be augmented by clients' apprehensions, if not corrected, that the communicative disorder will adversely affect interpersonal relationships; prevent attainment of educational, vocational, and avocational goals; and cause others to regard them as unattractive or abnormal.

Anxiety consists of uncomfortable physiologic reactions (e.g., perspiration, nausea, increased heart rate, and so forth) to a perceived threat of approaching dangers and psychological reactions to the belief that one is powerless to prevent imminent dangers. These reactions distract clients from focusing on therapy goals and, if anxiety persists, may lead to clients convincing themselves that their clinicians also are powerless in preventing the perceived impending dangers. Clients may attempt to keep their anxiety hidden from their clinicians or deny its existence to themselves, which might only serve ultimately to intensify their anxiety and to extend it to other real and imagined threats. Clinicians should be vigilant for signs of a client's suppressed anxiety. Clients who ask questions that suggest worry about the future in general or about therapy outcome, exhibit a distracted demeanor in therapy, or develop physical behaviors associated with anxiety might be displaying signs of internalized anxiety. Clinicians should attempt to establish a clinical atmosphere of trust and unconditioned acceptance in which a client feels comfortable externalizing anxiety and, thereby, is able to place it in objective perspective and possibly resolve it.

In some cases, clients' anxiety about the present and future consequences of their communicative disorder might be displaced to clinicians and family members as vocal and nonvocal hostility. Such displays related to anxiety should not be punished or discouraged by clinicians or family; instead, they should be explored with the client to identify the perceived threats that are causing their fulmination or aggression.

Another way that clients might manifest anxiety is by speaking of it openly. Here again, clinicians should facilitate such self-examination and provide the setting, time, data, and empathy to help the client identify the nature and sources of anxiety that are having a negative influence on quality of life or progress in therapy.

Often anxiety associated with communicative disorders develops owing to a client having incomplete knowledge or inaccurate perceptions of the disorder or inappropriate attitudes about therapy. This anxiety might be allayed in short order if the clinician helps distinguish real from imagined threats by taking ample time at the start of therapy to discuss all aspects of the relevant disorder and of the proposed treatment for it. This discussion should be repeated occasionally to confirm that a client has acquired adequate and accurate knowledge about the disorder and therapy and has adjusted personal attitudes and perceptions to facilitate the desired behavioral changes. Clients should also be allowed to ask questions about their clinicians and make suggestions about the plan of therapy, which might help to establish an equal partner relationship in therapy, rather than one of student-teacher or subject-technician.

The time required to achieve therapy goals is another factor that figures into how completely and quickly clients resolve anxiety. Anxiety is less likely to remain a concern with clients who readily have success in therapy. This does not ensure that all of the anxiety associated with their communicative disorder automatically remits with therapy success; they may, for example, be anxious that their therapy success will not last. The logical forecast to make is that anxiety will be less of a continuing problem with a readily successful client than with those for whom successful therapy comes slowly and with difficulty.

Passage of time might result in clients becoming progressively inured to anxiety, which could make it more difficult for them to identify the sources of their anxiety and to describe how it affects them. Some clients might never resolve nor become inured to their anxiety, with its intensity increasing across time and new sources of anxiety constantly being added to existing ones.

Rogers (1951) notes that a minimal level of client anxiety is a precondition for change to occur in therapy; client anxiety, in this sense, is the motivating force behind successful therapy. Anxiety that goes beyond minimum, however, can itself become debilitating and obstructive to any real progress in therapy. Clinicians should make every effort to keep clients' anxiety about their communicative disorder minimal. If a client's anxiety becomes disproportionate to the severity of the disorder, persists after appreciable time in therapy or after achieving therapy goals, or appears unrelated to the client's communicative disorder, that client should be referred for psychological evaluation or specialized counseling.

## GUILT

*Guilt* is an emotion associated with anxiety. These two emotions engender and intensify one another and might not easily be distinguished by clinicians. It is even somewhat difficult to differentiate semantically between guilt and anxiety. In a psychoanalytic context, for example, guilt is considered to be an anxiety localized in the ego due to perceived transgressions by the ego (unconscious impulses) against the authority of the superego (conscience and ego-ideal); guilt is the fear of retribution for those transgressions. Although guilt and anxiety are related, there are characteristics that distinguish one from the other. Persons experiencing either guilt or anxiety feel a prescience of approaching punishment or danger. But, whereas anxiety implies feelings of helplessness when confronted with fate, guilt is supported by the belief that one has the power to control fate and reality (Luterman, 1991). Clients and parents often experience guilt due to a belief that they could have prevented their or their children's communicative disorder by having (*a*) led more moral lives, (*b*) paid more attention and been more responsive to their or their children's health and development, or (*c*) been more knowledgeable about the causes and characteristics of speech, language, and hearing disorders. Feelings of guilt about present misfortune being a result of not having properly controlled past events might be indicated in client comments such as, "If only I hadn't . . .," "If I had it to do over . . .," "I never thought it might result in . . .," and "I feel badly that I didn't know. . . ."

Clients and parents also experience guilt when they perceive that they are not presently using their fate-control powers to improve the future status of their or their children's communicative disorder. These guilt feelings are revealed in such statements as, "If I would get off my . . ." and "I could do it if only I would. . . ." Guilt of this type is seen in clients who enroll in therapy and in parents who enroll their children in therapy because they would feel guilty if they did not do so. Once enrolled, however, they frequently miss therapy sessions or are noncompliant as to completion of therapy assignments and their noncompliancy reconstitutes the guilt that was assuaged by enrolling in therapy. Most typically, guilt is a feeling tied to past events, whereas anxiety is present- and future-oriented. To accomplish therapy goals efficiently, clinicians should help clients and parents direct their problem-solving to the present and to be concerned with *how* best to modify their speech, language, or hearing, rather than trying to determine *why* they or their children were fated to develop a communicative disorder. Shipley (1992) makes this point well:

> Involving people with guilt in certain treatment activities can be helpful for these people as concern becomes focused on the present. Individuals experiencing guilt often benefit when they are made to feel part of the *solution* rather than part of the *problem*. (p. 63)

Guilt is prevalent among parents of children with disabilities (Webster, 1977); Luterman (1991) suggests, that of the emotions of clinical significance, guilt tends to be the most prevalent among these parents. However, guilt can be experienced by both child and adult clients irrespective of whether parents and significant others are experiencing it and intentionally or unintentionally projecting it on the clients. Guilt can be "real," in instances where it is associated with violation of a moral, social, legal, religious, or ethical code. It can also be imagined (e.g., when it is adduced to an external event to mask repressed guilt that is connected to id impulses and societal taboos). Guilt can be conscious, as with real guilt, or unconscious, as with imagined guilt. Unconscious guilt most often manifests in a client's expressions of a lowered sense of personal worth. Guilt can be "normal" or neurotic. Everyone experiences guilt—it is an emotion that helps societies maintain some level of control. Referral for psychological evaluation is indicated if a client's guilt becomes so profound as to affect adversely interpersonal relationships, daily responsibilities, homeostasis, or therapy, or if it is disproportionate to the perceived infraction or transgression producing it.

Speech-language pathologists and audiologists should attend to both the real and imagined guilt their clients might be experiencing. Conscious guilt might be openly revealed by clients and quickly worked through; or, it might be indicated tacitly in comments and behaviors such as those discussed. A client's unconscious guilt can only be surmised by clinicians, but if indications of its existence are observed (e.g., professions of guilt for numerous acts that do not reasonably seem to constitute even minor offenses against any code) consultation with a clinical psychologist or psychiatrist is appropriate. Guilt, as with anxiety, can lower the quality of life for clients and their families. It can come between relationships and contribute to parents' and clients' feelings of isolation. Parents experiencing guilt over their belief that the onset or development of their child's communicative disorder is their fault might attempt to expiate their guilt by becoming overly protective parents, by treating their communicatively disordered child with more attention and understanding than they do their other children, or by placing unrealistic expectations, either too low or too high, on their disordered child. In some cases, they might even reject their child as a way of denying guilt by discontinuing contact with or responsibility for the perceived source of their guilt feelings.

Regardless of how guilt is manifested or directed by parents and clients, it is an especially important emotion for clinicians to be sensitive to throughout the course of therapy. It might be present at the first session and subsequently resolved through counseling, only to appear later in therapy perhaps because of minimal therapy progress for which parents or clients blame themselves. Feelings of guilt can change into depression or exacerbate an existing state of depression; both are characterized by a loss of self-esteem. As is the case with the other relevant emotions in therapy, clinicians can help parents and clients resolve their guilt by establishing nonjudgmental, trusting clinical relationships and by permitting parents and clients the opportunity to explore and objectify their guilt feelings. Guilt is often predicated on superstitions, beliefs, myths, or inaccurate information; clinicians should help parents and clients develop realistic, objective understanding of the relevant communicative disorders. At the same time, clinicians should be careful not to create guilt inadvertently, to show approbation for guilt feelings, or to reinforce the guilt of parents or clients. Comments such as, "What have you done before now for your child's language disorder?" and "She hasn't been seen by an audiologist before today?," can be perceived as imputations that parents have been less than exemplary in attending to their child's communicative disorder. Such seemingly benign, empathic statements like "I understand fully," in response to parents' or clients' expressions of guilt, can be interpreted as clinician approval of their guilt feelings.

ISOLATION

*Isolation* is not just a physical state of social alienation that is either self-imposed or due to ostracism, it is also a feeling state. It is a feeling often experienced by persons with communicative disorders and one, as with the previously discussed feelings, that can lessen a client's motivation and focus in therapy. A client may experience isolation by rejecting contact with others or by behaving in ways that cause others to reject them, although not necessarily for reasons directly appertaining to communicative disorders. Isolation develops from various cognitive and affective reactions of clients to their disorders which they describe in counseling as perceptions that they are unattractive, inadequate, incompetent, or undeserving. Clinicians should take note of verbal and nonverbal behaviors that suggest low self-esteem and explore with the client the reasons for it. If clients translate their feelings of isolation into action, they might isolate themselves, psychically if not physically, from friends, family members, teachers, and clinicians with the likelihood that they will be less than effective in their roles of parent, spouse, significant other, student, employee, and client.

All the emotions discussed above can be implicated in a client's developing feelings of isolation: In essence, denial is isolation from reality. Anger is an isolating emotion; it puts clients in conflict rather than in correspondence with the world, causes others to break off relationships, and isolates clients from their emotions and from their rational selves. Anxiety can lead to isolation through avoidance behaviors; the anxiety that prompted avoidance subsequently is increased by added fear that the avoidance behaviors will be discovered and confronted by others. Feelings of isolation are perhaps most influenced by the emotions of depression and guilt, and conversely they by them. The loss of self-esteem that characterizes depression leads also to feelings of isolation; the feelings of isolation can in turn result in a deepening of depression. Parents or clients who are experiencing guilt can consciously or unconsciously impose isolation on themselves as penance for perceived wrongs they have committed. Although guilt is the reason why some parents or clients isolate themselves, subsequent feelings of isolation make it only more difficult for them to resolve their guilt.

Clients sometimes use isolation in a preemptive sense. That is, they isolate themselves, figuratively or literally, before others have the opportunity to isolate them through rejection. Deliberate or voluntary isolation also can result from thoughts that one is unique. Parents of a child with a communicative disorder, for example, might believe that no one has had their experience or has felt their emotions; in essence, they feel that no one can be fully or truly congruent to a relationship with them that is based on their child's problem. Attempts by clinicians to be congruent might be seen as patronizing or condescending.

The insular state of isolation can seem oddly comforting to parents and clients, existing in bittersweet symbiosis with depression and guilt. This sense of protection-in-isolation can cause parents and clients to be particularly resistant to abandoning their isolated states of feeling or being. Isolation is a condition that is especially obstructive to effective counseling, owing to the difficulty it presents in establishing an honest, open, client-counselor relationship. A client who is experiencing isolation as a positive state is also less likely to be motivated to work on a speech, language, or hearing problem, as effective communication negates isolation.

To determine if a client is experiencing a sense of isolation, clinicians should observe both physical and attitudinal indices of isolation. For instance, clients might isolate themselves physically by not dating, not joining social organizations, living alone, not forming friendships, and so forth. Or they might exhibit all of the acts of socialization, yet feel isolated—the "I am never more alone than when in a crowd" feeling. If clinicians suspect that their clients are experiencing isolation, confrontation often is the most effective and time-efficient technique to use in helping clients to resolve their sense of isolation. Being an empathic listener might not begin to get the job done, as it plays into the hands of isolation by not forcing communication. Confronting a client's isolation brings it into conscious focus, in terms of the degree of rationality behind it, the factors maintaining it, its relevance to success or failure in therapy, and the ways in which it might be resolved. In addition to confrontation, other ways in which a client's feelings of isolation might be resolved are:

1. Successful treatment of communicative disorders despite emotional overlay.
2. Information and insights imparted that afford more accurate and realistic internal self-perceptions and perceptions of self relative to external objects, events, and persons.
3. Support groups wherein clients cannot avoid admitting that they are not unique or alone in their present dilemma of whether to face the discomforting reality of a communicative disorder or to avoid reality through isolation.

## SELF-CONCEPT AND COMMUNICATIVE BEHAVIOR

The clinically relevant emotions discussed in this chapter are more easily resolved by clients who have positive, strong self-concepts and high levels of self-esteem. These emotions, however, can erode self-esteem, even in such clients, and can result in their developing adversely altered self-concepts, which would not augur well for therapy outcome. It is important, therefore, for clinicians to be concerned about both a client's self-concept throughout therapy and the various emotions that can affect self-concept.

An individual's self-concept is affected by speech, language, and hearing status. It could be reasoned that self-concept, self-esteem, and persona (as described by Jung, 1923) are all determined by or symbolized in how individuals are able or choose to communicate with themselves and with their environment. If this reasoning is accurate, it would follow that appreciable changes in an individual's self-concept, self-esteem, or persona might effect to varying degrees corresponding changes in communicative capabilities or behaviors, in either healthy or disordered directions. The reverse effect would also then be feasible; changes in an individual's communicative status may precipitate changes in attitudes about self, losses or gains in ego strength, and redesigns, whether consciously or unconsciously, of the face presented to the world. It is therefore critical for speech-language pathologists and audiologists to understand that whenever they enter into a client-clinician relationship to help change a client's communicative behavior, they may also inadvertently promote change in the client's self-concept.

It is well for clinicians to counsel their clients to the possible reciprocal relationship of self-concept and communicative disorders. First, through counseling, a client might be able in therapy to increase self-esteem or adopt a more realistic persona even with minimal success in modifying speech, language, or hearing problems. Second, prognosis for successful modification of a client's communicative problem is improved by increases in self-esteem, resolution of self-concept conflicts, and abandonment of a contrived, defensive persona. Third, counseling can be used to help a client comprehend self-concept concerns and to develop strategies for resolving those concerns by establishing, regaining, or maintaining coping ego functions.

It should be noted that successful therapy outcomes do not guarantee an automatic healthy shift in self-concept, particularly when a client's experiences with communicative disorders have been particularly intense or long-standing. This is not to suggest that all individuals with communicative disorders have or tend to develop problems with self-concept; communicative disorders, however, do place them at risk to develop self-concept problems and clinicians should be alert to that possibility.

If self-concept is manifested in communicative behavior and communicative behavior is representative of self-concept and changes in either might influence the status of the other, should both be addressed in therapy? The answer unequivocally is yes, but clinicians should keep in mind the continuum model of counseling and psychotherapy and refer clients whose self-concept problems are more intrapsychic than interpersonal in nature. Development of concept of self is discussed in Chapter 3.

## HOLISTIC APPROACH TO COUNSELING

Should speech-language pathologists and audiologists regard their clients' communicative disorders as problems *in vitro,* isolated problems to be "fixed" using technical, standardized, impersonal protocols? Or, should they see their clients as persons with unique role, self-concept, or relationship problems related to their communicative disorders; debilitating levels of emotions (e.g., anxiety, guilt, anger, and depression) as a direct or indirect result of their communicative disorders; or who deny their communicative disorders or resist change in the status of their speech, language, or hearing? If, through counseling, clinicians assess and address these affective, cognitive, and interpersonal dimensions of their clients' speech, language, and hearing problems, their clients are more likely to accept responsibility for minimizing their disorders and maximizing their communicative potential. These clients will enter into partnerships with their clinicians to achieve the maximal benefits of therapy and will become whole persons independent of the ultimate status of their communicative disorders. The general goal of a holistic approach to therapy is the same as the basic goal of counseling. For self-healing to be maximally effective, individuals must take responsibility for making the decisions that will result in life-enhancing changes in all aspects of being—physical, emotional, mental, existential, and spiritual (Vaughn, 1985). The idea that the interrelationships among body, cognition, emotion, and perception affect the wellness states of each other, as well as the wellness of the combined whole forms the basis of holistic thought. Dossey, Keegan, Kolkmeier, and Guzzetta (1989) define this concept of holism:

> Holism is a philosophy that views everything in terms of patterns of organization, relationships, interactions, and processes that combine to form a whole. Wholeness can be present when one has high levels of wellness and also when one has a known disease/disability or is in the process of dying. Wholeness is a process and is present when we view ourselves as an open living system in a tapestry of relationships and events. Our actions have an effect on our body-mind-spirit. Because of the holistic aspect of our being, each dimension has a direct effect on the other. . . . (p. 5)

The holistic approach to therapy is in line with Gestalt psychology principles in which images are held to be perceived whole patterns or configurations, gestalten, which cannot be explained by the characteristics of their components; the whole of a perceptual experience is more than a sum of its parts. In this view, the organism responds to gestalten with a whole response, rather than with summative responses to specific elements within the gestalten. Gestalt therapy is discussed in Chapter 4.

In this whole person sense, communicatively disordered clients can be viewed as interacting with the world in gestalt fashion, with their speech, language, or hearing problems and their reactions to those problems being part of the intricate experiential configurations of their perceived reality. These configurations can figure for or against a successful outcome of therapy, depending on how closely they correspond to clinicians, parents, and significant others' perceptions of reality. Each client's perception of reality can be explored and possibly altered through counseling, to create enhanced attitudinal states that benefit the individual by increasing overall wellness and improving the prognosis of therapy.

## REFERENCES

Arnold, M. B (1960). *Emotion and personality: Vol. I and II.* New York: Columbia University Press.
Barbara, D. A. (1954). *Stuttering: A psychodynamic approach to its understanding and treatment.* New York: Julian Press.

Barbara, D. A. (1958). *Your speech reveals your personality.* Springfield, IL: Charles C. Thomas.

Bloodstein, O. (1987). *A handbook on stuttering.* Chicago, IL: National Easter Seals Society.

Bowlby, J. (1969). *Attachment and loss. Vol. I: Attachment.* New York: Basic Books.

Bowlby, J. (1973). *Attachment and loss. Vol. II: Anxiety and anger.* New York: Basic Books.

Bowlby, J. (1980). *Attachment and loss. Vol. III: Sadness and depression.* New York: Basic Books.

Brill, A. A. (1923). Speech disturbances in nervous and mental diseases. *Quarterly Journal of Speech Education, 9,* 129–135.

Bristor, M. W. (1984). The birth of a handicapped child—A holistic model for grieving. *Family Relations, 33,* 25–32.

Coriat, I. H. (1928) Stammering: A psychoanalytic interpretation. *Nervous and Mental Disease Monograph, 47,* 1–68.

Dossey, B. M., Keegan, L., Kalkmeier, L. G., and Guzzetta, C. E. (1989). *Holistic health promotion: A guide for practice.* Rockville, MD: Aspen Systems.

Engel, G. L. (1964). Grief and grieving. *American Journal of Nursing, 64,* 93–98.

English, H. B., and English, A. C. (1958). *A comprehensive dictionary of psychological and psychoanalytical terms.* New York: David McKay Company.

Fenichel, O. (1945). *The psychoanalytic theory of neurosis.* New York: WW Norton.

Gemelli, R. J. (1982a). Classification of child stuttering. Part I: Transient developmental, neurogenic acquired, and persistent child stuttering. *Child Psychiatry and Human Development, 12,* 220–253.

Gemelli, R. J. (1982b). Classification of child stuttering. Part II: Persistent late onset male stuttering, and treatment issues for persistent stutterers—psychotherapy or speech therapy, or both? *Child Psychiatry and Human Development, 13,* 3–34.

Glauber, I. P. (1958). The psychoanalysis of stuttering. In J. Eisenson (Ed.), *Stuttering: A symposium.* New York: Harper & Row.

Hartbauer, R. E. (1978). *Counseling in communicative disorders.* Springfield, IL: Charles C. Thomas.

Johnson, W., and Knott, J. R. (1936). The moment of stuttering. *Journal of Genetic Psychology, 48,* 475–479.

Jung, C. G. (1923). *Psychological types or the psychology of individuation.* Orlando, FL: Harcourt Brace Jovanovich.

Kroeber, T. C. (1964). The coping functions of the ego mechanisms. In R. W. White (Ed.), *The study of lives.* New York: Atherton.

Kubler-Ross, E. (1969). *On death and dying.* New York: Macmillan.

Kubler-Ross, E. (1975). *Death: The final stage of growth.* Englewood Cliffs, NJ: Prentice-Hall.

Luterman, D. M. (1991). *Counseling the communicatively disordered and their families* (2nd ed.). Austin, TX: Pro-Ed.

Moses, K., and Van Hecke-Wulatin, M. (1981). A counseling model re: The socio-emotional impact of infant deafness. In G. T. Mencher, and S. E. Gerber (Eds.), *Early management of hearing loss.* New York: Grune & Stratton.

Moses, K. L. (1985). Dynamic intervention with families. In E. Cherow (Ed.), *Hearing impaired children and youth with disabilities.* Washington, DC: Gallaudet College Press.

Nacht, S., and Racamier, P. C. (1960). Symposium as "depressive illness" II. Depressive states. *International Journal of Psycho-Analysis, XLI,* 481–496.

Rogers, C. R. (1951). *Client-centered therapy.* Boston, MA: Houghton Mifflin.

Rollin, W. J. (1987). *The psychology of communicative disorders in individuals and their families.* Englewood Cliffs, NJ: Prentice-Hall.

Shipley, K. G. (1992). *Interviewing and counseling in communicative disorders: Principles and procedures.* New York: Merrill.

Sheehan, J. G. (1953). Theory and treatment of stuttering as an approach-avoidance conflict. *Journal of Psychology, 36,* 27–49.

Tanner, D. C. (1980). Loss and grief: Implications for the speech-language pathologist and audiologist. *ASHA, 22,* 916–928.

Van Riper, C. (1982). *The nature of stuttering* (2nd ed.). Englewood Cliffs, NJ: Prentice-Hall.

Vaughn, F. (1985). *The inward arc.* Boston: Shambhala Publications.

Webster, E. J. (1977). *Counseling with parents of handicapped children: Guidelines for improving communication.* New York: Grune & Stratton.

West, R. (1931). The phenomenology of stuttering. In R. West (Ed.), *A symposium on stuttering.* Madison, WI: College Typing Company.

Wolman, B. B. (1989). *Dictionary of behavioral science* (2nd ed.). New York: Academic Press.

# 3. Theories of Personality

Thomas A. Crowe

---

| | |
|---|---|
| **Importance of Theory** | **Personality Theory** |
|    Building a Personal Theory of Counseling |    Freud's Classic Psychoanalytic Theory |
|    Evaluating Theory |    Ego-Analytic Theory |
| **Personality Defined** |    Self Theory |

---

Theories relevant to the practice of counseling are presented in this chapter and in Chapter 4. As mentioned in Chapter 1, accountable professional counseling is that which is based on theory. The theories presented herein are only several of the many that have been put forward to explain personality and approaches to its modification. The theories discussed in this chapter, however, have been some of the most influential ones in the evolution of contemporary personality theory and contain some of the most widely adopted strategies used in modern counseling practice.

## IMPORTANCE OF THEORY

Generally, it is agreed that it is essential to base counseling practice on a theoretic base that includes, foremostly, personality theory (Bischof, 1964; Hall & Lindzey, 1978; Pepinsky & Pepinsky, 1954; Ryckman, 1978; Schultz, 1976). Theory provides practical frameworks on which clinicians can order the strategies they use in counseling with clients. Theory lends a sense of logic and order to processes and events that constitute each counseling encounter. Just as speech-language pathologists and audiologists base both their views of normal communication development and behavior—from language development to auditory perception—and their assessment and programmatic treatment of communication disorders on theory, so too should their counseling intervention be based on theory. If not, there is danger of counseling being based on clinician bias about human behavior, bias not based on scientifically interpreted empirical data, as is a theory, but only on indistinct assumptions. That is not to say that assumption is not a part of theory. But the assumptions on which a theory is based must be stated clearly and be explicitly relevant to the empirical events to which the theory is related. If a clinician's assumptions about human behavior on which counseling practice is based are implicit, vague assumptions, his or her approach to counseling will be one that does not generate empirical consequences such as predictions and hypotheses that can be tested and thereby enhance the clinician's counseling effectiveness. The inference-to-hypothesis-to-theory progression should also work in reverse; that is, a theory should ideally lead to deductions that can be stated as testable hypotheses. Thus, in time, theory should become more clinically useful and generate predictions about client behavior that prove to be accurate through empirical verification. Hall and Lindzey (1978) suggest that *verifiability* is one determinate of the utility of a theory, another being its *comprehensiveness*. The more inclusively theories predict the empirical phenomena that are relevant to them, the more useful they are. These inclusive predictions become generalizations that enable the clinician to understand comprehensively each client's thoughts, emotions, and behaviors relative to specific problems and across clients. These generalizations also serve to guide clinicians in their counseling with clients to modify their thoughts, emotions, and behaviors.

## Building a Personal Theory of Counseling

In developing personal philosophies of counseling, speech-language pathologists and audiologists might be inclined, on studying personality and counseling theories, to reject certain theories out of hand. They may have preconceived notions about their verifiability or comprehensiveness or have initial impressions of whether particular theories will be useful in their clinical practice. Clinicians should thoroughly study and seriously contemplate as many personality, behavior change, and counseling theories as possible prior to forming their own. They will be able then to cull from the various historical and contemporary theories appreciable aspects that have utility in their practice of counseling.

Bischof (1964) suggests that students of theory move through three stages in constructing their own theories or philosophies. The first stage, the *purist* stage, is a myopic period in which students ascribe explanation of diverse, even unrelated phenomena to a single theoretic construct. Experience and study, however, eventually lead students to the realization that one or a limited number of theories cannot be used to explain all events. Students move next to the *synthesis* stage, which represents their first attempt to assemble a personal theory. In this stage, numerous concepts and details from various theories are assimilated into a complex network of assumptions and empirical definitions that can be used to answer many more questions about people and events than in the purist stage. The problem with this stage is its tangled fabric of theory parts; the parts are so interwoven that they do not lend themselves easily to individual examination. *Inductive* problem-solving is more useful in the synthesis stage of theory formation than is *deductive* problem-solving. Attempts to extract single theoretic fibers for study or application might cause the unraveling of the complete fabric of a synthetic theory. Thus, students often move on to a third stage of personal theory formation, the *eclecticist* stage. In this stage, various theoretic constructs are used to form personal theories and philosophies as in the synthesis stage, but here the constructs are more fully understood individually and are more compartmentalized within the personal theory amalgam. Rather than a tangle of bits and pieces, as in the previous stages, students now have a personal theory that, in essence, is a framework on which substantive theoretic insights can be hung, as are windows in a house. Together, the framework and theoretic "windows" represent a complete structure of personal philosophy; taken singly, the "windows" offer different views of the landscape of human personality and behavior; at times, a single window is useful with a client and at times windows are used in diverse combinations. The theoretic positions constituting the eclectic amalgam of personal theory can also be tested and criticized individually, without necessary risk to the cohesiveness of personal theory in general.

## Evaluating Theory

What are the characteristics that define a personal theory or philosophy as good or clinically useful? Some of the characteristics of a good theory, personal or not, already have been discussed. A summary of those characteristics and a few other are listed below. A theory should:

1. Have *utility*. It should relate to the empirical events with which it is associated.
2. Have high *verifiability*. It should yield predictions that can be empirically tested and proved accurate.

3. Be *comprehensive.* It should be inclusive of the empirical phenomena with which it is concerned.
4. Lead to the *formulation of generalizations* about emotions, behavior, and events that can be used as a means-end road map in counseling.
5. Be *heuristic* in that it lends itself to the process of derivation in which empirically testable hypotheses are generated.
6. Be formed specifically on which to base counseling and should itself be *based on theories of personality, maladaptive behavior, and behavior change.* It should also include an end-product that is the target of counseling (Hansen, Stevic, & Warner, 1982). In counseling with persons with communicative disorders, the desired end-product might be correction or control of the disorders. Or, for some clients, the desired end-product might be establishing coping control of their ego functions to help them become self-actualizing and experience a high quality of life despite communicative disorders persisting after therapy.
7. Include *techniques* for achieving the desired end-product of counseling. Their applicability to the theory in general and their appropriateness for clinical use should have been established through empiric observation and testing and through trial-and-error use.
8. Bring *order* to assumptions, definitions, empiric data, and clinical insights that are drawn from various sources. This is the framework function of a theory; it should both incorporate and synthesize various bits of thought and knowledge.
9. Bring the *cause and effect* of phenomena into focus. It should serve to enhance knowledge about a topic by clarifying and expanding that knowledge.
10. Include all of the above in *lucid, logical language.* It should not be stated in a recondite manner in which its clinical practicality is obfuscated in erudite disputation.

Unfortunately, theories of personality do not score very high marks on the foregoing ten-point theory appraisal checklist. In particular, the assumptions upon which personality theories mostly are based lack the explicitness that leads to derivation of hypotheses and their empirical verification. This in turn makes it difficult on the bases of these theories, to formulate generalizations about client behavior that are used to guide clinical technique. But personality theories are useful in orienting clinicians to consideration of personality as an influencing factor in the success of the clinical encounter. Personality theories also stir healthy debate and prompt scientific inquiry, albeit often informal science, into the role personality plays in the health and happiness of clients. And, as was noted in Chapter 2, there is close correspondence between personality and communication ability; changes in one typically is reflected in changes in the other. Clinicians' personal theories of counseling therefore should include conceptualizations of what personality is, how it develops, how it can become maladjusted, and how personality maladjustment can adversely affect the course of therapy.

## PERSONALITY DEFINED

What is personality? The definition of personality depends to a large extent on the theory or theories used to define it. Because each theory is composed of a unique array of assumptions and empirical definitions (not that taken individually, all the assumptions and empirical definitions comprising a theory are exclusive to it), the description rendered personality by each also is unique, although not necessarily radically or appreciably different from one another. Yet some general statements can be made about what personality is and how to define it in a general sense.

Perhaps the most economic and possibly simplistic way to define personality is to state how it is recognized as a distinguishable part of one's being at any given point in time. In this regard, personality is recognized as *trait patterns,* with each person's pattern being unique. The traits comprising the patterns are psychological characteristics that manifest as observed behavioral consistencies or are inferred as behavioral dispositions (Wolman, 1989). The behavioral attributes that constitute personality may be implicit (e.g., thoughts, emotions, and perceptions) or explicit (e.g., physical behavior or spoken language).

Attempts have been made to define personality based on *nomothetic* approaches in which general laws are sought through the study of discrete personality units that will ultimately reveal universal commonalities or links in personality. In contrast, the *ideographic* approach holds that personality cannot be divided into discrete units for empirical testing; individual personalities are unique; personality research should be designed to study individual persons rather than groups of persons or universal traits; and the hope of ever fully defining personality is unrealistic.

Allport (1937), in a landmark project, classified personality definitions in categories that indicated their primary philosophic, clinical, or scientific orientations. The *biophysical* category has definitions of personality according to its organic bases and social traits. *Biosocial* definitions regard personality in terms of its social effect; an individual's personality is defined, although not necessarily determined, by others' responses to it. The *unique* definitions category holds that no two personalities are alike. *Integrative* definitions describe personality as a system for mediating and organizing all stimuli that impact on an individual and the individual's responses to those stimuli. The *adjustment* category defines personality as a process for maintaining homeostasis; here personality is viewed as a system that is constantly attempting to resolve stress, anxiety, and moral or social dilemmas for the individual. As the name indicates, *differential essential* personality definitions are those concerned with the individualized traits of personality that essentially make one person different from another. The *omnibus* category is composed of personality definitions that do not fall into any of the above categories.

The inner and outer aspects of personality can be defined in terms of social reputation or in terms of social values and behavior developed through social interaction (English & English, 1958). In this regard, personality is based on others' perceptions or on others' values. In this social context, the inner self is regarded as the true self—the actual traits that comprise one's personality. The outer self can be true or false, a mask or persona presented to the world. In this sense, one's personality is similar to the concept of persona in theater (and as described in the analytic psychology of Jung, 1923), adopting guises consistent with the role one wishes to portray and to be perceived.

## PERSONALITY THEORY

The personality theories presented in this chapter are of more import in modern thought about personality than are any other. Based on broad concepts and voluminous literature, they have spawned numerous spin-off theories, scholarly criticism and challenge, and empirical inquiry. They have undergone rigorous scholarly debate and scientific inquiry on which extensive opinion has been reported. Each has led to the development of clinical techniques and strategies representing differing approaches to counseling and psychotherapy. It would require a book, if not books, for each theory to be fully explicated, which is not the intention here. Only brief summaries are presented for each theory. These summaries include:

- historical perspective on each theory's development
- definitions of the key concepts embedded in and unique to each
- delineation of each theory's explanation of personality and behavior development and of abnormal personality and maladaptive behavior
- applicability of each theory to counseling persons with communicative disorders

## Freud's Classic Psychoanalytic Theory

A study of Freud and his psychoanalytic theory is an experience heavy with irony. Freud's detractors have been legion, including both lay persons and professionals, from the moment he first published his ideas about humankind's mental nature to the present. At the same time, he is recognized, even those who speak disparagingly of him, as an almost mystic genius, who as a thinker with radical and provocative notions, like Darwin and Einstein, changed how humankind fundamentally conceptualizes its existence. And while many counselors and psychotherapists reject Freud's psychoanalytic theory in a broad sense, they partially embrace it, to varying degrees, and acknowledge him as the father of psychoanalysis. Most theories of personality and approaches to counseling and psychotherapy derive in some measure from Freud's theory and from his clinical strategies. Just as during the Roman Empire's days of grandeur when it was said that "all roads lead to Rome," all extant theories of personality and counseling in some measure lead to Freud. Hall and Lindzey (1978) note that classic psychoanalytic theory has had an appreciable influence on the social sciences, particularly a strong impact on the interpretation of art and literature.

The study of personality theories should begin with Freud because of his profound influence on modern thought about mind and behavior. Freud's theory leaves much to be desired if evaluated by the criteria of a good theory discussed earlier in this chapter. In particular, it is not grounded on explicit propositions that can be empirically tested nor does it readily permit the derivation of testable hypotheses. It has had heuristic influence, however, by stimulating debate and provoking challenge that has led to an increasingly scientific approach to the study of personality.

## Historical Perspective

Sigmund Freud was born May 6, 1856, in Freiburg, Moravia. His family moved to Vienna in 1860 when Freud was four years old; he resided in that city for most of his life, until the Nazi invasion of Austria. In 1938, Freud and his family fled to England with the help of the British psychoanalyst, Ernest Jones, who later wrote the definitive biography of Freud. Freud lived in London with his wife, Martha Bernays Freud, until his death on September 23, 1939. He died of jaw and palate cancer, which was attributed to frequent smoking of the cigars he loved. The last 15 years of Freud's life were spent in considerable pain, although they were productive years in terms of scholarship and awards. He received the Goethe prize for literature in 1930, was named an honorary member of England's Royal Society of Medicine in 1935, and was appointed to London's Royal Society in 1936; however the hoped-for Nobel prize in medicine eluded him.

Freud's ascension to the position of psychoanalysis's leading light surrounded by a coterie of disciples, all destined to become luminaries in their own right, followed an interesting, if lengthy, path. Space does not permit a full history to any degree of justice, but the defining events of his life can be mentioned. Excellent detailed accounts of Freud's personal life and professional career can be found in the biographies by Jones (1953, 1955, 1957) and Gay (1988).

Freud received his medical degree in 1881 from the University of Vienna. Interestingly, among the early courses Freud took at university, which helped turn his interest from law to medicine, was one on the physiology of voice and speech taught by the renowned physiologist Ernst Brücke who was later to become one of Freud's most influencing mentors. After graduation, Freud worked on neurological studies with Jean Martin Charcot in France and published papers on cerebral paralysis and aphasia. Charcot increased Freud's interest in psychology by demonstrating his cure of hysterical paralyses by hypnotic suggestion.

After studying with Charcot for 1 year, Freud returned to Vienna, started a private practice, and began his collaboration with another significant mentor, Josef Breuer. Freud was interested in Breuer's "talking cure" for cases of hysteria; in particular, the case of Anna O., whom Breuer had begun treating in 1880, prior to his collaboration with Freud. The Anna O. case study was included in *Studies on Hysteria*, which was published by Breuer and Freud in 1895 and which Freud considered the seminal work in psychoanalysis (Freud deferred the mantle of founding father of psychoanalysis to Breuer, although others have persisted in bestowing it on Freud). The collaboration with Breuer was productive for Freud; for example, Breuer's process of catharsis would evolve into Freud's classic psychoanalytic technique of free association. But Freud's relationship with Breuer, which had been in decline since 1891, dissolved entirely by 1896. The reasons their collaboration ended were both prosaic and philosophic—Freud's financial indebtedness to Breuer and Breuer's ambivalence about or tacit rejection of Freud's emphasis on the significance of sex as a causative factor in neuroses.

After parting with Breuer, Freud entered a period during which he worked alone and was ostracized by the medical community of Vienna. During this period he personally experienced psychological difficulties, for which he treated himself by analyzing his dreams. That experience led to the publication in 1900 of his *opus artificem probat, Interpretation of Dreams.* This work increased Freud's fame and psychoanalysis' credibility. In 1909 Freud was invited by G. Stanley Hall to lecture on psychoanalysis at Clark University in the United States; Freud felt that this was a validating event for himself and for his theory. The next year Freud, along with a distinguished circle of proteges, founded the International Psychoanalytic Association. Freud's disciples at that time included Alfred Adler, Otto Rank, and Wilhelm Stekel, of Austria; Carl Jung of Switzerland; Ernest Jones of England; Sandor Ferenczi of Hungary; and A. A. Brill of the United States. Many of these early students of Freud would later desert his camp to form their own theories of personality and schools of psychotherapy.

Although Freud's last years were painful ones—33 surgeries for his cancer—they were also peaceful. He had persevered through many trials, from ostracism at university because he was a Jew to ridicule of his theory by both the general populace and his professional colleagues. Freud was ultimately recognized before his death for his genius as a writer and thinker and his theory of personality was accorded historical preeminence; however, both the man and the theory remain foci of controversy and challenge.

## BASIC CONCEPTS

The concepts basic to Freud's classic psychoanalytic theory of personality are in a very real sense basic to personality theories that have been developed since. Some theorists have established schools of thought on personality that take direct opposition to Freud's basic concepts. Others have modified Freud's concepts to fit personality constructs similar to his in process but different in philosophy. Freud's ideas about levels of awareness, components of personality, stages of personality development, defense mechanisms, and so forth appear in some form in most extant personality theories. At times, Freud's basic concepts are attributed to him when they appear in other theories and at times they are semantically disguised and presented as original thought.

### Assumptions

The basic assumptions about personality and behavior that Freud formed while treating patients with psychosomatic illnesses in his private practice can be briefly summarized. Following are the basic assumptions that underlie Freud's classic psychoanalytic theory of personality.

1. The first 5 years of life are the most critical to the development of normal and abnormal adult behavior. Although behavior may be modified superficially by the vicissitudes of living, Freud felt that an individual's basic personality or tendencies to behave in certain patterns are established during the preschool years. This is one reason why Freud's treatment of neuroses was focused on revisiting and analyzing events that occurred during the patient's preschool years. Other theories agree with this opinion as will be seen later in this and following chapters.
2. Adult behavior is determined in part by *psychosexual events* that occurred during the first 5 years of life.
3. Behavior exhibited in the present is in part determined by *emotional events* from the past.
4. Behavior is determined in part by the need to gratify biologic urges, the two chief basic urges being *sex* and *aggression.* Sex, in this sense, is inclusive of physical pleasures generally.
5. Individuals are not in actual control of their present behavior because of the control exerted by past sexual and emotional events and by the need to gratify basic urges. Freud termed this concept *psychic determinism.*
6. The events from the past and the urges of the present that shape behavior operate on *the unconscious* level of awareness.
7. As to basic character, humankind is *selfish* and *amoral;* as to their cognitive nature, people in general are *irrational.*

Levels of Awareness

To Freud, personality is an abstract structure consisting of contrasting functions (Hampden-Turner, 1981). One contrast can be seen in his levels of awareness construct. In Freud's view, personality development and present behavior are affected by three levels of awareness: conscious, preconscious, and unconscious.

The *conscious* level of awareness consists of those experiences, cognitions, and emotions of which one is aware at any given moment. It includes the act of selective attention, enabling heightened focus on specific tasks.

The *preconscious* level of awareness involves those cognitions, perceptions, and feelings that lie just below the conscious level. Stored here are information and impressions that can be volitionally called to the conscious level, given time for thought. The preconscious is an indexing and filing system of accessible memory. It is possible to retrieve items stored there, as in recalling someone's name or in recollecting the essence of a past experience. Awareness of sensory stimuli can also be held in check at the preconscious level, as in the case of "tuning out" intrusive or extraneous auditory stimuli from conscious awareness.

Freud's third level of awareness, the *unconscious,* is one of the mainstays of his theory proper. Behavior, according to Freud, is controlled by mental activity in the unconscious, which in effect is a dumping ground for bothersome, painful, and taboo thoughts and experiences. Jung (1959) later described a collective unconscious, which in addition to a personal unconscious, consists of inherited motives and memories. Individuals are unaware of what is locked away or repressed in their unconscious minds and equally unknowing how unconscious thoughts and feelings affect their behavior. Nor do they want to know, according to Freud. The classic example is of a man who hates his mother but does not permit that thought to enter his conscious awareness and is unaware that he is repressing the thought. Psychic energy must constantly be expended to keep the lid on the unconscious; that, in turn, can lead to an individual experiencing stress and anxiety, although their cause is unknown. The unconscious basically represents an internal conflict in which unwanted, denied thoughts and feelings located therein continually strive to break through to conscious awareness and the individual constantly attempts to keep them from doing so. Freud used the example that thoughts and feelings repressed in the unconscious are like unruly students ejected from the classroom. Although the door is locked against them, they pound on the door in an effort to gain readmission, only to be ignored by the instructor. But the instructor's ignoring of the students' clamor requires expenditure of psychic energy, which creates tension and stress, which have potential adverse consequences for the psyche and behavior of the instructor.

Personality Systems

The systems comprising personality in Freud's theory also are set in contrasting functions as are the levels of awareness. These systems—the id, the ego, and the superego, interact in different patterns and relative strengths for different people. It is the way in which they interact, in Freud's view, that determines an individual's essential personality.

The *id* is the only system of personality that is present at birth. It is the reservoir of sexual energy, or *libido* (Jung, 1916) and it operates as the agent of the *pleasure principle.* The pleasure principle dictates that the id keep the individual in a state of low-tension, which is achieved by immediate gratification of instinctual needs, including hunger and thirst as well as the basic sex and aggression impulses. The id is demanding and can be unrealistic in its uninhibited insistence to have urges satisfied. One tends to think of a hungry infant, rigid and red-faced, screaming for succor as the embodiment of the id. It is, in fact, but the id is controlled by the pleasure principle throughout life and can be the dominant system in an adult's personality. A person who spends money beyond their means because they cannot wait to purchase an item they badly want is an example of a person in id control. Id impulses operate on the unconscious level of awareness, coming into consciousness only when the ego is in a weakened state.

In contrast to the id, or "it," is the *ego,* the "I" system of personality. The ego operates as the agent of the *reality principle* and thereby serves to mediate between id impulses and external realities. The ego develops as the infant begins to interact with the environment at about 6 months of age. It develops owing to the need for the infant to match internal mental images and physical and emotional feeling with external reality. This involves a process known as *identification,* wherein the infant learns to differentiate impulses from objective reality through a secondary process, or means-end thinking. Thus, a hungry infant at first will attempt to consume any object within reach but will eventually learn to identify certain objects in the environment that satisfy hunger and understands that delay may be required to obtain those objects. Although the ego serves the id by helping reduce the organism's tension through impulse gratification, it does so with a reality orientation. The ego operates on both the preconscious and unconscious levels of awareness.

If the ego can be described as realistic in its orientation, the *superego* can be described as moralistic. As the child has its needs met by caretakers, it learns early on that some behaviors meet with approbation and reward whereas others do not. The superego develops out of this experience, between 3 and 6 years of age. It eventually becomes an internal personalized system which arbitrates right and wrong; it is a value system based on the beliefs and values of significant others and on the laws and mores of society. This system serves both to control id impulses and to help the individual grow. There are two subsystems that comprise the superego—the *conscience* which represents the individual's moral codes and the *ego-ideal* which is concerned with achieving aspirations and full potential. Both of these superego subsystems are often in conflict with id demands.

Hall (1954) refers to the id, ego, and superego as the personality's hedonistic, executive, and judicial branches, respectively. The ego strives to maintain a tight balance between the id and the superego so that individuals who tend to be id dominant are not excessively impulsive and if they tend to be superego dominant they are not overly moralistic. At times, the ego might become overwhelmed by this responsibility if it were not for defense mechanisms.

Defense Mechanisms

During psychosexual development, an individual experiences tension and anxiety attributable to four sources (Hall & Lindzey, 1978): physiological growth, frustrations, conflicts, and threats at each developmental stage that challenge the ego. In the early stages of development these sources of tension might be external to the self (e.g., threats from a bully) and later become internal (e.g., threats to the superego by repressed aggressive impulses). As its major role, the ego attempts to allay this tension and anxiety so that the individual can function productively within the environment and move positively and uneventfully through the developmental stages of personality. The ego can accomplish this in two basic ways: by using problem-solving strategies or by constructing defense mechanisms. The use of problem-solving is the conscious realistic approach to tension reduction and results in ego enhancement. Defense mechanisms, which operate in the unconscious, are used to deny, falsify, and distort reality (Nystul, 1993) and do not enhance the personality. In fact, they have the potential to impede personality growth. Following are brief descriptions of the defense mechanisms described by Freud.

*Identification* is used by the individual early in psychosexual development to form the ego and superego. In adult life, it tends to resemble imitation, whereby an individual, by trial-and-error, incorporates into his or her personality the traits and behaviors of others. The adopted characteristics that effectively reduce tension are retained; those that do not are abandoned.

*Displacement* involves transfer of psychic energy from one object to another when the original object has lost its ability to reduce tension or is regarded as an unsafe object on which to vent emotions. Sexual and aggressive impulses are thus directed toward secondary, safer targets, such as arguing with one's spouse owing to conflicts at work.

*Sublimation* is a socially acceptable form of displacement. Sexual and aggressive impulses are directed in positive, creative directions, (e.g., writing or painting) to redirect excessive libidinal energy.

*Reaction formation* is a way to cope with a stressful impulse by an opposite emotional reaction to it. For example, if a man hates his mother, he may profess great love for her in order to deny the reality of his true feelings.

*Projection* is the attempt to externalize the source of one's anxiety so that it might be attributed to another and thereby, unconsciously, serve to reduce the anxiety. The man who feels an aggressive hatred toward his mother might deny that feeling and project it onto her, saying, "My mother hates me." This helps him deal with the anxiety emanating from the shame and guilt associated with his true feelings. Projection is used to enhance one's self-esteem at the expense of others.

*Repression* occurs when an individual deals with an anxiety-producing impulse by denying its existence. Conscious confrontation with the impulse is avoided by forcing it into the unconscious. Repression is often a factor in the strict, rigid behavior of individuals whose personalities are superego dominate.

*Fixation* relates to an individual's progression through the psychosexual stages of development. If an individual experiences excessive anxiety at any stage, transition to the subsequent stage might be delayed or prevented by fear of encountering new anxiety-producing challenges. Or, although a developmental stage might be fraught with frustrations, the individual might not want to leave it because the behaviors it entails are self-gratifying and represent a type of security. Fixation at any one stage is most usually incomplete and temporary.

*Regression* occurs when individuals revert to a stage of psychosexual development through which they passed earlier and in which they felt secure. An individual tends to regress to a stage where fixation once occurred. For children, regression delays progression through developmental stages; for adults, it returns them to childhood behavior. Regression helps individuals avoid unpleasant reality by symbolically returning to comfortable stages of their development, by way of exhibiting associated patterns of behavior. As with fixation, regression usually is incomplete and temporary.

PERSONALITY DEVELOPMENT

Freud assumed that everyone passes through the same sequence of psychosexual stages in personality development. Three of these stages, the oral, anal, and phallic, occur during the first 5 or 6 years of life, followed by a latency stage that lasts until puberty. The final stage, the genital, occurs during puberty and adolescence. With the exception of the latency stage, one body area is the focal point of sexual gratification in each stage of development. As an individual passes from one stage to another, attention to specific body areas shifts. Freud assumed that personality disorders were the result of failing to complete this sequence or were due to problems encountered while completing it.

The *oral stage* occurs during the first 12 to 18 months of life. Freud believed that the oral behaviors of infants (e.g., sucking breast or bottle, exploring their environment by incorporating objects into their mouths, gnawing their fists during teething, and so forth) in this stage are not only performed for life-sustaining reasons, but for pleasurable erotic feelings they evoke in the infant as well. The infant who finds too much security and pleasure in this stage, might become overly dependent on the mother and fixate, possibly later becoming an adult whose personality is chiefly characterized by dependency. On the other hand, if gratification of oral impulses is insufficient, the infant may proceed into the following stages with feelings of insecurity due to unfulfilled latent needs. Later in life, he or she may unconsciously use symbolic displacement—thumb sucking, nail biting, smoking, over-eating—in attempts to diminish the anxiety resulting from unresolved oral needs.

The *anal stage* of psychosexual development in Freud's theory occurs between 18 months and 3 years of age. In this stage, the oral region of the body as the source of psychic and physical attention and gratification is supplanted by the anal region. In the anal stage the child first begins to experience self-control and control over the environment. Toilet training is a very significant activity in this stage and if the child's experiences with it are extreme in any regard, his or her adult personality might reflect that. For example, an anal-explosive personality characterized by aggressive behaviors might develop for children who use the need for frequent toileting to maintain parental attention. Anal-retentive personalities, characterized by parsimony, rigid behavior, obstinacy, and spitefulness, might develop if the child is disciplined too harshly during toilet training.

An especially important stage, according to Freud, is the *phallic stage,* which occurs from 3 to 5 years of age. It is in this stage that self-stimulation of the genital area receives the focused attention of the child, which leads to events that determine whether adult behavior will be normal or maladaptive. *Castration anxiety* and *penis envy* can arise from guilt associated with masturbation in this stage and can cause the child continuing unconscious concern past this stage, especially if these concerns are addressed in a ridiculing or punitive manner by parents. The *Oedipus complex* (the son's sexual interest in his mother) and *Electra complex* (the daughter's sexual interest in her father) also occur in this stage and in

Freud's opinion were the most influential childhood experiences that shape adult attitudes toward authority figures and the opposite sex. If a son's possessive behavior toward his mother is met with threats from his father, he might unconsciously fear castration and owing to his fears be unable to successfully resolve the Oedipus complex. Similarly, a daughter must resolve the Electra complex without experiencing the extremes of rejection by or incest with the father for it not to influence personality development beyond this stage.

From age 5 until the onset of puberty the child is in the *latency stage.* These might be thought of as the golden years for the child, during which he or she works at acquiring intellectual skills without the intrusion of anxiety from pregenital sexual impulses. This stage is important to the development of social skills also. It is a stress-free time for learning, unless the child did not develop successfully through the earlier stages of psychosexual development.

In the *genital stage* the individual becomes fully socialized and self-interest or narcissism turns into interest in and romantic attraction to others. Freud's idea of the person with normal personality at this stage was of one who was interested in opposite-sex relationships, had successfully resolved the fears and complexes of the phallic stage, and did not derive gratification from autoeroticism.

ABNORMAL PERSONALITY

Freud held that deep structures were involved in personality maladjustment. The id-ego-superego interaction is upset by excessive tension and anxiety emanating from internal and external sources. The ego is unable to cope with this tension through problem-solving strategies and resorts to the use of defense mechanisms. Repression is the first and most typically used defense in such instances. The tension producing impulses are forced into the unconscious, unresolved, only to resurface later in life to create even more tension and anxiety for the individual.

As an individual moves through life and encounters stressful situations that the ego is unable to deal with successfully, he or she might tend to regress to an early stage of psychosexual development for help in dealing with the tension, only to encounter the impulses repressed when that stage was first experienced. The stress experienced by the individual is thus increased. More defensive behaviors might be adopted by the ego and more psychic energy must be expended to cope with the tension in increasing amounts each time this pattern is repeated. The individual becomes preoccupied with this struggle, which hinders his or her ability and energy to function creatively and contentedly in life. Neurotic behaviors begin to appear, the ultimate configuration of which is determined by the psychosexual stage to which regression occurs, the types of defense mechanisms adopted, and early learned behaviors used to control sexual and aggressive impulses.

Psychoanalysis attempts to uncover these repressed impulses and to bring them into conscious awareness. A nonevaluative atmosphere is created for the client in which impulses can be confronted, defensive behaviors examined, and more positive coping strategies learned. Psychoanalytic techniques include *dream analysis,* which is used to analyze the unconscious symbolic significance of dreams; *transference* in which emotions felt earlier toward a parent or other person is directed toward the therapist in order to confront and resolve it; *free association,* which essentially involves encouraging the client to talk freely about whatever is on his or her mind in order to discover sources of tension and "talk through" resolution strategies; *confrontation and clarification,* which are used to provide feedback to the client about a problem and the course of treatment; and *interpretation,* which is used to help the client understand information revealed through the use of the foregoing techniques to strengthen the ego and establish healthy id-superego balance.

RELEVANCE TO SPEECH-LANGUAGE PATHOLOGY AND AUDIOLOGY

At first glance it might seem that Freud's psychoanalytic theory with its focus on id urges, the unconscious, and neurotic behavior has little utility to speech-language pathologists and audiologists. On closer examination, however, it might be found to have some, albeit limited, relevance other than historical.

First of all, the causes of some communicative disorders are attributed to conversion hysteria, which is a neurosis characterized by the psychic conversion of repressed conflicts into physical symptoms when there is no physical or physiological explanation for them; conversion aphonia and conversion deafness are two such disorders. Understanding Freud's psychoanalytic theory helps the clinician conceptualize, from one point of view, how these disorders develop. Stuttering is another communicative disorder that has been explained from a psychoanalytic perspective by Freud and his followers, Brill (1923) and Coriat (1943), for instance. In their views, stuttering is seen as a behavior that serves unconsciously and symbolically to gratify sexual or aggressive impulses associated with the psychosexual stages of personality development or that is used consciously for epinosic gains. Little credence or practical value is given such theories of stuttering causality by speech-language pathologists, but attempts to explain stuttering in Freudian terms have persisted to current times (e.g., Gemelli, 1982a, 1982b).

Freud's theory of personality can also be used to help clinicians recognize and understand client behaviors that might assist or prevent progress in therapy. For instance, id-dominant clients might skip therapy on a whim or quit altogether if therapy is not pleasurable to them. Superego-dominant clients might assiduously attend therapy but rigidly resist behavior change. Understanding the psychosexual stages of personality development might help clinicians understand the reasons, from Freud's point of view, for dependent, narcissistic, and obstinate behavior in clients. The critical importance of socialization to normal personality development and to success in therapy is also made evident in psychoanalytic theory. Socialization is especially important to address in holistic treatment of communicatively disordered children, particularly those in the latency stage of psychosexual development.

The presence and purpose of a client's defense mechanisms are particularly important for clinicians to comprehend. Defense mechanisms frequently exhibited by clients in therapy might impede its progress. They often serve to translate a communicative difference into a communicative disorder or communicative handicap, yet they are often unobserved or ignored by clinicians. For example, a child might say to his or her clinician, "I can tell you don't like me," and reiterate that projection to his or her parents, when the truth is that the child does not like to attend therapy, wants to be permitted to quit, and does not want to experience reproof or guilt for having done so. The attempt should be made by speech-language pathologists and audiologists to recognize defensive behaviors in their clients and to counsel with them or their parents about those behaviors.

A governing principle of psychoanalytic theory is that maladjustment results from excessive anxiety and tension. Many persons with communicative disorders exist in daily states of high stress that generate anxiety and tension. Their communicative disorders contribute appreciably to and sometimes are the sole causes of that anxiety and tension. Anxiety and tension, in turn, exacerbate the communicative disorders. Psychoanalysis, speech-language therapy, and aural rehabilitation all seek the same end, albeit by different means, in counseling with clients to help them identify and control sources of stress and to improve prognosis both for treatment of their communicative disorder and for improvement in the quality of their life.

## Ego-Analytic Theory

As mentioned earlier, Freud ignited the imaginations of other theorists, many of whom modified his original psychoanalytic theory into new, or "neo-Freudian," theories of their own. These neoanalysts—Carl Jung, Alfred Adler, Otto Rank, Erich Fromm, and Karen Horney, among others—drew liberally from Freud's basic concepts. Many of these personality theories became prominent in their own right and led to associated approaches to psychoanalysis and shorter term psychotherapy and counseling. They typically do not ascribe as much importance to sex in personality development as did Freud. They also hold different views on id-ego-superego dynamics and on the stages and temporal aspects of personality development. These theories cannot all be summarized here. However, the ego-analytic theory, one such theory that bridges psychoanalysis and psychology and which has application to several disciplines, including speech-language pathology and audiology, will be discussed.

### HISTORICAL PERSPECTIVE

Heinz Hartmann (1894–1970) is regarded as the father of ego psychology (Hall & Lindzey, 1970)—the major school of thought on which the ego-analytic theory of personality is based. Although Hartmann's landmark work, *Ego Psychology and the Problem of Adaptation*, was published in 1939 and received widespread acclaim, including from Anna Freud, ego-analytic theory is also chiefly attributed to the works in the 1950s of Erik Erikson (1902–1995) and David Rapaport (1911–1960).

Particularly influential were Erikson's works *Childhood and Society* (1963a) and *Identity: Youth and Crisis* (1968). Erikson, who is best known for his epigenetic model of ego development, which is a counterpart of Freud's psychosexual stages model, left Germany for the United States in 1933 as the Nazis rose to power. He had earlier been befriended by Anna Freud and while in training as a psychoanalyst underwent psychoanalysis with her. She was one of the first psychoanalysts to specialize in children and Erikson later also specialized in analysis of children. He devoted much of his long, prolific career to studying the personality development of children from various cultures. He demonstrated that ego development is appreciably influenced by social structure and that the character of ego is bound up with historical changes in social structure (Erikson, 1946). During his career, Erickson was affiliated with the Harvard Psychological Clinic, the Yale Institute of Human Relations, the University of California's Institute of Child Welfare, and the Western Psychiatric Institute in Pittsburgh, Pennsylvania. He was the winner of both the Pulitzer Prize and the National Book Award.

### BASIC CONCEPTS

In Freudian theory the id is considered the reservoir of psychic energy and, therefore, the force behind personality development. In Freud's view, the ego develops out of the id's energy in response to the need to bring id impulse gratification into alignment with environmental reality; the behavior of the ego is controlled by the impulses of the id. The ego psychology position is that the ego develops independent of the influence of id impulses and, once formed, resists assimilation into the id (Hartmann, 1967). Ego-analysts do not see the id and ego as existing in a necessarily co-dependent interrelationship. Rather, they hold that in a healthy personality the ego is an independent structure with its own psychic energy source and, as Freud held, reality oriented. Other basic concepts in ego-analytic theory follow.

Assumptions

1. The instinctual determinants of personality are not as important in ego psychology as they are in classic psychoanalytic theory. Instead, more importance is given in ego psychology to the role that learned responses to environmental events play in ego development, rather than to the role played by biologic variables. The emphasis placed on the role of learning in personality development suggests that an individual's behavior is determined by rational, conscious planning; it is perhaps this aspect of ego-analytic theory that most distinguishes it from classic psychoanalytic theory (Ford & Urban, 1963).
2. A similar amount of influence is assumed to be exerted by society on the nature of an individual's personality as by the individual's personality on the nature of society. Society thus is held by ego-analysts to play a major role in personality development, along with inherited traits and instinctual impulses emphasized by Freudian psychologists.
3. Because it has a source of psychic energy exclusive of the id, the ego generates its own goals and interests.
4. In Freud's theory, the goals of the ego are to help the id gratify its sexual and aggressive impulses. Ego-analytic theory, in contrast, purports the primary goals of the ego are socialization of the individual (Fromm, 1947) and intellectual growth.
5. The ego serves to help the individual exist productively within society by developing coping behaviors discovered through trial-and-error learning in various situations.
6. Normal personality development is emphasized over abnormal personality. Ego-analysts are suspicious of Freud's assumptions about normal personality because they were based largely on his observation and treatment of abnormal personality.
7. Personality is believed to develop across the life span rather than occurring essentially during the first 5 years of life. In ego-analytic theory, as much importance is given to the adult stages of personality development as to the pregenital stages.
8. The ego is thought to consist of inherited traits, instinctual impulses, and environmental influences (Hartmann, 1964).

Ego Functions

Kroeber (1963) established three categories of ego function: impulse economics, cognitive functions, and controlling functions. Ego mechanisms are viewed as serving both defensive and coping purposes that are not mutually exclusive. But coping behaviors are regarded as neurosis-free and the degrees of autonomy and normality of the ego depend on the number of coping behaviors used by the individual relative to the number of defense mechanisms used. In ego-analytic theory, the ego's defense mechanisms are viewed as being oriented to the past, characterized by rigidity, and protective of the ego through unconscious denial or falsification of reality. Coping functions of the ego are present and reality oriented, characterized by flexibility, and protective of the ego through conscious problem-solving. Ego flexibility denotes absence of fixed, rigid patterns of behavior and thought and the presence of freedom to learn from experience, to change positively with constantly changing internal and external conditions, and to think and act adaptively in various situations (Kubie, 1961).

*Impulse economics* include the ego mechanisms of impulse diversion, impulse transformation, and impulse restraint. Defense mechanisms associated with impulse economics include displacement, reaction formation, and repression; the respective impulse economics coping strategies are sublimation, substitution, and suppression. Impulse economics generally concern the individual's ability to recognize impulses as such and to respond to them with productive, socially acceptable behavior. Weak impulse economics can result in negative introjects that are perceived as feelings of personal inadequacy.

*Cognitive functions* include the ego mechanisms of discrimination, detachment, and means-end symbolization. Isolation, intellectualization, and rationalization are the defense mechanisms associated with cognitive functions and correspond to the coping behaviors objectivity, intellectuality, and logical analysis. The ability to exercise unbiased evaluation of people, objects, and events; to think freely without internal or external restrictions; and to analyze events, anticipate outcomes, and make appropriate choices all require normal development and coping use of cognitive functions.

The third functional component of the ego, *controlling functions*, includes the ego mechanisms of selective awareness, sensitivity, delayed response, and time reversal. Defense mechanisms associated with this ego function are denial, projection, doubt and indecision, and regression. Associated coping behaviors, respectively, are concentration, empathy, tolerance of ambiguity, and playfulness. Healthy development of controlling functions enables the individual to focus on tasks without emotional interference, exist in the present and be forward-moving, and be flexible and open to experience. Controlling functions used mainly as defense mechanisms can lead to obsessive behaviors that might limit the individual's sensitivity to another's needs, feelings, and ideas that in turn adversely affect interpersonal relationships, even at an early age.

Role of Language

Ego-analysts consider normal language acquisition and healthy language use by a child to be the foundation for rapid growth of a normal ego (King & Neal, 1968). Healthy language use includes language skills used to *formulate abstractions* to discriminate between symbols and their corresponding objects. This gives the child a sense of what is real and what is not; what gratifies an impulse and what only symbolizes that gratification; and also permits the child to have experiences vicariously, without risk to the self and in socially acceptable ways.

Language is used in the same sense by the child to differentiate among objects and between object and event on different levels of abstraction. This enables the child to experience ever-changing reality without fear or confusion and to *avoid overgeneralizing* opinions and feelings (e.g., if upbraided unfairly by a parent on one occasion, a child with healthy language use will tend to avoid assuming all adults are unfair to children all of the time).

Language also helps the child *learn to delay* in making judgments until he or she has time to distinguish verbal description from verbal inference. Learning to delay helps the child resist forming conclusions about the environment that later might become regarded as facts before verification input from the environment enters conscious awareness. The child might form prejudicial "truths" about himself or herself or about his or her environment that are based on inferential conclusions only. Being able to delay also pertains to an ability to delay gratification of impulses by remembering similar past situations in which gratification had to be delayed but was eventually obtained. Delay helps the child both avoid inappropriate social behaviors that create tension and anxiety and maintain ego identity through behavior identity (i.e., behavior continuity that satisfies one's needs and is understood and accepted by society) (Erikson, 1946).

PERSONALITY DEVELOPMENT

The stages of ego development designed by Erikson (1963a), "*the eight ages of man*" or the "*life cycle*" as they are called, are perhaps most representative of the ego-analytic theory of personality development. Erikson based his epigenetic model on the ideas of both Freud and Hartmann. From Freud he borrowed the basic idea of a sequential stage model of personality development. In fact, Erikson's first five stages are similar to Freud's five stages and, as with Freud's model, the first four stages are controlled by unconscious impulses. But Erikson's last four stages are characterized by learning through conscious problem-solving. And, whereas Freud's developmental stages are defined in terms of a psychosexual perspective of personality development, Erikson uses a psychosocial context to describe the process of ego development.

From Hartmann, Erikson borrowed the idea of an environment of predictable events or stages (e.g., experiences associated with the cradle, family, school, and so forth) that sequentially steer an individual through life, from one environmental event to another. Each environmental event represents some form of challenge to the individual which, if met with successfully, prepares him or her for the next stage. For instance, success with interpersonal relationships at the stage in which peer group identity is paramount is predictive of success at the next stage in which marriage typically occurs. Erikson held that although the number and sequence of environmental stages in the life cycle may vary from culture to culture, a sequence does exist that defines the culture and determines the ego-identity for persons within a culture.

Erikson's general model of personality development consists of eight psychosocial stages through which individuals pass in ego development. Each stage involves challenges or crises the individual attempts to surmount before passing on to the next stage: "...psychosocial development proceeds by critical steps—'critical' being a characteristic of turning points, of moments of decision between progress and regression, integration and retardation" (Erikson, 1963a, pp. 270–271). Success at any stage augurs well for success at the following stage; failure at any stage might make progress to the next stage more difficult. Failure, however, does not necessarily prohibit progress, although it may have to be resolved in later stages for ego development to reach its maximal positive potential. Success meeting the challenges confronted in each stage is largely a matter of striking a balance between the contrasting traits that represent each stage (Erikson, 1963a). In the first stage, for instance, trust versus mistrust, it is hoped that the child would achieve both characteristics in a realistic sense. To have complete trust in one's environment is both irrational and dangerous; complete mistrust in one's environment encourages self-alienation from society and inhibits the learning experiences that result in ego identity.

*Ego identity* is one of Erikson's principal concepts. It is the defining state the individual aspires to obtain in ego development. Ego identity is essentially a sense of continuity in the behavior, represented in the ego functions, that an individual uses to gratify needs. It also involves an awareness that the ego functions maintain continuity in how an individual is perceived by others. Basically, ego identity consists of predictable behavior patterns that can be depended on to relieve tension and anxiety and society's identification of the individual by those behavior patterns.

A late addition that Erikson made to his developmental model was eight *virtues,* or accomplishments, that correspond to a psychosocial stage. The virtues represent what Erikson viewed as the optimal emotional, behavioral, and intellectual outcomes of crisis resolution at each stage; each virtue is an essential inherent strength that helps ensure mental health for the individual and a productive life cycle. Erikson did not elaborate on these virtues to the extent he did on other aspects of his model.

The first stage in Erikson's model is *sensory-anal,* which occurs in early infancy between birth and 1 year of age. The challenge or crisis faced by the infant in this stage is *trust versus mistrust* and centers around the infant's relationship with its mother or caretakers. How the infant resolves the crisis in this stage and in the first three stages depends on the nature of the child's relationship with its caretakers and on the strategies for crisis resolution, which are largely determined by a caretaker's culture, provided to the child by the caretakers. In this stage, the infant must depend on these others for primary needs satisfaction. If its needs are met with continuity and affection by the caretakers, the infant tends to develop trust for both its providers and for its environment. Erikson viewed the development of trust at this stage to be the cornerstone of healthy personality development and a critical factor in the infant achieving full crisis resolution in subsequent psychosocial stages. If it trusts caretakers and environment, the infant will tend to develop a healthy sense of what is and what is not self, a realistic awareness of what is ego and what is non-ego. The virtue Erikson associated with successful resolution of this stage is *hope*. Failure at this stage, due to neglect or abuse by caretakers, can result in the infant developing regressive behaviors, childhood schizophrenia (held by some to include early infantile autism), and depression.

In late infancy, between 1 and 3 years of age, the child experiences the challenge of *autonomy versus shame and doubt*. This is the *muscular-anal* stage of psychosocial development and, as in Freud's anal stage, toilet training is a central event in this period. If a child is made to feel public humiliation while trying to gain control of the most socially private of bodily functions he or she might form a life-long conviction that all bodily functions, including sex, are dirty and shameful. Additionally, further trial-and-error learning from the child's interaction with the environment might be inhibited owing to the child's wish to avoid additional humiliation. On the other hand, if the child feels respectful support from caretakers as he or she attempts to gain self-control, a sense of autonomy will develop, manifested in the virtue, *will*. If shame and doubt are experienced by the child, anal-retentive traits might develop, as well as obsessive-compulsive behavior, especially regarding those behaviors associated with cleanliness.

The crisis of *initiative versus guilt* is encountered by the child in the *locomotive-genital* stage in early childhood between 4 and 5 years of age. In this stage physical growth and development of motor skills enable the child to explore and interact more actively with the environment (Hartmann, 1964). If caretakers encourage the child to use imagination to cope with environmental realities, the child will embark on a trial-and-error learning process that is enhanced by his or her sense of initiative. Language skills and their healthy use facilitate problem-solving through imagination and initiative, which in turn can lead to the child's acquisition of the virtue, *purpose*. Emerging language skills can also be used by the child for secret fantasies during this stage, as with the Oedipus and Electra complexes. Guilt administered by the superego punishes the child for these fantasies. In attempting to atone, the child might become unnaturally obedient to caretakers, so overcontrolled by the superego that the ego is obliterated, develop regressive behaviors, and form life-long resentments toward caretakers if children do not see the same obedience to conscience exhibited by their caretakers as by themselves. In adulthood, failure at this stage might manifest as hysterical denial and repression of superego demands, which results in inhibited, impotent behaviors or as over-compensatory "showing off" behaviors, both of which can lead to psychosomatic disease (Erikson, 1963a).

The fourth stage in Erikson's model is the *latency* stage, which involves the crisis of *industry versus inferiority*. This stage occurs from 6 to 11 years of age in middle childhood and is roughly equivalent temporally and characteristically to Freud's latency stage. Erikson (1963a) calls this stage "the lull before the storm of puberty" (p. 260). The child enters school during this period and puts aside needs for impulse gratification to concentrate on developing problem-solving skills. The acquisition and productive application of these skills, in itself, will bring the child recognition and satisfaction (Hartmann, 1961). Erikson notes that even if the school is a field or jungle rather than a formal classroom, some form of systematic instruction occurs for all children at this stage and the skills learned through that instruction become represented in his or her ego boundaries. Play gives way to problem-solving; fantasy gives way to accomplishment. For children in this stage to come to value accomplishment, however, they must early on identify with the industrious students in their school. If earlier family life has failed to prepare children to do so or if children find their teachers and school environment are not ego reinforcing, they might regress to earlier conflict stages and have difficulty both in developing skills and in identifying with their peers. These children will be subject to feelings of inadequacy, failure, and incompetence and will have to struggle daily against feared humiliation for their incompetence. Children who are successful in this stage will experience the virtue, *competence.*

The crisis of *identity versus role confusion* occurs between the ages of 12 to 20 years, during Erikson's *puberty and adolescence* stage of psychosocial development. As the result of rapid growth during this period and the development of genital maturity, adolescents question the sameness and continuity of behavior patterns that formed their ego identity through the earlier stages. They feel that they must find a new sameness and continuity, a final ego identity, by revisiting old conflicts and often fighting them out with unwitting antagonists. If adolescents are successful in resolving these conflicts by integrating childhood identifications with their libido fluctuations, endowed talents, acquired skills, and social opportunities, then their adult identities will emerge. They will feel confident that their past sameness and continuity matches the sameness and continuity of their meaning to others, which is Erikson's basic definition of ego identity. Failure to coalesce the variables mentioned above can result in role confusion for the adolescent. If this lack of sameness and continuity is due to strong sexual identity doubts, Erikson (1963b) contends that delinquency and psychotic episodes might result. However, if as is most often the case, the cause of role confusion is difficulty in forming a career direction or identity, adolescents may react by attempting to over-identify. They form cliques, join groups, and develop prejudices toward others to strengthen their group identities. This results in further diffusion of the ego, which adolescents attempt to clarify by falling in love and projecting their ego onto a romantic other so that it might be reflected and discussed in lengthy, soulful conversations; an interest in others replaces narcissism. Loyalty in these love matches and in the group experiences, although sometimes hurtful to self and others, leads in this stage to the virtue, *fidelity.*

For continued growth to occur, the ego identity tumultuously formed during adolescence must be placed at risk in the next crisis, *intimacy versus isolation.* This *early adulthood* stage occurs when individuals willingly commit to permanent intimate alliances that will test their ego identities through personal sacrifice and interpersonal compromise. Experiences must be embraced that require some measure of self-abandon, such as in melding one's ego identity with another's in an intimate relationship or modifying one's ego identity as the result of a mentoring experience. Self-abandon is also required in competitive and combative situations that arise during this stage. If an individual can resist the fear of identity loss in relationships that are both intimate and competitive and can distinguish between the two experiences, true intimacy and an ethical commitment to the intimate partnership are realized and the virtue, *love,* is attained. The ethical sense associated with intimacy is held by Erikson to be a defining characteristic of the adult ego. If individuals avoid situations in this stage that call for self-abandon, they might instead become self-absorbed. Self-absorption can lead to self-imposed exile from personal contacts and experiences that lead to intimacy. Rather than intimacy, isolation (or distantiation) is experienced and aggression is displayed toward persons and experiences that threaten one's ego identity. Erikson (1963a) notes that experiencing isolation can be manifested as serious "character-problems."

Stage seven, occurs in *middle adulthood*. The generativity versus stagnation conflict that occurs in this stage is considered by Erikson to be the central challenge of the adult stages. Here the intimate relationships developed in the preceding stage produce children and the parents become teachers as well as learners. These events are critical in both psychosexual and psychosocial frameworks of personality development. Productivity and creativity are aspects of generativity but are not wholly synonymous with it; one can be personally productive and creative without influencing the next generation. Generativity essentially is the establishment and guidance of the next generation. It is important to note that having children does not guarantee successful resolution of the crisis at this stage. Parents must be able to act as effective guides for their children and be open to guidance from their children as well. The virtue, *care,* is achieved by this symbiotic relationship between generations. Failure to achieve such a relationship can lead to feelings of being unfulfilled and stagnant. Regression to a need for an adolescent-type love can occur in such cases, along with obsessive self-indulgence. Excessive self-concern also can develop; it is often displayed as unfounded or exaggerated psychological or physical invalidism.

The final stage in Erickson's life cycle of personality epigenesis is *late adulthood,* with the crisis of *ego integrity versus despair.* A state of self-actualization is reached in this stage by individuals who, to some degree, have developed the ego characteristics that represent successful resolution of the foregoing seven crises and whose egos are an integration of the outcome virtues ascribed to each stage. These individuals will exhibit the final virtue, *wisdom,* and will feel the dignity that comes with accepting and defending their ego identities and their life cycles, their successes and their failures, and the products of their generativity. They will approach death with an integrity of spirit and mind and without fear, which encourages the younger generation not to fear life. One is reminded of Ralph Waldo Emerson's observation that: "Nothing is at last sacred but the integrity of your own mind" (1950, p. 148). Individuals who cannot accept their ego identities and who reject their life cycles will fail to achieve this ego integrity. They will despair of life and fear death because it is too late for them to start again the process of ego development and to salvage what little integrity they have brought forth from the process. Their despair will be expressed as disgust—disgust with themselves, with others, and with life.

ABNORMAL PERSONALITY

The development of abnormal personality and disordered behavior was discussed in the foregoing section relative to each of the stages in the life-cycle model of ego development. In more general terms, ego-analysts hold that maladaptive behavior occurs when control of ego functions shift from conscious ego control to unconscious id control (Rapaport, 1958). More specifically, patterns of behavior that have been formed through the ego functions to cope with situational challenges break down if the anxiety and tension associated with the challenges become too intense. Defense mechanisms might then supplant coping behaviors to separate the individual from reality and neurotic behavior might replace problem-solving patterns of behavior. This loss of coping control does not necessarily occur in all of the ego functions at once; some ego functions may continue to operate with normal coping patterns of behavior, whereas others have lost control of behavior (Kroeber, 1963).

The ego-analysts contend that the ego's proclivity to relinquish control of ego functions to the id in times of intense anxiety typically is due to unsuccessful or incomplete resolution of one or more of the psychosocial stages of personality development. Rapaport (1958) suggests that removal of a reward for a behavior that was successfully established at a developmental stage also can lead to behavior becoming unconsciously controlled by the id. If an individual develops intimacy at Erikson's stage seven, for example, he or she will exhibit intimacy for others as long as this intimacy is accepted and returned. But if attempts at intimacy are repeatedly rebuffed or if affection is suddenly not reciprocated after a period of having been returned, the behaviors associated with intimacy might then be replaced with the unconscious defensive behaviors associated with isolation. Behavior patterns developed in the other psychosocial stages might remain in the conscious control of the ego even though the individual's loss of intimacy might result in maladaptive behavior associated with that specific stage.

Id control of the personality also can occur for individuals who experience psychosocial development without the support and reinforcement of caretakers; in stressful or threatening environments that are outside the mainstream societies of their cultures; without opportunities for intimacy and friendship; and with emotionally distressing burdens of illness and personal tragedy. For example, healthy ego development and its maintenance are especially challenging for individuals who:

- must virtually raise themselves on the streets, who grow up in orphanages
- spend their adolescence in juvenile correctional facilities or in adult prisons
- have war or prisoner-of-war experiences
- live in areas that are geographically isolated from society
- are creative and economically prosperous one day and bereft of talent or homeless the next
- are born with mental or physical disability or who acquire disability or disease at any point in life

The stages of ego development in Erikson's model might be encountered in different sequences by these persons and some stages might not be experienced by them at all. In such instances, patterns of behavior learned at various stages might develop as or have the tendency to change to inflexible, defensive patterns of behavior.

Counseling practiced within an ego-analytic framework is generally of shorter term than is classic psychoanalysis, owing to its usual focus on a limited number of ego mechanisms rather than on the personality as a whole. Ego counseling is oriented to the present rather than to the past and addresses environmental reality rather than the symbolism in behavior. Its goals are to help clients develop or re-establish ego integrity and ego flexibility so that their maladaptive behavior will be replaced by adaptive goal-oriented behavior. Rather than trying to find clues to present behavior in unconscious memories of the past, ego counseling attempts to assist clients in building new ego functions or in shoring up weakened ones so they might become more socialized, generative individuals.

RELEVANCE TO SPEECH-LANGUAGE PATHOLOGY AND AUDIOLOGY

It was mentioned above that circumstances that are both within and outside the control of individuals can cause the order or completeness of stages in the epigenesis of psychosocial development to be adversely altered. Disorders of speech, language, and hearing frequently qualify as examples of these circumstances. Infants born with severe physical or physiological conditions (e.g., cleft palate, cerebral palsy, profound hearing loss) are faced from birth with unique sets of challenges in personality development relative to the crises that typically mark each epigenetic stage. For instance, basic trust in the environment might come with more difficulty to infants who to varying degrees are separated from it by their physical and communicative problems. Autonomy and initiative often are not as readily achievable to children with communicative disorders as they are to others. The school years of middle childhood might not be carefree to children attempting to cope with a speech, language, or hearing disorder; instead, developing a sense of inferiority is a very real possibility for them during these years.

Erikson's model is useful both in considering the problems in ego development that children with congenital disorders might face and in predicting problems that children with adventitious and developmental communicative disorders might encounter. Children who stutter, for example, might successfully develop through the preschool stages and then abandon trust for mistrust, autonomy for shame and doubt, and initiative for guilt in the latency stage if they encounter ridicule from peers, unreasonable expectations from teachers, and disappointment from parents. Erikson (1963a) notes that ego characteristics achieved at any given stage are not necessarily permanent and are subject to change with the vicissitudes of life.

It is perhaps during puberty and adolescence, Erikson's identity versus role confusion stage, that children and adolescents with communicative disorders face their greatest challenges. At the time when the pregenital ego is in the throes of transformation to adult ego, adolescents with communicative disorders might be distracted from this process by the anxiety and tension associated with their disorder. They may find it difficult to form identity-reflecting adolescent love relationships, to be accepted into identity-giving groups and cliques, and to envision themselves in careers or intimate relationships that lead to generativity. It is clinically accountable for the speech-language pathologist or audiologist to address these issues with their adolescent clients; such issues might well be the potential catalysts in determining whether or not speech, language, and hearing differences and disorders become life-long handicaps.

Communicative disorders also can adversely impact on the adult stages of ego development even if ego identity and ego flexibility are established by early adulthood. Intimate relationships might be more difficult to establish for individuals with communicative disorders owing to avoidance of such relationships because of others' rejective reactions to their disorders or simply because of difficulty with effective interpersonal communication, which they attribute to their disorders; instead, isolation, as discussed in Chapter 2, might be experienced by these individuals. The generativity of middle adulthood can be delayed, decreased, or diverted by a communicative disorder; for example, a professional singer who develops vocal nodules might have to put a career on hold while receiving treatment for the nodules and, if the premorbid status of the voice cannot be re-established, settle for a less successful or an alternative career. In late adulthood, there are many potential challenges to ego integrity. Acquired hearing loss, particularly presbycusis, often carries with it an examination of and reckoning with one's self-image; it also serves as an unsubtle harbinger of decline and death. The ego's continuity also can be threatened by direct brushes with death, as in the case of persons with aphasia and laryngectomies.

Speech-language pathologists and audiologists should consider in their intervention with persons with communicative disorders any impact the speech, language, and hearing disorders is having on a client's ego development. It is not the type or severity of a communicative disability that is most relevant; instead, it is the client's and caretakers' emotional reactions to the disorders that most influence success or failure in ego development. As noted in Chapter 2, emotional responses to communicative disorders can be debilitating in themselves. Counseling should be used to ensure that the potential emotions associated with communicative disorders do not impede or unravel the client's ego development process. The quality of life for clients is determined by their ego identity and ego flexibility as well as by the status of their speech, language, and hearing; communication and personality are closely bound and one appreciably influences the other.

In particular, as mentioned earlier, normal language development is a critical prerequisite to normal personality development. By assisting with a client's language development, speech-language pathologists and audiologists also are inadvertently facilitating the client's normal acquisition of the ego functions. To help their children develop "health-sustaining language usage" (King & Neal, 1968), which is not necessarily normal language skills, parents should help them understand that words are not the objects they represent and that facts are not temporally absolute. Parents should also help their children learn to resist forming conclusions about the environment until adequate information enters conscious awareness. On this point, Wendell Johnson, who was a general semanticist and pioneer in the field of speech-language pathology, is frequently cited in the ego psychology literature. He (1946) suggests that parents can facilitate circumspective language use by their children by using extensional phrases—"to me," "in my opinion," "from my point of view"—when discussing persons or events with them. Thus, children become conscious of the tendency to project and are better able to resist the tendency to introject the projected, untested values of others in lieu of their own organismic values.

Ego functions should also be considered by speech-language pathologists and audiologists to be important to clinical success and to posttherapy carryover and generalization of that success. Clients with a strong sense of ego identity and flexible egos and in coping control are better able to achieve and maintain successful behavioral modification of their communicative disorders than are those whose egos are defensive and inflexible. For instance, Crowe (1995) opined that perhaps the greatest ironic issue in therapy for stuttering is that the client can master the clinical techniques to produce fluent speech and can use them to achieve asymptotic behavior in therapy, yet stutters without control outside of the clinical setting, particularly after termination of therapy. Crowe suggests that the reason for this frequent outcome to stuttering therapy is that the client's ego functions might be in defensive rather than coping control because those functions do not have the ego strength to deal effectively with the shifting and buffeting demands of reality.

Finally, ego-analytic theory and ego psychology is of relevance to speech-language pathologists and audiologists because of the manner in which ego-analysts maintain conscious control of the ego can be lost and abnormal behavior result: by absence, removal, or reduction of reward for particular behavior patterns. If an individual perceives that attempts at adaptive patterns of communicative behavior are not receiving reinforcement from the environment or if, in fact, the reinforcement cannot get through as with individuals experiencing severe hearing loss, maladaptive communicative behavior patterns might be substituted for coping behaviors. The maladaptive patterns might represent a communicative disorder in and of themselves or they might exacerbate the disordering effects of an existing speech, language, or hearing problem. In either case, the process of socialization (i.e., identifying with others in the environment to acquire behavior patterns that satisfy primary and interpersonal needs) becomes a more formidable challenge. Paradoxically, in such cases, clients can become less motivated for therapy owing to a mistrust of the environment, a sense of isolation from society, and the quick but false security in the falsification of the reality that both their communicative effectiveness and the socialization process are not critical to their sense of well-being.

## Self Theory

Since the 1930s, a number of theorists have turned discussion of personality development from the ego as the *primum mobile* of personality to the *self*. Although some contemporary theorists have used the terms ego and self interchangeably, most tend to draw distinctions between the two. The term ego is sometimes defined, in particular by nonpsychoanalysts, as a set of processes involving thought, problem-solving, memory, and intuition. The self, on the other hand, is often defined as an individual's concept of self or self-image (i.e., all of the impressions, perceptions, attitudes, feelings, and judgments that one holds about himself or herself as an entity or *object*) (Hall & Lindzey, 1978). In some theorists' views, however, the ego is properly defined in knowledge sense and the self in process terms. Other writers choose to speak of either the ego or the self as involving both a set of psychological *processes* that actively guide and regulate behavior (ego/self as process definition) and an array of perceptions of self (ego/self as object definition).

Modern discussion of the definitions of the ego and the self and of their relationship to each other was initiated by William James. James (1890) termed the self the *"Empirical Me"* and defined it as consisting of three aspects: the constituents of the self, perceptions of self, and the process of self-actualization. The self's constituents include material, social, and spiritual identities and the ego. The ego according to James is the stream of consciousness that symbolizes an individual's overall, unique identity.

Snygg and Combs (1949) approach the definition of the self from a phenomenologic position. They hold that all of an individual's behavior is determined by his or her phenomenal field; the phenomenal field is all experiences, represented in thought and feeling, of which an individual is consciously aware at the moment of response. The experiences in an individual's phenomenal field that are characteristic of "I" or "me" become differentiated into a *phenomenal self*. Because, according to Syngg and Combs, the phenomenal field controls an individual's behavior and a differentiated portion of it represents attitudes and perceptions of self, it can be said that the phenomenal self is defined as both process and object. Buhler (1962) later proposed that individual's possess a *core self* in addition to the phenomenal self. The core self is defined as a process whereby the self performs executive functions much as does the ego in classic psychoanalytic theory. Buhler's phenomenal self is defined in object terms composed of self-knowledge.

Mead (1934) defines the self as object only that is formed through social encounters. He describes the self as an awareness that one is an object because other individuals respond to him or her as one, just as he or she responded early in life to others as objects. Once the individual forms a sense of self as object, self-attitudes and judgments begin to accrue, determined by how others react to him or her in social settings. Mead holds that one may develop numerous selves, each representing the differing reactions of various social settings—family, school, work, and so forth. Individuals tend to respond to themselves in each unique setting in accordance with how others in those settings respond to them.

Sarbin (1952), as with Mead, does not view the self as being process. He identifies three selves: a *somatic self* that forms first and consists of an awareness and perceptions of one's body; a *receptor-effector self*, which is an awareness of individual sensory and motor systems; and a *social self* that develops last and consists of one's awareness of others and how to interact with them. Sarbin maintains that these three selves develop through experience and ultimately combine to become a unified cognitive structure. Chein (1944), in contrast, suggests that the self is the content rather than the object of awareness; that is, the self is the knowledge represented in self-awareness. According to Chein, the self is passive, protected, and developed by ego action and the ego, not the self, is a cognitive structure.

There have been many other formulations of the self and of the self relative to the ego (e.g., Allport, 1943; Bertocci, 1945; Hilgard, 1949; Jung, 1953; Koffka, 1935; Lundholm, 1940; Sherif & Cantril, 1947; Stephenson, 1953; Sullivan, 1964) that contributed to the evolution of self-theory. It is Carl Rogers' contributions to self-theory, however, that are generally regarded as most profound in terms of the modern text of self-theory and its wide practical applicability. Rogers' theory of personality development will be discussed here and his method of nondirective counseling, which derives from the theory, will be discussed in Chapter 4.

Rogers, as with Freud and others, based his personality theory on his clinical experiences with individuals he saw for counseling and psychotherapy. Drawing from an abundant number of these therapeutic relationships, Rogers developed a personality theory within a self-theory framework, a theory of interpersonal relationship, and his nondirective or person-centered approach to therapy. Although all three aspects of his overall theory—personality, interpersonal relationships, and therapy—are framed within a client-centered context (Rogers, 1959), it is rather like a chicken-or-egg conundrum to determine whether his opinions of personality development evolved from empirical data collected from his client-centered therapeutic relationships or if client-centered therapy was built on a rudimentary personality theory he had yet to articulate. His first publications dealt with therapy and his writings on personality theory followed later. Since then, both theory and therapy have evolved together, and continue to evolve through new interpretations and evaluation of his personality theory. It is this aspect of Rogers' theory that is perhaps most noteworthy. Although others have tended to regard their theory as immutable, in formulation if not in fact, Rogers often revised his on the basis of data from extensive, ongoing scientific testing. He encouraged the testing of his theory, welcomed challenges to it, and did not resist modifications to it in the face of new insight. This is in sharp contrast to many of his predecessors. Rogers' extensive research publications and his awards for research attest to his seriousness about scientific validation of his theories. His 24-year career as an academician perhaps engendered and maintained his counselor-as-scientist approach to therapy.

When Rogers and B. F. Skinner debated in 1956, the two became lastingly identified as the standard bearers for the humanistic and behavioristic camps of psychology. Rogers' humanistic approach to counseling has been embraced both by psychologists and by many professionals not trained in psychoanalysis or behavior modification principles but who use counseling in their professional practices. Psychoanalysis, behaviorism, and humanism can be viewed as representing the three major approaches to modern counseling or psychotherapy. The humanistic school of psychology, with Rogers most typically recognized as its leading light (Bugental, 1967), was founded by Abraham Maslow; its theoretical origins are in existentialism and phenomenology. Counseling based on humanistic psychology emphasizes holism, creativity, free choice, client and clinician spontaneity, and, especially important in Rogers' theory, self-actualization, which also is a concept developed by Maslow. Rogers' humanistic view of personality is in marked contrast to both classic psychoanalytic and behavioristic views. Whereas Freud viewed humankind with pessimism and as inherently bad, Rogers views it with optimism and as innately good. Those who see behaviorists as tending toward an impersonal, coldly objective consideration of human personality and behavior, prefer Rogers' warm, personal approach to counseling.

HISTORICAL PERSPECTIVE

Carl Rogers (1902–1987) was born in Oak Park, Illinois, to a close-knit and "almost fundamentalist" religious family (Rogers, 1959, 1961). The fourth of six children, Rogers was taught to value a strict work ethic. When he was 12 years old, Rogers' family moved to a farm where he developed an interest in the agricultural sciences, which prompted an interest in biologic and physical sciences during his early undergraduate years at the University of Wisconsin. On graduation with his baccalaureate degree, he enrolled in New York City's Union Theological Seminary. Here he was afforded a more liberal perspective on religion and later transferred to Columbia University's Teachers College where he earned his master's degree in 1928 and his doctorate in clinical psychology in 1931. Important mentors for him at Columbia were Edward Thorndike; John Dewey; and Leta Hollingworth, who introduced Rogers to clinical psychology.

The first clinical experience Rogers obtained was at the Institute for Child Guidance in New York in which treatment practice was based on Freudian concepts. Rogers had difficulty consolidating the subjective Freudian thought at the Institute with the objective, statistical Thorndikean orientation at Columbia.

On graduating from Columbia with his doctorate, Rogers accepted a clinical position with the Child Guidance Center in Rochester, Minnesota. During his years at the Center, Rogers was influenced by the writings of Otto Rank, who had formulated his own concepts of personality and behavior after starting out as a follower of Freud. Rogers eventually became the director of the Center and while there published his first book, *The Clinical Treatment of the Problem Child* (1939).

In 1940 Rogers left the clinical setting for an academic one at Ohio State University where he explicated his philosophy of psychotherapy in *Counseling and Psychotherapy* (1942). Rogers accepted a position in 1945 on the faculty at the University of Chicago and embarked on one of the most productive decades of his professional life. It was here that he first used the term "client-centered" to describe his style of counseling and published his classic work on nondirective counseling and psychotherapy, *Client-Centered Therapy* (1951), which included a chapter on his newly formulated personality theory. Roger's research activities were prolific at Ohio State and later at the University of Wisconsin where he accepted an appointment in 1957. At the University of Wisconsin, Rogers conducted research on the effects of psychotherapy on institutionalized persons with schizophrenia.

Rogers left academia in 1964 for a position as resident fellow at the Western Behavioral Sciences Institute in La Jolla, California. In 1968 he helped establish the Center for Studies of the Person in La Jolla and remained there until the end of his career.

BASIC CONCEPTS

Rogers' personality theory, although largely original, does derive in part from the concepts of other theorists to whom he readily acknowledges his indebtedness. In Rogers' theory can be seen Rank's (1945) humanistic influence; Gendlin (1962) and Standal's (1954) self-theory interpretations; Angyal's (1941) organismic theory; Lecky's (1945) concept of the self; Maslow's (1943) holistic-dynamic theory; Sullivan's (1953) interpersonal theory; and Snygg and Comb's (1949) concepts of the phenomenal self and the human tendency for self-actualization (also seen in Maslow's theory). Rogers (1951) notes that his theory is basically a phenomenological one that is explained by heavy reliance on the concept of self.

Assumptions

In 1951, in his book *Client-Centered Therapy*, Rogers set forth nineteen propositions concerning the uniqueness of the individual or self; he later (Rogers, 1959) added three additional propositions. Those twenty-two propositions are the framework of his personality theory. The following eight assumptions are salient aspects of Rogers' propositions about human personality.

1. Individuals are inherently good, rational, and goal-directed socialized beings. This is in direct contrast to Freudian views of the innate character of humankind.
2. Individuals have the basic capacity to control their destinies and themselves, given adequate conditions in which to grow and develop.
3. Individuals respond to events in accordance with their internal frame of reference to the phenomenal field.
4. Individuals' internal frame of reference forms from their perceptions of the environment; it is their perceptions of reality, rather than reality itself, that chiefly determine their behavior.
5. Individuals' behavior can best be understood through knowledge of their unique internal frame of reference.

6. Most of the behaviors adopted by individuals are consistent with their sense of self.
7. The one basic tendency or drive of individuals is to actualize. The need to self-actualize involves enhancing and maintaining the organism: "the urge to expand, extend, develop, mature" (Rogers, 1961, p. 351).
8. All behavior is purposeful and in response to perceived reality.

Personality Constructs

Rogers' personality theory is conceptualized essentially as process constructs. That is, he places most of his emphasis on growth and change, the drive toward self-actualization, and the conditions necessary to facilitate positive forward-moving change in the individual. But Rogers' theory also contains three important structural constructs: the organism, phenomenal field, and the self.

The *organism* is the totality of an individual—all of the psychological and physiologic characteristics that constitute the total awareness an individual has at any given moment which, in turn, determines how the individual will behave. The organism is a holistic construct, composed of emotions, thoughts, attitudes, and physical attributes that reacts to the phenomenal field as a unified whole. A change in any part of the organism, psychological or physiologic, might cause changes to occur in other parts, so that the organism can continue problem-solving effectively to maintain and enhance itself. This tendency toward self-actualization, according to Rogers, is the most basic characteristic of the organism, "its tendency toward total, organized, goal-directed responses" (Rogers 1951, pp. 486–487).

The *phenomenal field* is the totality of an individual's subjective perceptions of reality which may or may not match external reality. It is these perceptions that determine how the individual behaves in trying to maintain and enhance itself: "Behavior is basically the goal-directed attempt of the organism to satisfy its needs as experienced, in the field as perceived" (Rogers, 1951, p. 491). The phenomenal field constitutes an *internal frame of reference* to reality for the individual and can be only partly known to others through empathic inference; to understand an individual's behavior, one must attempt to regard it from that individual's internal frame of reference. The phenomenal field provides security to individuals by representing their world in tested hypotheses that lend predictability to living. But the phenomenal field is also composed of untested perceptions that can influence behavior with as much authority as can the tested perceptions (Rogers, 1951). Both conscious and unconscious experiences also make up the phenomenal field. The conscious experiences are those symbolized in awareness and effect learning and growth for the individual. The more open individuals are to experience and the more experiences that are permitted to become symbolized in awareness, the more enhanced is their drive toward self-actualization.

The *self* develops out of the organism's interaction with the phenomenal field. The phenomenal field is ever dynamic and the self constantly changes in response to altering landscapes of experience. The self is a part of the individual's perceptual field and becomes differentiated from the total field in infancy as perceptions of "me" and "I." Although the self changes as the organism moves through the world of experience, it nonetheless attempts at all times to remain organized and consistent in its internal perceptions and its influence on behavior. It accomplishes this by valuing experiences and incorporating these values into the structure of self. The organism may directly experience these values or introject the values of others, distorting them to be perceived as direct experience. Experiences that are consistent with the patterns of self-perception are symbolized in awareness. Experiences that are not consistent with the organism's sense of self are either denied or are distorted before being admitted to awareness.

PERSONALITY DEVELOPMENT

As discussed, Rogers holds that "the organism has one basic tendency and striving—to actualize, maintain, and enhance the experiencing organism" (Rogers, 1951, p. 487). This tendency is present in infancy and continues throughout life. The infant's behavior is not random but is purposeful toward the goal of self-actualization. The infant interacts holistically with the phenomenal field and evaluates experiences it has therewith according to how consistent the experiences are with its sense of self and with its need to actualize. Experiences perceived as meeting those criteria are assigned positive values and are symbolized in awareness. Experiences perceived as being inconsistent with those needs are given negative values; they are denied, distorted, or avoided. The operable word in the *organismic valuing process* (Rogers, 1959) is "perceived." Experiences are evaluated according to the infant's internal frame of reference, which is formed from its perceptions of reality. The infant will give positive values to experiences it perceives as enhancing its concept of self, whether or not they actually do, and negative values to those perceived as threats, whether or not they in fact are. Rogers (1951) contends that the infant engages in this valuing process with certitude, although it may not yet have developed the language skills to conceptualize experiences verbally. But nonverbal concepts about the structure of self, the environment, and the infant's relationship to the environment are formed early and become the guiding principles for the infant's behavior. Never fixed, these values are under constant evaluation by the organism and are subject to change.

As the infant matures into early childhood, the phenomenal field expands to include social experiences. This brings an external evaluation to bear on the child's behavior. The child's organismic valuing of experiences is augmented by others' evaluations of him or her, in particular parents or primary caretakers. The child "perceives himself as lovable, worthy of love, and his relationship to his parents as one of affection" (Rogers, 1959, p. 499). These perceptions are satisfying to the child and represent an important central element of the developing structure of self. Soon the child develops a *need for positive regard*, a need to be regarded as a lovable person by others in his or her perceptual field, especially by significant others (Meador & Rogers, 1973). The child begins to learn that certain of his or her behaviors are consistent with the concept of self as lovable in that they elicit loving, satisfying responses from parents and others, whereas other behaviors are met with reproof and, therefore, are not consistent with their concept of self. To maintain and enhance a sense of self which is dependent on positive regard, the child begins to incorporate the values others place on behavior into his or her self-structure. Experiences that receive positive regard are symbolized in awareness; whereas experiences that do not fulfill the need for positive regard, although they may be satisfying to the child in other ways, are denied or symbolized in a distorted manner to protect the emerging concept of self from perceived threats. For example, rather than accurately symbolizing "I perceive my parents as experiencing this behavior as unsatisfying to them," the child might distort the symbolization to "I perceive this behavior as unsatisfying" (Rogers, 1959, p. 500).

Thus, the child eventually comes to have two loci of evaluation of his or her behavior: 1) an internal locus of evaluation—the organismic valuing process and 2) an external locus of evaluation that involves the values others place on behavior. At this point the child develops a *self-regard need* that is dependent on the evaluations of others. The child learns a sense of self based on his or her perceptions of the regard received from others (Meador & Rogers, 1973). If a healthy balance exists in the child's use of organismic valuing and the values of others in meeting the need for self-regard, the potential exists for normal personality development. The child will judge him- or herself positively or negatively, primarily on organismic values, but also on the introjected values of others, and will behave in ways that are both innately satisfying and favorably responded to by others.

Rogers (1959) suggests that certain conditions are necessary for the child to develop congruency between the organismic valuing process and the needs for positive regard and self-regard. Most important is that the child receive *unconditional positive regard* from parents or caretakers. This does not mean that significant others must approve or accept all of a child's behaviors. Instead, it means that when significant others express disapproval of a child's behavior, the goodness or worth of the child's concept of self is not brought negatively into question. If the child perceives the unconditional positive regard of parents and caretakers, he or she will develop *unconditional self-regard* and will not perceive the negative responses of others to specific behaviors as threats to his or her basic self-structure that is grounded chiefly on organismic values.

If the child can establish and maintain unconditional self-regard, he or she will develop toward adolescence and adulthood as a *fully functioning* person. In Rogers' (1951, 1959) view, a fully functioning individual is:

- open to and aware of experiences
- free of defense mechanisms
- socialized, living with others in harmony
- able to symbolize experiences accurately
- in possession of unconditional self-regard
- adaptive in a continually changing phenomenal field

The concept of self as a fully functioning person is undergoing constant change in response to new experiences, but behavior consistently moves toward the goal of self-actualization.

## ABNORMAL PERSONALITY

At the time that the child develops a need for self-regard, there exists the tendency for introjection of others' values into the self-structure, particularly if unconditional positive regard from significant others is not perceived by the child. If the child's behavior becomes controlled by these introjected values, he or she is said to have developed *conditions of worth*. The child believes that in order to be perceived as worthy, he or she must subjugate organismic values to the values of others. The child who has developed conditions of worth avoids experiences that would be innately satisfying and distorts experiences inconsistent with the conditions of worth rather than accurately symbolizing them in awareness. This leads to *incongruence* between reality as experienced by the organism and reality as experienced by the self. The individual becomes torn between the two disparate dictates of organismic values and introjected conditions of worth, behaving at times in response to one set of values and at times in response to the other. Such incongruity sets the stage for psychological maladjustment and maladaptive behavior.

Conditions of worth can also lead to the individual experiencing incongruity between perceived subjective reality and actual external reality, as well as incongruity between the self and the ideal self. Conditions of worth can begin to develop early in childhood, as the structure of self starts to form from an awareness of self-experiences. Or, conditions of worth can develop at any point in life owing to changes in one's phenomenal field or sense of self. These changes can be brought on by any number of circumstances (e.g., illness, geographic relocation, occupational changes, financial insecurity, or interpersonal relationships). In a marriage, for example, a wife's need for positive regard might be stronger than her husband's need. Until marrying she might have been true to her organismic values but now can only have positive self-regard if she is true to the values of her husband. She introjects his values into her self-structure and behaves in ways to which he will respond favorably, but not necessarily in ways that are innately satisfying to her. At this point she has developed conditions of worth and must falsify her own values to perceive them as being consistent with those of her husband and to maintain his positive regard.

If the individual is in a state of congruence, the experiences in the phenomenal field will match the symbolized experiences that constitute the perceived self. The individual will be free of anxiety and will perceive no threat in the phenomenal field. Behavior will be based on realistic thinking and will serve the process of self-actualization, making this individual fully functioning, free of external control, and forward-moving (Rogers, 1959). If incongruity exists between the perceived self and the organism's experiences, the individual may also develop incongruent behavior. The individual's behaviors will be inconsistent, at times serving the process of self-actualization and at other times serving conditions of worth. Behaviors in response to conditions of worth to fulfill the need for self-regard will cause the self to feel threatened and to experience anxiety and tension. To preserve itself and to maintain a low-tension state for the organism, the self will falsify, distort, or deny experiences that are not consistent with its values rather than symbolizing them accurately in awareness. The classic defense mechanisms described by Freud are methods by which individuals maintain consistency between the perceived self and actual experience (Combs & Snygg, 1959; Rogers, 1959). If in any instance an individual's defense mechanisms are not adequate to maintain this consistency, the individual will feel anxiety and tension to a degree relative to the perceived threat to the concept of self.

Defense mechanisms protect the self through deception. But they do not work effectively in all situations nor do they change the behaviors and experiences that are the sources of the individual's anxiety and tension. The individual develops more defensive behaviors in response to recurring and increasing threats to the self. Owing to the inaccurate symbolization of experiences in awareness, the individual's behavior becomes rigid and irrational; he or she is less open to experiences and has difficulty reacting adaptively to changing reality. Such a person is not forward-moving or fully functioning owing to the avoidance of some experiences and the inaccurate symbolization of others, which limits enhancement of the self. Client-centered counseling was designed by Rogers (1951) to help the maladjusted individual establish or re-establish congruency between the self and experiences and to shift from an external locus of control to an internal one; this process is discussed in Chapter 4.

## RELEVANCE TO SPEECH-LANGUAGE PATHOLOGY AND AUDIOLOGY

Roger's client-centered approach to counseling is amply relevant to therapy with persons who have speech, language, or hearing disorders, as is discussed in Chapter 4. In fact, it has been applied to more disciplines that involve counseling than any other approach to counseling. Rogers' personality theory also has clinical relevance for speech-language pathologists and audiologists; in particular, the constructs of internal frame of reference, conditions of worth, congruence versus incongruence, and locus of behavior evaluation and control.

In Rogers' view each person exists in a unique phenomenal field in which reality consists of perceptions derived from an internal frame of reference. The only way to understand an individual's thoughts, feelings, and behavior is to understand this internal frame of reference. This is important to keep in mind in counseling persons with communicative disorders or with their parents and significant others. Everyone involved in the counseling encounter—the client, the father, the mother, the spouse, the friend, the teacher, the physician, and the speech-language pathologist or audiologist—may view the problem from an appreciably different frame of reference. For instance, one individual may see the

client's communicative disorder as not being a problem, whereas another sees it as a handicap. One individual might view therapy as a waste of time, whereas another believes it is
critical to personal well-being. Individuals may have different cognitive and affective reactions to a communicative disorder, reactions that are based on their differing perceptions
of reality, and on their varying degrees of factual data about the disorder. For therapy to be
maximally effective, the internal frame of reference of all those meaningfully involved with
the client must be as closely aligned as possible, in regard both to the client and to the communicative disorder. This facilitates clinically meaningful client-clinician, family-clinician,
client-family, and clinician-other professional interactions, especially when everyone's
perceptions are in alignment with one another and if these perceptions closely match external reality.

Attempting to understand the client's internal frame of reference also helps the clinician understand the emotional ramifications occasioned by the communicative disorder.
For example, a client may perceive certain communicative situations as threatening and try
to avoid them, even when successfully modifying the disorder. An understanding of a
client's internal frame of reference helps the clinician comprehend and address such barriers to total communicative rehabilitation and be more effective in helping clients personally adjust to communicative disorders to become fully functioning individuals despite
the continued presence of a disorder.

Individuals with communicative disorders are at risk for developing conditions of
worth. Often they view the positive regard from others as affirmation of their acceptability, effectiveness, and worthiness. Their organismic values in such instances are not as-
serted and they tend to behave in ways to which others respond favorably, even if the behavior is not innately satisfying to them. If persons with communicative disorders perceive
that to be deemed worthy by others and, thus, fulfill a need for self-regard, they must
adopt the values of others and give positive value to some experiences that are not innately
self-satisfying and negative values to satisfying ones, their communicative disorder becomes a handicap as their perceptions of it and of others' reactions to it have diminished
the quality of their lives.

A further danger associated with the introjection of conditions of worth by persons
with communicative disorders is that the incongruity between the perceived self and
environmental experiences for them become so significant as to result in maladaptive
behavior. They may develop general feelings of anxiety and tension in reaction to this
incongruity that appreciably exceed what might be considered an understandable concern
about their communicative disorder. In an attempt to cope with this anxiety and tension,
they may assemble defense mechanisms that distort their awareness of the reality of their
world of experience and their place in that world as socialized individuals. The prognosis
for successful (re)habilitation (i.e., establishing something that has not existed) of their
speech, language, or hearing problem will be guarded for such individuals. Their feelings
of anxiety and tension may become increasingly distracting and, as additional defense
mechanisms are erected, their behavior may become increasingly maladaptive. In such a
state, their behavior will be inflexible and they will have difficulty developing adaptive behaviors and accurately symbolizing new experiences in awareness.

Therapy is quite difficult for clients with communicative disorders who are not fully
functioning and who have developed maladjusted behavior as a result of introjected conditions of worth. They are not forward-moving and have difficulty setting, achieving, and
maintaining therapy goals. In effect, they might not be in control of their lives if they have
placed the locus of evaluation and control of their behavior external to their self-structures.
Their perceptions of external reality may be distorted to the extent that they are ineffective

communicators with actual reality, irrespective of their speech, language, and hearing problems.

Speech-language pathologists and audiologists can help such clients, through counseling, to (re)enter the process of self-actualization. For this to occur, the experiences and behaviors that led to a client's anxiety and tension must be identified and changed. Maladaptive behaviors must be abandoned and new behaviors learned that facilitate the client becoming fully functioning. Rogers (1951) suggests that the goals for developing congruence between the self and experience should be individualized for clients and determined by the clients themselves, as well as the methods for achieving those goals. Clinicians should provide general goals only and establish the conditions conducive to a client's effecting behavior changes. One such condition is the clinician's unconditional positive regard for clients as discussed earlier, but there are others described in Chapter 4. If these conditions are met, clients move forward under their own momentum, with clinicians helping them discard defense mechanisms that distort their perceptions of external reality and regain congruence between their concept of self and their organismic values.

## REFERENCES

Allport, G. (1937). *Personality: A psychological interpretation.* New York: Henry Holt and Co.

Allport, G. W. (1943). The ego in contemporary psychology. *Psychological Review, 50,* 451–478.

Angyal, A. (1941). *Foundations for a science of personality.* New York: Commonwealth Fund.

Bertocci, P. A. (1945). The psychological self, the ego and personality. *Psychological Review, 52,* 91–99.

Bischof, L. J. (1964). *Interpreting personality theories.* New York: Harper & Row.

Breuer, J., & Freud, S. (1955). Studies on hysteria. *Standard edition, 2,* 1–305. London: Hogarth Press. (Originally published 1895).

Brill, A. A. (1923). Speech disturbances in nervous and mental diseases. *Quarterly Journal of Speech Education, 9,* 129–135.

Bugental, J. F. T. (Ed.). (1967). *Challenges of humanistic psychology.* New York: McGraw-Hill.

Buhler, C. (1962). Genetic aspects of the self. In E. Harms (Ed.), Fundamentals of psychology: The psychology of the self. *Annals of the New York Academy of Sciences, 96,* 730–764.

Chein, I. (1944). The awareness of self and the structure of the ego. *Psychological Review, 51,* 304–314.

Combs, A. W., & Snygg, D. (1959). *Individual behavior.* New York: Harper & Brothers.

Coriat, I. H. (1943). The psychoanalytic conception of stammering. *Nervous Child, 2,* 167–171.

Crowe, T. A. (1995). Counseling for fluency disorders: Rationale, strategy, and technique. Paper presented as part of short course with W. H. Manning, & G. W. Blood at the American Speech-Language-Hearing Association Convention, Orlando, FL.

Emerson, R. W. (1950). B. Atkinson (Ed.), *The selected writings.* New York: Modern Library.

English, H. B., & English, A. C. (1958). *A comprehensive dictionary of psychological and psychoanalytical terms.* New York: David McKay.

Erikson, E. H. (1946). Ego development and historical change. In A. Freud et al. (Eds.), *The psychoanalytic study of the child,* Vol. 2. New York: International Universities Press.

Erikson, E. H. (1963a). *Childhood and society* (2nd ed.). New York: WW Norton.

Erikson, E. H. (Ed.). (1963b). *Youth: Change and challenge.* New York: Basic Books.

Erikson, E. H. (1968). *Identity, youth, and crises.* New York: WW Norton.

Ford, D. H., & Urban, H. B. (1963). *Systems of psychotherapy.* New York: John Wiley & Sons.

Fromm, E. (1947). *Man for himself: an inquiry into the psychology of ethics.* New York: Holt, Rinehart & Winston.

Freud, S. (1955). *Interpretation of dreams.* London: Hogarth Press. (Originally published 1900.)

Gay, P. (1988). *Freud: A life for our time.* New York: WW Norton.

Gemelli, R. J. (1982a). Classification of child stuttering. Part I: Transient developmental, neurogenic acquired, and persistent child stuttering. *Child Psychiatry and Human Development, 12,* 220–253.

Gemelli, R. J. (1982b). Classification of child stuttering. Part II: Persistent late onset male stuttering and treatment issues for persistent stutterers—psychotherapy or speech therapy, or both? *Child Psychiatry and Human Development, 13,* 3–34.

Gendlin, E. T. (1962). *Experiencing and the creation of meaning.* New York: Free Press of Glencoe.

Hall, C. S. (1954). *A primer of Freudian psychology.* New York: World Publishing.

Hall, C. S., & Lindzey, G. (1978). *Theories of personality* (3rd ed.). New York: John Wiley & Sons.

Hampden-Turner, C. (1981). *Maps of the mind: Charts and concepts of the mind and its labyrinths.* New York:

Macmillan.

Hansen, J. C., Stevic, R. R., & Warner, R. W. Jr. (1982). *Counseling: Theory and process* (3rd ed.). Newton, MA: Allyn and Bacon.

Hartmann, H. (1958). *Ego psychology and the problem of adaptation.* New York: International Universities Press. (Originally published 1939.)

Hartmann, H. (1961). The mutual influence in the development of the ego and the id. *Psychoanalytic Quarterly, 20,* 31–43.

Hartmann, H. (1964). *Essays on ego psychology.* New York: International Universities Press.

Hartmann, H. (1967). Psychoanalysis as a scientific theory. In T. Millon (Ed.), *Theories of psychopathology.* Philadelphia: WB Saunders.

Hilgard, E. R. (1949). Human motives and the concept of the self. *American Psychologist, 4,* 374–382.

James, W. (1890). *Principles of psychology.* New York: Henry Holt.

Johnson, W. (1946). *People in quandaries.* New York: Harper & Brothers.

Jones, E. (1953; 1955; 1957). *The life and work of Sigmund Freud.* New York: Basic Books (Vol. 1–3.

Jung, C. G. (1916). *Analytical psychology.* New York: Moffat, Yard.

Jung, C. G. (1923). *Psychological types or the psychology of individuation.* Orlando, FL: Harcourt Brace Jovanovich.

Jung, C. G. (1953). Psychology and alchemy. In *Collected works.* Vol. 7. Princeton, NJ: Princeton University Press.

Jung, C. G. (1959). The concept of the collective unconscious. In *Collected works.* Vol. 9, Part I. Princeton, NJ: Princeton University Press.

King, P. T., & Neal, R. (1968). *Ego psychology in counseling.* Boston, MA: Houghton Mifflin.

Koffka, K. (1935). *Principles of gestalt psychology.* New York: Harcourt, Brace, & World.

Kroeber, T. C. (1963). The coping functions of the ego mechanisms. In R. W. White (Ed.), *The study of lives.* New York: Atherton.

Kubie, L. S. (1961). *Neurotic distortion of the creative process.* New York: Noonday Press.

Lecky, P. (1940). *Self-consistency.* New York: Island Press.

Lundholm, H. (1940). Reflections upon the nature of the psychological self. *Psychological Review, 47,* 110–127.

Maslow, A. H. (1943). Dynamics of personality organization. *Psychological Review, 50,* 514–539, 541–558.

Mead, G. H. (1934). *Mind, self, and society.* Chicago, IL: University of Chicago Press.

Meador, B. D., & Rogers, C. R. (1973). Client-centered therapy. In R. Corsini (Ed.), *Current psychotherapies.* Itasca, IL: F.E. Peacock.

Nystul, M. S. (1993). *The art and science of counseling and psychotherapy.* New York: Macmillan.

Pepinsky, H. B., & Pepinsky, P. N. (1954). *Counseling: Theory and practice.* New York: Ronald Press.

Rank, O. (1945). *Will therapy and truth and reality.* New York: Alfred A. Knopf.

Rapaport, D. (1958). *The structure of psychoanalytic theory: A systematizing attempt.* New York: International Universities Press.

Rogers, C. R. (1939). *The clinical treatment of the problem child.* Boston, MA: Houghton Mifflin.

Rogers, C. R. (1942). *Counseling and psychotherapy.* Cambridge, MA: Riverside Press.

Rogers, C. R. (1951). *Client-centered therapy.* Boston, MA: Houghton Mifflin.

Rogers, C. R. (1959). A theory of therapy, personality, and interpersonal relationships as developed in the client-centered framework. In S. Koch (Ed.), *Psychology—A study of science Vol III, Formulations of the person in the social context.* New York: McGraw-Hill.

Rogers, C. W. (1978). *On becoming a person: A therapist's view of psychotherapy.* Boston, MA: Houghton Mifflin.

Ryckman, R. M. (1978). *Theories of personality.* New York: D. Van Nostrand.

Sarbin, T. R. (1952). A preface to a psychological analysis of the self. *Psychological Review, 59,* 11–22.

Schultz, D. (1976). *Theories of personality.* Monterey, CA: Brooks/Cole.

Sherif, M., & Cantril, H. (1947). *The psychology of ego-involvements.* New York: John Wiley & Sons.

Snygg, D., & Combs, A. W. (1949). *Individual behavior.* New York: Harper & Row.

Standal, S. (1954). The need for positive regard: A contribution to client-centered theory. Unpublished doctoral dissertation, University of Chicago.

Stephenson, W. (1953). *The study of behavior.* Chicago, IL: University of Chicago Press.

Sullivan, H. S. (1953). *The interpersonal theory of psychiatry.* New York: WW Norton.

Sullivan, H. S. (1964). *The fusion of psychiatry and social science.* New York: WW Norton.

Wolman, B. B. (Ed.). (1989). *Dictionary of behavioral science* (2nd ed.). New York: Academic Press.

# 4. Approaches to Counseling

Thomas A. Crowe

---

**Counseling Approaches Derived from Psychoanalytic Theories**

Psychoanalytic Approaches Other than Adler's

- *Freud's Psychoanalysis*
- *Analytic Psychology*
- *Ego-Analysis*

Individual Psychology

- *Historical Perspective*
- *Basic Concepts*
- *Counseling Techniques*
- *Outcomes of Counseling*
- *Relevance to Speech-Language Pathology and Audiology*

**Cognitive-Behavioral Approaches**

Cognitive-Behavioral Approaches other than Ellis'

- *Transactional Analysis*
- *Behavior Therapy*
- *Reality Therapy*
- *Cognitive Therapy*

Rational Emotive Behavior Therapy

- *Historical Perspective*
- *Basic Concepts*
- *Counseling Technique*
- *Outcomes of Counseling*
- *Relevance to Speech-Language Pathology and Audiology*

**Experiential Approaches**

Experiential Approaches Other than Rogers'

- *Existential Therapy*
- *Gestalt Therapy*
- *Creative Arts Therapy*

Person-Centered Therapy

- *Historical Perspective*
- *Basic Concepts*
- *Counseling Technique*
- *Goals of Therapy*
- *If-Then Conditions*
- *Progress of Therapy*
- *Outcomes of Counseling*
- *Relevance to Speech-Language Pathology and Audiology*

---

In constructing their personal theory of counseling, clinicians should incorporate a philosophy of counseling process into a framework that includes theories of personality development and abnormal personality, human growth and development, fundamentals of learning, and principles and processes of behavior change. Just as with personality theory, through eclectic study clinicians might develop a composite philosophy of counseling process or adhere to one approach to counseling, becoming increasingly skillful across time in its use with various clients and with various types of client problems. However, whether speech-language pathologists and audiologists base their personal approach to counseling on multiple theories or essentially on one theory only, their approach should be flexible enough to meet the challenges of counseling with various clients of different ages, from various cultures, with various communicative disorders, and with various secondary concerns related to their communicative disorders.

Numerous modern concepts of how best to approach counseling have been advanced, beginning with the psychoanalytic approach of Joseph Breuer and Sigmund Freud in the late 19th century to the neo-analytic theories of Freud's psychoanalytic descendants in the early 20th century, through the guidance movement theories of the mid-20th century, to current theories of general and specialized counseling and psychotherapy. It is not possible in the space of this chapter to discuss every historical and extant approach to counseling. Instead, brief descriptions of leading approaches that represent the three major camps of counseling theory—psychoanalytic, cognitive-behavioral, experiential—are provided along with expanded descriptions of three seminal approaches to counseling: (*a*) Alfred Adler's individual psychology, which represents approaches derived from psychoanalytic theories; (*b*) Albert Ellis' rational emotive behavior therapy, representing cognitive-behavioral approaches to counseling; and (*c*) Carl Rogers' person-centered therapy, which represents experiential approaches.

## COUNSELING APPROACHES DERIVED FROM PSYCHOANALYTIC THEORIES

The individual psychology approach to counseling developed by Alfred Adler is discussed at length in this section to represent counseling approaches derived from psychoanalytic theory. Adlerian psychology has had far-reaching influences on all schools of psychology, with neo-Freudians, cognitive-behaviorists, and humanists alike drawing liberally from Adler's ideas when formulating their own theories (Mosak, 1989). Other approaches to counseling have been developed within a psychoanalytic framework that also have been influential in determining the current status of counseling technique. These include Freud's classic psychoanalytic approach to counseling, Jung's analytic psychology, and ego-analysis.

### Psychoanalytic Approaches Other Than Adler's

FREUD'S PSYCHOANALYSIS

Freud's *classic psychoanalytic theory* of personality was discussed in Chapter 3. His approach to counseling, which is true of psychoanalytic approaches in general, seeks to reconstruct the client's personality by identifying, analyzing, and resolving intrapsychic conflicts. This is typically not simple to accomplish so therapy may be of long duration. Arlow (1989) identifies four phases of psychoanalysis:

1. An *opening phase* that can last up to six months, during which a detailed history of the client and his or her problem is obtained.
2. A *development of transference* phase during which the client projects feelings about his or her significant others onto the analyst and by so doing gains insight into interpersonal relationship problems (countertransference also can occur during this phase).
3. A *working through* phase involving further analysis of the client's transference.
4. A *resolution of transference* phase in which the client is prepared for therapy termination and independent functioning. Techniques used by the psychoanalyst throughout these phases include *free association, confrontation, dream analysis,* and *interpretation.*

ANALYTIC PSYCHOLOGY

Carl G. Jung (1875–1961) was an early associate of Freud, as was Adler. As with Adler, Jung soon differed with Freud on theoretic issues, chief among which were Freud's emphasis on the role played by sexuality in personality development and Jung's belief that science and religion could be compatible. Jung dissociated himself with the Freudian movement in 1914 by resigning as the first president of the International Psychoanalytic Association and establishing his own school of psychology, which he named *analytic psychology.* Jung's view of humankind was more positive than was Freud's; he held that individuals possess an innate tendency to achieve wholeness, uniqueness, and self-realization (Jung, 1916).

This process, which Jung termed *individualization,* contains the basic elements of Freudian theory—conscious and unconscious levels of awareness, the libido, and the mediation of personality by the ego protected by defense mechanisms. It is, however, distinguished by Jung's own concepts of personality development, some of which tend toward the metaphysical (Hall & Lindzey, 1978). Jung's concepts include:

1. The idea of a *collective unconscious* containing universal thoughts passed from generation to generation that have a strong influence on an individual's personality and behavior.
2. *Archetypes,* which are the universal thoughts in the collective unconscious and include: the *persona* or public self; the *animus and anima* concept that individuals possess both male and female personality characteristics in a Yin-Yang sense; the *shadow* or evil side of personality that individuals deny; and the *self,* which unifies and stabilizes the personality, typically emerging during middle age when the conscious ego and unconscious processes achieve integration.
3. *Personality types* that are distinguishable by two types of attitude—*introverted* and *extroverted*—and by four types of function—*thinking, feeling, sensation,* and *intuition.* According to Jung, individuals rely on all four personality functions to deal effectively with the challenges of living, but one function that varies from person to person typically becomes better developed than the other functions; individuals tend to prefer using this function and an auxiliary function to react to most situations.

Based on these concepts, the primary goal of analytic psychology is to assist the client in developing the systems of personality necessary for the self to emerge. Once the self has emerged, the process of individualization is enhanced and the client can be more fully functioning in his or her movement toward self-realization. This goal might be achieved by helping clients become aware of the various dimensions of their personality, for instance becoming more aware of both their male and female sides. Jung's discussion of specific techniques of counseling and psychotherapy was limited. He advised that (*a*) techniques should be tailored to the unique challenges presented by each client, (*b*) clinicians should be flexible and creative in designing therapy techniques, and (*c*) practically any technique was satisfactory if it helped clients effect the desired changes in their personality and behavior.

EGO-ANALYSIS

*Ego-analysis,* or ego-counseling, is another approach to counseling and psychotherapy that is psychoanalytic in its foundations. Whereas ego-analysis is in some measure predicated on classic Freudian concepts, its ideas of personality development and human behavior are drawn more from the principles of ego-psychology (e.g., Erikson, 1963; Rapaport, 1958). The ego-analytic concepts of personality development and maladaptive behavior and the manner in which these concepts differ from Freud's are discussed in Chapter 3. Ego-counseling does not attempt to reconstruct the client's entire personality but instead is designed to help the client modify a limited number of specific ego problems that are responsible for maladaptive behavior. The goal of ego-counseling is to help clients replace maladaptive behavior with adaptive patterns of behavior that promote growth (Kroeber, 1963) and to establish ego flexibility and ego-integrity as described in Chapter 3. Owing to the limited nature of the goals of ego-counseling, its process typically is not as intense or as long as Freudian psychoanalysis, often requiring less than ten sessions.

Technique in ego-counseling does not consist of specified, prescribed strategies only. It chiefly involves clinician skills used to help clients develop new patterns of behavior while respecting their right to be individuals (Hummel, 1962) and experience freedom in the counseling relationship, particularly in the early stages of therapy (Bordin, 1955). The clinician maintains control of the counseling relationship and of the client's focus on therapy goals while conveying commitment and warmth to the client. *Ambiguity* is one way in which the clinician can both maintain control and create a climate in therapy in which clients can openly express their thoughts and feelings. With the use of nondirective techniques, the clinician permits therapy to be minimally structured and therefore clients tend not to interact rigidly with their clinician. If therapy becomes so ambiguous that no progress is being accomplished, the clinician can reduce ambiguity in the relationship by employing more directive techniques. Other strategies used in ego-counseling include *transference, diagnosis,* and *interpretation,* which are used in most other psychoanalytic approaches.

## Individual Psychology

As mentioned, Alfred Adler's theory of individual psychology has had considerable influence on the formulation of other psychoanalytic approaches to counseling and psychotherapy. Neo-Freudians, frequently without acknowledgment, have borrowed more from him perhaps than from any other source in formulating their own theories (Ellenberger, 1970). For example, Adler's influence can be seen in the theories of Karen Horney and Harry Stack Sullivan (Mosak, 1989). His influence also crosses the boundary separating the psychoanalytic approach to counseling from other schools of counseling and psychotherapy. Adler's influence on Albert Ellis and Carl Rogers, leading representatives of the other two primary schools of psychology, is discussed later in this chapter. His early contributions to humanistic psychology are noted by Ellis (1970), Maslow (1970), and May (1970). Adler's adherence to a holistic concept of humankind and the early support of his ideas by Gestalt psychologists are noted by Dreikurs (1960). The opinion that Adler was a founder of the existential psychology movement is expressed by Bottome (1939), Ansbacher (1959), and Frankl (1970), among others.

Adler's individual psychology can be viewed as practically the antithesis of Freud's classic psychoanalytic theory (see Mosak, 1989, p. 70, for a point-by-point comparison of the theories of Adler and Freud). In Adler's theory emphasis is placed on social rather than sexual urges and behavior, on conscious rather than unconscious determinants of personality and behavior, and on the ego rather than the id as the *primum mobile* of behavior. Adler is considered a founder of the specialty of ego-oriented social psychology. His espousal of a social orientation to personality and behavior caused his irrevocable break with Freud and Freud's coterie of pioneer psychoanalysts.

HISTORICAL PERSPECTIVE

Alfred Adler was born in Vienna in 1870 and died in 1937 in Aberdeen, Scotland, while on a lecture tour, two years after having moved from Austria to take up residence in the United States. As did Freud, he attended the University of Vienna where he received a medical degree in 1895, the same year Breuer and Freud published *Studies on Hysteria.* Adler specialized in psychiatry after first practicing ophthalmology and general medicine. In 1902, Adler entered a productive although brief professional relationship with Freud. They co-founded the *Journal of Psychoanalysis* as the journal of the Vienna Psychoanalytic Society and served as its co-editors. In 1910, Adler was elected president of the Vienna Psychoanalytic Society, of which he was a charter member. One year later, in 1911, Adler was required by the Vienna Society to articulate in full his theory on personality and behavior, in particular those ideas that did not correspond to Freud's. He did so and was consequently asked by Freud to resign as president of the Vienna Society and as co-editor of its journal. Adler resigned and dissociated himself from Freudian psychoanalysis (Ansbacher & Ansbacher, 1956, 1964; Jones, 1955). Soon after he formed his own school of psychoanalytic thought which he called "individual psychology."

After World War I, in which Adler served as a medical officer, he became interested in the problems of children and in 1922 established a child guidance clinic in the Vienna public school system; this clinic was successful and led to the establishment of more than 50 child guidance clinics in Europe that were modeled on it (Dinkmeyer & Dinkmeyer, 1985). In 1935 Adler fled the political upheaval in Europe and accepted a faculty position at the Long Island College of Medicine in the United States for what were to be the last 2 years of his life. Adler published an extensive volume of work during his career and lectured untiringly, being one of the first counselors to demonstrate counseling technique with an actual client before an audience. As a result of his prolific scholarship, innovative concepts, and departure from Freudian psychology, Adler's individual psychology has influenced numerous disciplines other than counseling and psychotherapy and has attached adherents from many professions, many more than has Freud's psychoanalytic theory (Munroe, 1955; Allen, 1971).

BASIC CONCEPTS

The essential concepts of individual psychology are limited in number and can be briefly described. Detailed descriptions of Adler's basic concepts of personality and behavior can be found in Adler (1969) and Ansbacher and Ansbacher (1956, 1964). Adler's theory of personality and his approach to counseling is "social, teleological, phenomenological, holistic, ideographic, and humanistic" (Mosak, 1989, p. 106). According to its basic assumptions, each individual is unique, self-consistent, responsible, creative, and in control of his or her own behavior and destiny. Description of other basic assumptions follow.

Fictionalism and Finalism

Adler modified Vaihinger's (1925) idealistic "as if" philosophy, a premise that individuals live in accordance with fictional notions they hold that cannot be validated in reality; for instance "you shall reap what you sow." These *fictions* help individuals live harmoniously and productively with one another and can be discarded or augmented with other assumptions in response to the changing circumstances of living. Adler used this philosophy as his subjective psychology response to Freud's objective psychology concept of psychic determinism. Freud held that an individual's present behavior is determined by past emotional events; Adler, on the other hand, held that an individual's behavior is determined more by future goals than by past emotional experiences, although not in a teleologic sense that implies predestination. In particular, the final goal held by an individual serves to explain the psychological events he or she experiences and the behavior he or she exhibits in striving to reach that goal, even though it might be unattainable or fictional. According to Adler, the normal person can abandon the pursuit of fictional goals when reality demands it, whereas the neurotic person cannot.

Principle of Inferiority

An early concept Adler posited to explain human behavior was that of *organ inferiority* (Adler, 1917). Adler held that everyone was born with a potentially weak organ (which can break down under stress), or develops early in life a defective organ of one type or another. This causes individuals to experience feelings of incompleteness or inferiority and to spend their lives attempting to *compensate,* or overcompensate, for their hereditary or developmental abnormality. One of the examples Adler used to illustrate this principle is familiar to most speech-language pathologists and audiologists, that of Demosthenes not only controlling his stuttering by placing pebbles in his mouth when speaking but overcompensating for stuttering by becoming a celebrated orator. Although Adler believed that an individual's behavior is driven and determined by attempts to compensate for painful feelings of inferiority, he did not believe such compensation necessarily replaced painful feelings with pleasurable ones; this was because he assumed that perfection rather than pleasure was the final life goal for most individuals (Hall & Lindzey, 1978).

### Principle of Superiority

According to Adler (1930) the primary, in fact the only, drive that motivates human behavior is the *desire for superiority*. This drive exists owing to the feelings of inferiority discussed above and the two principles are part and parcel of one another. The superiority drive is universal and is experienced by both men and women. Adler initially presented the idea that striving for superiority was *"masculine protest"*—a protest by both men and women against being associated with the weakness inherent in femininity and for the power inherent in masculinity. Adler later abandoned this concept and stated instead that men and women strive for superiority simply to overcome their feelings of inferiority which are not necessarily related to gender. To Adler, striving for superiority did not mean attempting to gain self-esteem through mastery of or power over others; that is how the superiority striving of the neurotic individual would be manifested (Hall & Lindzey, 1978). Rather, Adler held that the normal individual is chiefly in self-competition, striving for superiority over himself or herself (Bischof, 1964). In this sense, the desire for superiority described by Adler is similar to the drive for self-actualization described by other humanists.

### Social Interest

In early formulations of his theory, Adler held that individuals have a life-long desire for power and status in society as compensation for their feelings of inferiority. He later modified this position and argued instead that individuals are born with an innate *social interest* and with the desire to work harmoniously with others in the society to attain an ultimate goal of the perfect society. Adler regarded the degree to which the individual develops this social interest to be a measure of his or her mental health. Although social interest is innate, according to Adler, it requires guidance and training to be developed. If it develops normally, the individual gives higher priority to society's interests and gains than to self-interests and self-gains.

### Style of Life

*Style of life* (Adler, 1929) is perhaps the defining concept of individual psychology. It is with this principle that Adler explained both how personality develops generally and how individual or unique personalities are developed. Everyone has a style of life and no two individuals share the same one; this is the primary ideographic concept in Adler's theory. The style of life is formed by the age of five and consists of innate, inner drives (the primary one being striving for superiority) and assimilated environmental experiences which to a limited extent determine how the goal of superiority will be pursued. After age five it is difficult to change an individual's style of life as it has come to represent compensation for his or her organ inferiority. The style of life includes not only the life goals of the individual, but also all of the personal and social conditions required for the individual to feel secure while pursuing goals (Mosak, 1989). The individual arranges his or her style of life in careful detail to compensate maximally for an inferiority. For instance, a physically disabled person might have an intricately patterned style of life as an intellectual; an intellectually challenged individual might develop a highly self-disciplined style of life as an athlete; and

so forth. Style of life, which is one of Adler's later concepts, is considered the most important to his theory.

Creative Self

Hall and Lindzey (1978) state that the concept of *the creative self* is Adler's crowning
achievement. Yet it is difficult to describe. It is an active inner sense or force that serves to
create a unique, individual self that is more than hereditary abilities or environmental impressions (Adler, 1935). It is an interpretation of experience that determines an individual's
relationship to society. The creative self is the invention of a unique subjective self from the
individual's inherited traits, his or her unique desire for superiority, and his or her mechanical style of life.

Family Influences

Adler held that certain family constellation factors contribute to the personality a child develops and to his or her behavior as an adult (Adler, 1931). He observed that *birth order* was
one such factor, explaining why children from the same family can develop appreciably
different personalities. The oldest child in a family, in Adler's view, is at risk to develop
neurotic maladaptive adult behavior (e.g., dislike of people, insecurity) owing to having
been abruptly displaced as the center of parents' attention and affection on the birth of a
second child. Adler felt that proper preparation by the parents of the first born for this
event might help him or her develop a sense of protection and responsibility for the new
sibling, rather than resentment and rejection. The middle child is typically the best adjusted of the children in a family, according to Adler, although they do tend to be rebellious and envious of the older siblings, constantly attempting to out perform them. The
youngest child is the most likely to be spoiled and, if spoiled, most likely next to the oldest child to develop a maladaptive personality.

   A second factor related to early childhood and the family that Adler felt was a key determinant of personality and behavior is *early memories.* He believed that an individual's
style of life can be understood by interpreting the significance of earliest memory.

   Adler was also concerned about other influences in early childhood that can lead to
maladaptive behavior as an adult. He identified three categories of children who are at risk
to have difficulty interacting appropriately and effectively with society:

1. *Children with mental or physical disabilities.*
2. *Children who have been spoiled* by parents or caretakers.
3. *Children who have been neglected* by parents or caretakers.

Adler noted that with the help of supportive parents, children with disabilities can be successful in compensating for their disabilities and can lead productive adult lives as contributors to society. But he believed that spoiled or pampered children pose a real threat to society in that they tend not to develop social interest. Rather, pampered children tend to grow
up to be self-centered adults who are concerned only with their own interests and needs and
who expect society to attend to their interests and fulfill their needs. Whereas pampered children might become manipulators of society, Adler believed that neglected children were at
risk to become society's enemies owing to a desire for revenge for having been neglected.

COUNSELING TECHNIQUE

Mosak (1989) notes that there are four aims of Adlerian counseling: (*a*) to establish a positive client-clinician relationship; (*b*) to understand the client's lifestyle; (*c*) to interpret the
client's lifestyle to him or her; and (*d*) to reorient the client's behaviors.

Establishing a Positive Client-Clinician Relationship

The characteristics of a positive client-clinician relationship within an Adlerian counseling context are:

1. Client *faith* in the clinician and in therapy. Client faith is fostered by the clinician's demeanor, which should convey egalitarian, noncritical acceptance of the client, and a permissive nonjudgmental clinical atmosphere. This concept was a harbinger of the ideas on the clinical relationship fundamental to Rogers' person-centered therapy.
2. Client *hope* for change. Mosak (1989) notes that hope often translates into self-fulfilling prophecy, prompting clients spontaneously to move toward desired change. The clinician's responsibility, therefore, is to keep client hope high.
3. Client perception of *love*. The client should feel the genuine concern and care of the clinician (Adler, 1964). Care must be taken by the clinician, however, not to become patronizing or overcaring. One technique advocated by Adler for demonstrating caring was empathic listening—another key technique in Rogers' approach to therapy.
4. Client perception of *freedom*. The client should understand that he or she is free to choose whether to be in therapy or not and whether to be concerned with self-interests or social interests (Ansbacher & Ansbacher, 1956).
5. Therapy is an *educational process*. The primary goal of therapy is to help the client learn the "basic mistakes" in his or her style of life and change inappropriate, nonproductive social values (Dreikurs, 1957). This is accomplished by helping the client (*a*) reduce feelings of inferiority, (*b*) maintain motivation for positive change, (*c*) realize his or her equality to other individuals in society, and (*d*) develop social interest and contribution (Dreikurs, 1971).
6. Therapy must be a *relationship of cooperation* between client and clinician. Mosak (1989) notes that this relationship is achieved through an alignment of goals as perceived by the client and clinician. One caution here is that clinicians should be aware of "scripts," an Adlerian term that basically means clients have the tendency to manipulate clinicians into responding to them in the way they have come to expect—clinician responses that indicate client goals are not valued or respected. The clinician should be alert to this client tendency and respond in ways to maintain competence and caring in the client's eyes.

Understanding the Client's Lifestyle

In the analysis or assessment aspect of counseling, Adlerians attempt to understand the client's style of life and to determine how the style of life is affecting the client's present behavior as regards his or her life-goals. Assessment of the client's lifestyle begins with the first session and is designed to ascertain the *basic mistakes* in the client's lifestyle that are interfering with his or her progress toward goals. Mosak (1989) calls the lifestyle a personal mythology because, as with mythology in general, it is comprised of both truths and partial truths; the partial truths are an individual's basic mistakes because partial truths are confused with truth and, although they are irrational ideas, can affect behavior to the extent that truth can. Adlerians identify five types of basic mistakes:

1. *Overgeneralizations:* "Life is always unfair." "People are only interested in themselves."
2. *Unrealistic goals of security:* "You have to keep up your guard constantly." "I have to be everything to everybody."
3. *Misperceptions of life and life's demands:* "Life is so unfair." "Life expects too much of me."
4. *Minimization or denial of one's worth.* "No one really cares about me." "I'm useless." "I'm not very bright."

5. *Faulty values.* "I must be the best, whatever it takes." "Let everyone else look out for themselves; achieving my goals is all that matters to me."

In addition to identification of the client's basic mistakes, assessment is used to determine both the personal assets the client already recognizes and assets the clinician perceives but which the client may be unaware of possessing. The basic mistakes and assets, along with family constellation information and a summary of early recollections, are then compiled into a summary presented to the client.

Interpreting the Client's Lifestyle

After assessment has been completed, the client's lifestyle is interpreted to him or her so that the client can develop the self-insight that Adlerians feel is necessary to effecting and maintaining long-term change. Insight is the client's identification of cognitive, affective, and behavioral roadblocks to personal growth and attainment of goals. Adlerians define insight as an understanding that translates into positive, purposeful action. Insight is an understanding that clients gain of the faulty apperceptions that underlie their behavior and of the role those apperceptions and behavior play in movement toward their life goals. Adlerians do not distinguish between intellectual and emotional insight but instead regard insight in a holistic sense. Adler (1964) notes that clients who gain intellectual insight only often are not serious about changing their behavior to achieve life goals but merely want to make a game of therapy by playing "yes-but"—"Yes, I want to change, but . . . ".

Various techniques used by Adlerian clinicians to help clients' gain insight (Alexander & French, 1946; Corsini, 1953; Dinkmeyer & Dinkmeyer, 1985; Mosak, 1989) are used in other approaches to counseling as well. These techniques include *role playing; giving advise,* being careful not to create client dependency on the clinician; *interpretation,* in which purpose, movement, and use are emphasized so that the client recognizes how to cope with life; *encouragement,* exercising caution not to become moralizing; *abreaction;* and *catharsis.* In Adlerian counseling the clinician avoids trying to out-reason the client through rational argument, which qualifies Adlerian counseling as one of the first, and pre-Rogerian, nondirective approaches to counseling.

Reorientation of the Client's Behaviors

This is the action phase of counseling, wherein the client makes decisive movement toward correcting the basic mistakes that have been inhibiting growth. The clinician serves here as a model for appropriate social attitudes and behaviors by displaying humor, fallibility, genuineness, and caring (Mosak, 1967). Description of some of the techniques used by Adlerians in the reorientation phase follows.

1. *Task setting.* Adlerians believe in structured counseling wherein tasks designed to move the client gradually and progressively toward targeted goals are set both by the clinician and by the client. Homework assignments are used by clients to practice various possible types of new behavior. *Negative practice* is one type of task used by Adlerians, in which the client is instructed to display intentionally and exaggeratedly the behavior he or she is struggling to change; negative practice has long been used in some clinical approaches to treatment of speech disfluency and voice disorders.
2. *Acting as-if.* This procedure simply involves requesting the client to act how he or she would like to be (e.g., more out-going, more confident, more assertive). Typically, a time period is specified for the acting out to occur, which might be increased if the initial acting is a positive experience. It is hoped that by acting as he or she would like to

be and seeing that he or she is capable of behaving in such a way, the client will spontaneously assimilate those behaviors into the lifestyle.

3. *Creating images.* To foster a mind-set of the goals he or she is trying to attain, the client often is described in a phrase or term used as a reminder of those goals. For example, if a client has difficulty comfortably interacting with others in social situations because he or she feels intellectually inferior, the image "professor" might be used to remind him or her that not everyone is a scholar or an intellectual. The client might then humorously think of himself or herself as the "professor" when interacting with others to relieve the stress experienced due to perceived intellectual competition in interpersonal relationships.

4. *Catching oneself.* This technique consists of helping the client develop an ability to catch himself or herself whenever performing an old, undesired behavior and modify to the new behavior. In time the client may be able to catch an old behavior before it occurs by being able to predict situations that might induce it. For this technique to be successful, the client must be able to laugh at "being caught," rather than experiencing guilt or disappointment when relapses to old undesired behavior occur.

5. *The pushbutton technique.* To demonstrate to the client that he or she has control of emotional states, the client is requested to imagine both pleasant and unpleasant experiences and the emotions attendant to both. The client is then informed that he or she has the power to turn off the unpleasant emotions and turn on pleasant ones simply by "pushing a button;" in other words, by volitionally deciding what will or will not be thought and felt. This helps the client comprehend that he or she governs what emotions are experienced rather than the emotions being in control of experiencing.

6. *The aha experience.* When the client has progressed to the point in therapy where increased self-awareness and self-confidence have served to increase social involvement and progress toward goals, the client is helped to discover, on his or her own, solutions to problems that are preventing full involvement in the social process. When these discoveries occur, the client experiences an "aha" response, a reaction that in effect says "I can do this," "Now I understand," "I just thought of an even better way." As the client continues to have "aha" experiences, his or her determination increases to meet life's challenges independently.

## OUTCOMES OF COUNSELING

The desired outcomes of counseling within the framework of individual psychology have been indicated, in part, in the discussion of the reorientation phase of the counseling process. General goals of Adlerian counseling can be stated simply—clients develop faith in themselves, learn to trust others, and are able to love (Mosak, 1989). The ideal goal of Adlerian counseling is to help clients activate their self-actualizing drive to maximize their potential for personal growth and to develop social interest that ultimately benefits society in general.

## RELEVANCE TO SPEECH-LANGUAGE PATHOLOGY AND AUDIOLOGY

There is a considerable amount of relevance to speech-language pathology and audiology in all dimensions of Adler's individual psychology. A communicative disorder can change the fictions by which an individual lives and might interfere more with achieving goals than does the speech, language, or hearing disorder. Fictions can also either enhance or adversely affect the course of therapy; it would be well for speech-language pathologists and audiologists to explore a client's individually unique fictions, or at least to recognize them for what they are when the client expresses them, and to understand their potential influence on the outcome of therapy.

Adler's principles of inferiority and superiority seem of particular potential relevance to persons with communicative disorders. A congenital or acquired communicative disorder might represent an organ inferiority for which the child or adult attempts to compensate or overcompensate, if one believes Adler's assumptions to be accurate. This can augur well for therapy if the client is counseled to include modification of speech, language, or hearing as compensation. Clinicians should take care not to encourage their clients to overcompensate for a communicative disorder by setting unrealistic, unattainable goals.

The central emphasis in individual psychology on social interest as the primary motivation in human behavior is of significance in understanding the personal impact of a speech, language, or hearing problem on the communicatively disordered individual. Adlerians view human problems as primarily social problems; communicative disorders are in effect potential social problems, problems that can adversely affect interpersonal behavior. This suggests that communicative disorders can have dramatic influence on the client's style of life; in turn, the client's style of life can serve either to facilitate or inhibit effective socialization and communication.

Parents and caretakers of children with communicative disorders play major roles in therapy for those disorders. Adler's ideas about family constellation influences on child and adult behavior is germane to parent counseling by speech-language pathologists and audiologists. Clinicians should be mindful that personality develops during the preschool years, concurrent with (and influenced by, according to ego psychologists) emerging speech and language skills. Parents should be counseled on the critical roles that time, experience, language, environment, and the creative self-play in their child's developing communicative behavior, and in their child's general social behavior which, governed by personality, is the functional dimension of communication. To help their communicatively disordered child develop normal social interest, parents should be counseled not to show approbation of their child's maladaptive behaviors simply because he or she has a communication disorder; nor should they be excessively strict and critical of their child's communicative and general behaviors. They should respond to their communicatively disordered child in ways that are neither pampering nor that imply rejection or neglect. Parents' responses to their child with a communicative disorder should be in line with their responses to their other children. By responding in appropriate ways parents help ensure that their child develops normal personality, adaptive behaviors, and social interest, which also improves the prognosis for treatment of the child's speech, language, or hearing disorder.

The clinical techniques used by Adlerians are appropriate to counseling in speech-language pathology and audiology if they are modified to address communicative disorders and the interpersonal and role problems directly related to them. The characteristics of the ideal client-clinician relationship described by Adlerians are universally appropriate to counseling relationships. Alderian technique has appeared throughout the literature on counseling, applied to numerous other approaches (e.g., the pushbutton technique is used in rational emotive behavior therapy). Techniques used in Adlerian counseling also appear in the literature on speech-language pathology; for instance, humor as therapy technique is basic to Adlerian counseling and is described by Manning (1996) as a technique also useful in treatment of fluency disorders.

## COGNITIVE-BEHAVIORAL APPROACHES

Cognitive-behavior approaches to counseling are grounded in theories that stress the influence of cognition and behavior in personality development, maladaptive behavior, and therapy. Rational emotive behavior therapy (Ellis, 1962) is discussed in this section to represent the cognitive-behavioral approaches; it is considered by some authorities to be the seminal approach in this category of theories (Corey, 1986). Other cognitive-behavioral approaches also have gained prominence in the practice of counseling and psychotherapy. Four approaches in particular—transactional analysis, behavior therapy, reality therapy, and cognitive therapy—are widely used and are backed by an extensive literature. Brief descriptions of each of these approaches follow.

## Cognitive-Behavioral Approaches Other Than Ellis'

TRANSACTIONAL ANALYSIS

*Transactional analysis* (TA) was developed by Eric Berne (1910–1970). Berne (1961, 1964) proposed that individuals have the innate ability to control their lives and destinies but that few have adequate self-awareness to do so. He emphasized the role of preschool experiences on personality development, suggesting that parental messages, movies, fantasies, dreams, books, and so forth lead to a child developing a *life script* to which he or she adheres throughout life, unless it is altered by life-changing events or in therapy (Berne, 1972).

Basic concepts in TA include three types of *ego states:*

1. The *child ego state,* which corresponds loosely to Freud's id, is ruled by emotions and has two dimensions—the *free child,* who seeks pleasure and is uninhibited, and the *adopted child,* who is conforming although rebellious.
2. The *adult ego state,* which is not ruled by emotions and serves as the mediator between the other two ego states—Berne's adult ego state corresponds to Freud's ego.
3. The *parent ego state,* which represents the parents' beliefs and morals and has two dimensions as does the child ego state—the *critical parent* is judgmental and fault-finding, the *nurturing parent* is reinforcing and fosters independence and growth.

Berne (1961, 1964, 1966) identified other concepts basic to TA, including: (*a*) *analysis of the transactions between individuals—crossed transactions* are unexpected or inappropriate communications received from another's ego state, *complementary transactions* are expected and appropriately received communications, and *ulterior transactions* are confusing communications, possibly due to an overt message from one individual's ego state and a covert message from another individual's ego state being transmitted simultaneously; (*b*) *games,* which are ulterior, unconscious transactions among individuals that produce negative feelings but also payoffs for some of the participants; (*c*) *life positions,* which relate to life scripts and perception of self—"I'm OK, you're OK" (healthy ego state), "I'm OK, you're not OK" (an inaccurate perception of superiority or possible paranoia), "I'm not OK, you're OK" (low self-esteem), and "I'm not OK, you're not OK" (despair and possible suicidal tendencies); and (*d*) *strokes,* which are considered in TA to be the human need that promotes social interaction—reinforcements that can be positive or negative, conditional or unconditional; healthy emotional growth is promoted through the receipt of positive, unconditional strokes.

Counseling techniques used in TA include *structural analysis,* which is used to help clients recognize their three ego states and learn to make maximally effective use of all three; *transactional analysis,* which is used to help clients learn to communicate more effectively by using complementary transactions; *script analysis,* which helps clients understand their life scripts and use them more effectively; and *game analysis,* which demonstrates to clients the games they play and how those games interfere with personal growth and interpersonal relationships.

Transactional analysis basically is a cognitive approach to counseling, predicated on the role interpersonal communication plays in personality development and in normal and maladjusted behavior. One of its strengths is that it is described in lay language rather than in esoteric psychological terminology which has made it a popular self-help approach to emotional health.

## BEHAVIOR THERAPY

Behavior therapy is grounded in classic learning theories, namely classical conditioning (Pavlov, 1906) and operant conditioning (Skinner 1938, 1953), and more recently in social learning theory (Bandura 1974, 1986; Beck, 1976; Meichenbaum, 1977). In the classic and operant theories of learning, individuals are viewed as organisms reacting in response to environmental conditioning, without purpose or direction other than what their environment at any moment dictates. The newer theories of social learning propose that behavior can be self-directed and, to an extent, individuals can control their destinies, although personality and behavior are still subject to the forces of environmental conditioning.

Counseling based on behavior theory is designed to modify maladaptive behavior according to scientific method—specific behaviors to be eliminated are identified and behavior modification strategies are used to help clients establish and reinforce new patterns of behavior. Therapy goals are focused on observable, measurable behavior and objective techniques are used to modify maladaptive behavior systematically into new, productive patterns of behavior that support personal growth. Techniques used in behavior therapy include *systematic desensitization* (Wolpe, 1958), *cognitive behavior modification* (Meichenbaum, 1977), *assertiveness training, token economy* (Ayllon & Azrin, 1968), and *self-control* (Kaufer, 1975).

## REALITY THERAPY

*Reality therapy* was developed by William Glasser (b. 1925) and formally presented in 1965 with the publication of *Reality Therapy: A New Approach to Psychiatry.* The major tenet underlying reality therapy is *control theory,* which is in direct opposition to the learning theory concept that behavior is a conditioned response to the environment. According to Glasser (1986), the environment does not stimulate behavior in individuals; control comes from within individuals rather than from without. In the control theory framework, all behavior is seen as "our best attempt to control ourselves to satisfy our needs" (Glasser, 1986, p. 17). When individuals perceive that they do not have adequate control of their lives to fulfill their basic psychological and physiologic needs, their emotional well-being suffers; when they perceive they are in control of their lives, they are content and happy.

Glasser (1961, 1984) takes opposition to psychiatry as well with his control theory. He maintains that individuals can control their mental health by behaving in a manner that suggests control; for example, by saying "I'm depressing" rather than "I'm depressed." This idea further leads Glasser to maintain that there is no such thing as a mental disorder and, therefore, it can only be harmful to an individual to be labeled as mentally disordered.

Other concepts (Glasser 1965, 1976, 1984) in reality therapy include: (*a*) *success and failure identities*—individuals with a success identity can meet their basic needs without attempting to control others, whereas individuals with a failure identity interfere with the rights of others or behave in socially inappropriate or irresponsible ways when attempting to fulfill their needs; (*b*) *responsibility,* which is a primary goal of reality therapy used to encourage individuals to evaluate their behavior and take responsible control of it; and (*c*) *positive addiction,* which is the idea that negative addictions (e.g., smoking) can be replaced with positive addictions (e.g., jogging).

Reality therapy is a short-term approach to counseling and is present-oriented. It is an educational process built on a positive client-clinician relationship. The goal of reality therapy is to help clients recognize how they are not in control of their lives and how they can use control theory to establish or regain control in order to satisfy their basic needs in responsible ways. Glasser (1980) identified eight interrelated steps of reality therapy used in helping clients achieve their goals: establish a positive counseling relationship; focus on the client's present behavior; encourage clients to examine their behavior; develop a plan of positive action; have the client commit to the plan; do not accept client excuses; do not punish the client; and do not give up. Reality therapy and control theory are popular in a variety of clinical settings, particularly in schools (Glasser 1969, 1986, 1990).

Cognitive Therapy

Aaron Beck, an authority on depression and anxiety, developed cognitive therapy in the mid-1950s. According to Beck (1976), individuals are able to determine their behavior and destiny through cognition; if cognition is distorted then behavior will be maladaptive: "Cognitive therapy is based on a theory of personality which maintains that how one thinks largely determines how one feels and behaves" (Beck & Weishaar, 1989).

Cognitive therapy was developed originally to treat depression and anxiety (e.g., Beck & Emery, 1985; Beck, Rush, Shaw & Emery, 1979) but is now used to treat a wide range of personality and behavioral disorders. It is based on the premise that emotional distress, such as depression and anxiety, and maladaptive behavior result from individuals having distorted images of themselves and their environment and misinterpreting their experiences. Individuals develop susceptibility or *cognitive vulnerability* to misinterpret experiences because of *schemata,* which are beliefs and attitudes about the self and the environment that develop during the preschool years and are reinforced throughout life (Beck & Weishaar, 1989).

Dysfunctional schemata such as "I am basically not worth anything to anyone" can lead to individuals developing *cognitive distortions,* which are systematic distortions in processing information or interpreting experience. Types of cognitive distortions are (Beck & Weishaar, 1989):

1. *Arbitrary inference:* drawing conclusions without verification of information or in contradiction of facts.
2. *Selective abstraction:* attending to selected information in external situations and internal emotions and cognition while ignoring other information.
3. *Overgeneralization:* establishing a general rule based on limited events and applying that rule both to all related events and to unrelated events.
4. *Magnification* and *minimization:* assigning an inappropriate degree of significance to experiences.
5. *Personalization:* attributing responsibility for the occurrence of events to oneself when there is no evidence to support such attribution.
6. *Dichotomous thinking:* viewing experiences in dichotomous terms such as pleasurable or painful, good or bad, depressing or uplifting.

In cognitive therapy clients are helped to recognize their dysfunctional schemata and their patterns of cognitive distortion and to develop new patterns of thinking that serve to reduce psychological distress. Counseling techniques used in cognitive therapy include (Beck, 1976; Beck & Weishaar, 1989): (*a*) *reattribution,* which involves helping clients challenge unsupported personalization of causality by thinking of other possible causes of events than themselves; (*b*) *redefining,* which involves helping clients learn to refer to their problems in terms of action—of what can be done about them, rather than merely in terms of their existence; (c) *decatastrophizing*, which concerns the use by clients of decision-making and problem-solving skills to prepare for experiences about which they are anxious; and (d) *decentering*, which involves helping clients relieve the anxiety of feeling that they are the center of attention by observing that they are not the focus of others' reactions to most events.

## Rational Emotive Behavior Therapy

Rational emotive behavior therapy (REBT); until recently called rational-emotive therapy (Ellis, 1993, 1994), was developed by Albert Ellis in the 1950s owing to his opinion that psychoanalytic approaches to counseling were inefficient and tended at times to do more harm than good for the client (Ellis, 1979b). REBT introduced the use of logic and reasoning into counseling and is perhaps the most extreme approach in that regard (Patterson, 1966). REBT emphasizes thought, analysis, decision-making, and action. It is, as Corey (1986) notes, "highly didactic, very directive, and concerned as much with thinking as with feeling" (p. 209). Ellis drew from both humanistic and behavioral schools of counseling in formulating REBT and believes that to understand an individual's nonproductive, irrational behavior one must "understand how people perceive, think, emote, and act" (Ellis, 1989, p. 198).

Ellis credits Alfred Adler with developing the basic premise on which REBT is based—that an individual's cognitive fictions or beliefs influence emotions and style of life. Adler, according to Ellis (1989), "was the modern psychiatrist who was the main precursor to RET" (p. 202), although the idea that human emotions are ideogenic in origin had been expressed earlier by others including Stoic, Taoist, and Buddhist philosophers; Shakespeare; and even Freud. Mosak (1989) notes the many points of similarity between the theories of Adler and Ellis: Adler's basic mistakes are the same concept as Ellis' irrational beliefs. Both theorists assume that emotions are ideogenic and to change one's emotions, one must change his or her thinking. They view individuals as the creators, not victims, of their emotions. In therapy, they view the role of unconscious motivation similarly: confront the basic mistakes or irrational beliefs of clients, use counterpropaganda strategies, demand action of the clients, and place responsibility for change and growth with the client. Ellis (1989) suggests that, although there is significant overlap of REBT with individual psychology, REBT differs from Adlerian emphasis on early childhood memories, use of dream interpretation, and emphasis on social interest as the primary goal in therapy. Furthermore, according to Ellis (1984), REBT is much more direct in attacking the irrational beliefs of clients than is individual psychology and, in this regard, it corresponds more with general semantics theory than with individual psychology.

Ellis (1989) points out that REBT also is similar in many respects to Jung's analytic psychology. Commonalities between the two counseling approaches include a holistic view of the client, primary therapy goals of maximizing the client's potential for continuing personal growth in addition to symptom relief, and a regard for the individuality of each client. REBT departs, however, from the use in Jungian therapy of psychoanalytic technique which, according to Ellis (1989), "the REBT practitioner deems a waste of time" (p. 201).

HISTORICAL PERSPECTIVE

Albert Ellis (b. 1913) received his master's degree in 1943 and his doctorate in 1947 in clinical psychology from Columbia University. Early in his career he was interested in classic psychoanalysis, studied this approach to psychotherapy, and underwent analysis for three years. Ellis practiced psychoanalysis from 1947 to 1953, specializing in marriage and family counseling and sex therapy. Although most of Ellis' early career was spent in private practice he also held clinical positions in a state hospital and a state diagnostic center, an administrative position with the New Jersey Department of Institutions and Agencies, and teaching positions at Rutgers University and New York University.

By 1955, Ellis "had discovered the gross ineffectuality of psychoanalysis" (Ellis, 1977, p. 4). At that point he began to use what he viewed as more efficient counseling techniques, such as behavioral techniques, logic, bibliotherapy, information, confrontation, advice, and homework. Ellis founded the Institute for Rational-Emotive Therapy in 1959 in New York City and became executive director of the institute in 1960; the institute conducts nonprofit educational and scientific activities in REBT. In 1962 Ellis published the work that was the basis for REBT, *Reason and Emotion in Psychotherapy.*

To say that Ellis' scholarly output has been prolific throughout his career is an understatement; it has been prodigious. He has consistently published one or two books annually and 20 articles (Nystul, 1993). In addition to his scholarship, Ellis has seen as many as 80 clients a week for counseling and presented an average of 200 papers and workshops per year (Corey, 1986). Ellis remains professionally active, despite the facts that he is into his 80s and has had diabetes since his early 40s. He is appropriately identified as the founder of cognitive-behavioral counseling.

## BASIC CONCEPTS

The basic premise underlying REBT is that all people have the potential to behave rationally or irrationally. *Rational behavior* leads to happiness, self-enhancing behavior, and a productive style of life. *Irrational behavior* blocks happiness and leads to self-defeating behavior and a nonproductive style of life (Ellis, 1979c; Ellis & Harper, 1975). Descriptions of other concepts associated with the basic premise of REBT follow.

### Assumptions

1. Irrational thinking and behavior begin early in life and are reinforced by parents and others in the child's environment. Individuals possess an innate or biologic capacity at birth to be both irrational and rational.
2. According to Ellis (1989) individuals "tend to perceive, think, emote, and behave simultaneously" (p.198). These are interrelated processes and cannot easily be considered separately; thinking usually accompanies emoting and in course it becomes the emoting and the emoting becomes the thinking. Therefore, to understand a client's self-defeating behavior the clinician would need to understand how the client perceives, thinks, emotes, and behaves.
3. Emotional disturbance or self-defeating behavior, is caused by illogical, irrational, magical thinking.
4. Illogical, irrational thinking accompanies emotional disturbance and takes the form of *self-talk.* What individuals tell themselves in internalized phrases and sentences tends to become their emotions.
5. Self-talk consisting of irrational perceptions and attitudes about external reality serves to reinforce and maintain self-defeating behavior.
6. The basic goal of REBT counseling is to help the client replace illogical, irrational self-talk that is the source of emotional disturbance with logical, rational self-talk that does not promote self-defeating behavior or negative emotion.
7. REBT goals are achieved through highly cognitive, directive, and action- and discipline-oriented counseling. Because of this orientation, counseling goals in REBT are usually achieved with greater time efficiency and with more effectiveness than they are in therapies that are not thusly oriented.

8. It is not assumed in REBT that a warm open congruent client-clinician relationship is necessary or sufficient for positive change to occur in client behavior. This would suggest that Ellis does not completely embrace the existential concept of individuals having the innate tendency to move toward self-actualization given the right conditions, such as unconditional positive regard (Rogers, 1961; Standal, 1954). REBT, however, is in agreement with the person-centered therapy opinion that unconditional positive regard (i.e., full acceptance or tolerance in REBT) by the clinician for the client is essential in counseling; Ellis (1989) suggests that this might be the only point of agreement between REBT and person-centered therapy.

9. The client-clinician relationship in REBT is of a teacher-student nature, wherein the clinician teaches the client to think rationally by giving advice, information, interpretations, and homework assignments. The client is viewed as a student who must be committed to learning and to consistent practice of and vigilance with new ways of thinking and behaving.

10. The cause of emotional disturbance and self-defeating behavior is *blaming*. The potential for self-blaming occurs when individuals mistakenly define preferences—wishes to be accepted and loved, to succeed, and to achieve success—as needs.

## Irrational Beliefs

Ellis believes that the irrational beliefs individuals form early in life based on external experiences are what cause them to be upset, rather than external experiences controlling what they think and feel. These irrational beliefs are unable to be empirically validated and are individualized, although the emotional effect they have on individuals is universal. Individuals hold "thousands of specific irrational ideas and philosophies (not to mention superstitions and religiosities) which they creatively invent, dogmatically carry on, and stupidly upset themselves about" (Ellis, 1977, p. 4).

In REBT, irrational beliefs must be identified in order that they might be demonstrated to the client and replaced with logical thinking. One of the chief ways in which these beliefs are recognized is in verbalizations by the client of *should, must,* or *ought* (mustabatory) statements (Ellis, 1989). Rational ideas tend to be nonabsolutist; irrational ideas tend to be absolutist. Irrational beliefs are often expressed in "awful" statements or ideas that take the form of internalized *self-talk.* For example, a client might say to himself or herself, "I should do well in this job interview, if I don't, I'm not up to standards"; "I ought to be able to speak better, I just can't for some reason"; "I must wear my hearing aids at all times, even though I don't always want to, because if I don't I'm just no good."

According to Ellis (1989), individuals *musturbate* (absolutistically demand), because in childhood they learn and invent taboos, superstitions, and irrationalities which they use to *self-rate* their own worthlessness. Individuals reindoctrinate themselves throughout life with these irrational ideas through self-talk and thus continue to exhibit self-defeating behavior and reject logic.

As mentioned, specific irrational beliefs vary from individual to individual. Ellis (1962) posits, however, that there are eleven major ubiquitous, irrational beliefs producing widespread neurosis in Western civilization that can be identified. These beliefs are:

1. *It is essential for an individual to be loved or approved by every significant person in his or her community.* This is irrational because to be loved by everyone is an unattainable goal; the attempt to attain it leads to behavior that is not self-directing.

2. *To be worthwhile, an individual must be entirely competent, adequate, and achieving in all endeavors.* This belief leads to fear of failure and feelings of inferiority. The irrational individual sees all experiences as competitive rather than pleasurable.

3. *Certain people are bad, wicked, or villainous and should be blamed and punished for their behaviors.* Mistakes that people make are due to stupidity, ignorance, or emotional disorder rather than to inherent badness. Rational individuals recognize that everyone makes mistakes and that individuals do not become worthless by virtue of having made a mistake.

4. *It is a terrible catastrophe when circumstances are not as one wishes them to be.* It is one of life's realities that circumstances are not always as one would like them to be. The rational individual does not perceive this as a tragedy and instead tries to change the situation; if it cannot be changed, he or she accepts it.

5. *Individuals have no control over unhappiness, which is caused by circumstances external to them.* It is perceptions of and internalized verbalizations about events that are harmful to individuals (other than in the case of actual physical attack or deprivation) rather than the events themselves.

6. *Individuals should constantly be concerned about potentially dangerous or harmful things and dwell on them.* This is irrational because worrying about circumstances does not change them; in fact, worrying might lead to their occurrence and make them worse when they do happen. The logical individual assesses circumstances and takes decisive action to minimize danger or threat implicit in them.

7. *Difficulties and self-responsibilities are best run away from than faced.* The rational individual recognizes that avoidance of difficult situations does not change or eliminate them and that they ultimately must be faced.

8. *Individuals need others on whom to depend and someone stronger than themselves to rely on.* Dependency leads to insecurity and failure in actualizing the self. An individual who is dependent on others tends to become regulated by them rather than being self-directed.

9. *Past experiences cannot be changed and determine an individual's present behavior.* Rational individuals accept that past experiences may influence the present but recognize that present behavior is within their control. Their present behavior can be changed by questioning past beliefs and modifying those faulty beliefs to more logical thinking.

10. *Individuals should be concerned about and upset over other people's problems.* Rational individuals understand that they have no responsibility for others' problems and might exacerbate the problems or prove obstructive to their resolution by being upset about them.

11. *It is catastrophic if the correct and precise answer to every problem, which is always there, is not found.* There is no specific answer to every problem and searching for one might only produce frustration and anxiety.

## The ABC Principle

Ellis (1973) maintains that people in general are highly suggestible and that their suggestibility is greatest in childhood. Children prefer to receive love and approval from their parents and others in their environment and this preference soon becomes a need. Ellis holds that emotional disturbance is most typically due to individuals caring too much about others' opinions of them. Emotionally stable persons are those who establish a proper balance between their feelings and their concern about what others think of them. If parents help facilitate this balance through their interactions with their child, the child might develop a personality that is primarily composed of a rational belief system; if parents do not encourage this behavior then their child might develop a personality dominated by an irrational belief system. Ellis contends that most personalities are composed of both rational and irrational belief systems.

The ABC principle is used by Ellis (1977) to explain the process by which individuals develop their rational and irrational belief systems. The *A* in the acronym is an *activating* event that leads to an unpleasant *consequence, C.* Individuals can react to *C* in either of two ways of thinking or according to either of two *belief* systems, *B*—rational or irrational. A rational reaction would be for the individual to think "This wasn't a good experience. I didn't like it. I wish that it had not happened, and I'm angry that it did." An irrational response might be "I hated this experience. It was terrible and awful. It shouldn't have happened and I'm worthless because I didn't prevent it. I must not let it happen again and you ought not ever do it to me again. You're terrible for having done so." Ellis (1973) contends that such beliefs are irrational because they cannot be validated; they lead to unnecessary negative emotions, such as depression and anxiety, and obstruct the individual from appropriately resolving the original event, *A.* Irrational beliefs cannot be validated because:

1. The experiences with which they are associated can be withstood although they might not be pleasant.
2. The experiences, although unpleasant and unrewarding, are not awful—there is no real meaning for the term or concept.
3. Thinking that the experiences should not have happened is magical thinking in that it suggests that what individuals wish not to be should in fact not be.
4. The idea that one is worthless if he or she cannot prevent events occurring is in essence playing God by believing that it is possible and a personal responsibility to control the universe.

COUNSELING TECHNIQUE

The primary goal of REBT is to help the client shift from operating primarily on an irrational belief system to operating on the basis of their rational belief system. To achieve this, REBT counselors confront and attempt to change the client's whole irrational belief system, "the central self-defeating cognitions" (Ellis, 1989, p. 214), and help him or her develop a more realistic and tolerant pattern of thinking. If change does not occur in the central belief system, but occurs in the presenting symptoms only, Ellis maintains that in time the client will reindoctrinate himself or herself with self-defeating behavior through negative self-talk. The optional outcome of REBT is a change in the client's basic philosophies, not just change in certain behaviors.

To help the client achieve this change, the REBT counselor is direct, didactic, authoritarian, and confrontational. The REBT counselor uses an extensive armamentarium of techniques to teach clients that blaming is central to emotional disturbance and to help them learn how to dispute illogical thinking. These techniques include bibliotherapy, behavior modification strategies, homework assignments, audiovisual training aids, assertion training, role playing activities, humor, desensitization, suggestion, and support (Ellis, 1979a).

Unlike Rogers, who places critical emphasis on the client-clinician relationship in his person-centered approach to counseling, Ellis (1989) does not believe that a warm relationship between the client and clinician is a necessary condition for effective counseling. He does believe, however, as does Rogers, that the clinician must have unconditional, full acceptance of the client. Ellis (1989) notes that person-centered counselors and REBT counselors are virtually at opposite ends of the counseling continuum in some regards. Specifically, REBT counselors tend to be more challenging, persuasive, and didactic than person-centered counselors.

REBT addresses the client's cognitions, emotions, and behaviors. In the *cognitive dimension* of counseling clients are taught to identify their mustabatory behavior—shoulds, oughts, and musts—and to differentiate rational ideas from irrational ones. The clinician acts as a counterpropaganda agent who contradicts the client's illogical self-talk and encourages, persuades, and directs the client to think in patterns that serve as counterpropaganda against irrational behavior. Brief descriptions of a few specific counseling techniques employed in the cognitive phase of REBT follow.

1. *Bibliotherapy.* Use is made of instructional aids such as books, brochures, and audio and video tapes, to help clients learn about the aims and process of REBT and how to use their cognitive potential more effectively.
2. *Disputation of irrational beliefs.* This is probably the most common cognitive technique used in REBT. The clinician systematically refutes the client's irrational ideas, in particular absolutistic musts, to cajole the client into a more logical way of thinking. The clinician might ask such questions as "Why is it awful and terrible to have a child with a cleft palate?" "Why do you conclude that you are not a worthy parent simply because your child has a cleft palate?"
3. *Homework.* Assignments are given to REBT clients that afford them practice with positive, logical thinking in real-life, everyday situations outside the clinic setting. Negative self-talk is replaced with positive statements to produce a gradual change in the client's thoughts, emotions, and behaviors by creating positive self-fulfilling prophecies rather than negative ones. For instance, a stutterer might replace "I know I will be dysfluent and make a bad impression because of it" with "I will try to speak the best I can. I'm a good person regardless of how fluent I am. Not everyone understands stuttering, but that's their problem and not mine."
4. *Changing the client's language.* Language is considered in REBT to be the primary determinant of an individual's thinking and behavior. In the circular philosophy of REBT, language shapes thinking and behavior, and behavior and thinking shape language. Clients are taught to replace their shoulds, oughts, and musts with conveniences, preferences, and desirables. For instance, rather than saying "My voice must improve by the time the ceremony takes place this weekend," the client might be instructed to say in nonabsolutistic terms "It would be convenient if my voice improves by this weekend."
5. *Cognitive restructuring.* This is an extension of the ABC principle to the *ABCDE* technique (Ellis, 1989, 1991). It involves all of the techniques discussed above used in the attempt to have clients learn to *dispute, D,* their self-defeating thinking and bring about a more positive behavioral *effect, E.*

The second dimension of REBT is *emotive-evocative counseling.* In this phase, clients are taught to have unconditional acceptance of themselves regardless of their perceived shortcomings or disabilities. The basic value systems of clients are changed so that they are better able to distinguish between what is true and what is false (Ellis, 1973). Although catharsis is not encouraged (Ellis, 1984), other emotive-evocative techniques, such as humor and unconditional acceptance, are used, as well as the following techniques.

1. *Modeling.* This is one of the chief techniques used in the emotive-evocative phase of RET counseling. Clinicians demonstrate that they do not need the client's approval of their actions; that they are not controlled by shoulds, oughts, and musts; and that they do not mind putting themselves at risk in confrontation with the client.
2. *Shame-attacking exercises.* It is a general human tendency to believe that other people are always interested in and judgmental of one's behavior. These exercises involve assigning activities for clients to do outside of therapy that they would like to do but have refrained from in the past for fear of what others might think of them if they do not perform the activities well. The object of the exercises is to demonstrate to clients that others are not as interested in them as they might have believed and that their behavior should not be determined by their concern about the possible reactions of others.

3. *Imagery.* This technique is used to help a client change irrational ideas and self-defeating behavior by vividly imagining specific situations wherein those ideas and behaviors are experienced. The client then concentrates on using positive self-talk in these imagined situations to gradually change unpleasant, nonproductive feelings and behaviors to more pleasant and productive ones.

4. *Role playing.* Role playing affords the client the opportunity to challenge irrational beliefs by acting out feared situations with which the irrational beliefs are associated. For instance, a man with a newly acquired hearing aid might avoid going on job interviews because he fears that the interviewer will perceive him as unattractive or incompetent due to the aid and his hearing loss. By role playing interview situations, the client can work through the irrational idea that the hearing aid and hearing loss make him unattractive and incompetent by recognizing the emotions associated with those beliefs. The client's avoidance behaviors are ultimately modified and he develops more logical beliefs about his abilities, his worth, and his hearing loss.

*Behavioral techniques* are used in the third dimension of rational-emotive therapy to help clients adopt more appropriate patterns of thinking and behaving after they have identified their irrational beliefs in cognitive counseling and modified their belief system in emotive-evocative counseling. This is the direct action phase of therapy and numerous behavioral strategies are employed to teach clients new ways of thinking and behaving (Ellis, 1973). These strategies include operant conditioning, homework assignments, role-playing, instrumental conditioning, systematic desensitization, modeling, assertion training, biofeedback, and relaxation.

## Outcomes of Counseling

As mentioned, the primary goal of REBT is to help clients replace irrational ideas with rational ones and to minimize self-defeating behavior. As Ellis (1984) expresses it, the goal of REBT is to help the client acquire "a more realistic, tolerant philosophy of life" (p. 214). To achieve this goal as the ultimate outcome of counseling, other goals are specified for the client in REBT (Ellis, 1979a).

1. *Self-interest.* The client is encouraged to develop a healthy self-interest rather than engage only in self-blame and negative self-evaluation.

2. *Social interest.* Ellis (1989) departs from the Adlerian practice of "insisting that social interest is the heart of therapeutic effectiveness" (p. 200). It is suggested in REBT, however, that clients develop social interest to have maximally fulfilling and productive lives.

3. *Self-direction.* REBT encourages clients to develop independence in problem-solving and responsibility for their own lives, although they may accept the encouragement, advice, and support of others.

4. *Tolerance.* Emotionally healthy individuals realize and accept the fact that they and others will make mistakes. They do not self-blame or condemn others when mistakes occur.

5. *Flexibility.* REBT helps clients become flexible in their thinking and behaving in response to ever changing reality.

6. *Acceptance of uncertainty.* This relates to being flexible in an unpredictable existence. Emotionally healthy individuals are able to accept the fact that life is uncertain and maintain optimism and grow despite that fact.

7. *Commitment.* This goal relates to social interest. Clients are helped to develop interests and commitment to persons and projects other than themselves.

8. *Scientific thinking.* In REBT, clients are taught to think logically and rationally rather than in magical, unvalidatable ways, so that their behavior will become more productive, accountable, and fulfilling.

## RELEVANCE TO SPEECH-LANGUAGE PATHOLOGY AND AUDIOLOGY

The theoretic framework and practical techniques of REBT are appropriate and useful when applied to counseling in speech-language pathology and audiology. REBT takes a phenomenological approach to counseling and is both humanistic and holistic in its philosophy. In a holistic approach to treating an individual with speech, language, and hearing disorders, as in REBT, it is important to determine the client's beliefs and ideas about their own, their child's, or significant other's, disorder. Individuals who operate on an irrational belief system concerning their communicative disorder or concerning themselves, their child, or their significant other as a person with a communicative disorder, are not likely to be maximally successful in modifying, compensating for, or living with the disorder. These individuals might experience emotional distress because of their irrational beliefs about their disorder, rather than because of the disorder itself. They are not likely to be effective or comfortable in social situations, irrespective of their communicative disorder, and in life roles that place communicative demands on them. The idea that an individual's perceptions of his or her communicative behavior are at the core of the concept of self, as discussed in Chapter 2, suggests that the rational or irrational nature of the beliefs the client holds as a communicator significantly affects quality of life for the client.

It is specious reasoning to assume that improvement in, compensation for, or correction of a communicative disorder automatically dispels all irrational beliefs held by the person with the disorder and by his or her parents or significant others. It is equally specious to assume that those beliefs are not of equal importance in determining the effectiveness of an individual's communicative behavior as are his or her basic speech, language, and hearing skills. Therefore, it is important for speech-language pathologists and audiologists to confront the client's irrational ideas, within the context of the communicative disorder, and to help the client eliminate internalized self-defeating thinking and develop a logical belief system. If illogical thinking exceeds the contextual boundaries of speech-language pathology and audiology or if the client's irrational ideas about speech, language, or hearing problems have led to significant role problems, such as marital difficulty, then referral for specialized counseling is indicated.

One emphasis in REBT is that of placing responsibility for changes in thinking and behaving with the client. This is an important emphasis also in speech-language therapy and aural rehabilitation. The client's dependence on the clinician should be minimized for changes in the status of a client's speech, language, and hearing to occur, generalize, and stabilize. Clients will be able to act adaptively to the unpredictable demands that changing life situations place on them as communicators, regardless of whatever level of communicative competence they ultimately possess, only if they can establish and maintain responsibility for consistent change in their behavior and thinking.

Oftentimes individuals with communicative disorders or their parents and significant others experience an overwhelming sense of catastrophe owing to their speech, language, or hearing problem or that of their child, their spouse, or significant other. These feelings can, in turn, lead to irrational beliefs of personal worthlessness which diminish quality of life and inhibit positive change in the activating event—the communicative disorder (or, more precisely, the individual's reaction to the communicative disorder). Counseling in speech-language pathology and audiology can be designed to reveal and challenge these feelings and minimize the intrapersonal negative impact of communicative disorders.

In the same sense as perceiving catastrophe, the presence of a communicative disorder can lead to blaming—one's spouse or child, fate, or oneself—for its existence. Shoulds, oughts, and musts then have the tendency to develop, which can cause individuals to view themselves, their disorder, or their communicatively disordered significant other in an unrealistic, irrational, nonproductive manner. Speech-language pathologists and audiologists might explore each client's belief system, relative to the communicative disorder, to determine if mustabatory behavior is preventing the client from achieving the optimal benefit of therapy and leading a productive, contented life despite having to cope with a communicative disorder.

The clinical techniques used in REBT are adaptable to speech-language pathology and audiology and to other disciplines that include information and personal adjustment counseling as part of standard clinical procedure. The general didactic orientation of the techniques used in REBT does not require training in specific psychoanalytic technique or in specialized psychotherapy. The three types of counseling employed in REBT—cognitive, emotive-evocative, and behavioral—are all relevant in counseling persons with communicative disorders and can be easily modified to address each client's specific needs and concerns.

## EXPERIENTIAL APPROACHES

Experiential approaches to counseling are concerned with what the client experiences in the counseling or therapy encounter. These approaches tend to be optimistic regarding the human potential for change; individuals are viewed as positively motivated and socialized and having an inherent drive to self-actualize. In this section Carl Rogers' *person-centered counseling*, which introduced the experiential approach to counseling, is discussed. It is perhaps the most ascribed to of the experiential approaches, in regard to the total number of counseling professionals who include it in their personal theories, as well as to the number of different professional disciplines to which it is applied.

As in the case of counseling based on classic psychoanalytic approaches and cognitive-behavioral approaches, there are various important experiential approaches to counseling other than the one detailed in this section. Included among the experiential approaches are *existential therapy*, Gestalt therapy, and creative arts therapy. These experiential approaches to counseling are briefly discussed.

### Experiential Approaches Other Than Rogers'

EXISTENTIAL THERAPY

*Existential therapy*, or existential psychology, was "spontaneously" developed in the 1940s and 1950s, according to May and Yalom (1989), mainly by European psychologists and psychiatrists. Existential therapy is not predicated on formal theories of personality development and maladaptive behavior or on a specific array of clinical techniques. Mosak (1989) observes that "existential psychology is not a school but a viewpoint" (p. 72). The viewpoint of existential therapy can be traced to the existential concepts of philosophers and writers such as Soren Kierkegaard, Friedrich Nietzsche, Martin Heidegger, Jean-Paul Sartre, and Albert Camus. Important statements of the existential therapy approach are in works by James Bugental (1976), Viktor Frankl (1967, 1984), and Rollo May (1953, 1961, 1977).

The concern of existential therapists is with the client as an actual, existing, immediate individual rather than as "a composite of drives, archetypes, or conditioning" (May & Yalom, 1989, p. 399). This would seem to suggest that existential psychologists reject fundamentally the approaches to counseling and psychotherapy of Freud, Jung, and the behaviorists. But existential therapy was not developed to be an alternative to those or other therapies. Rather, it was developed to influence practitioners of other approaches to see clients as they actually exist, instead of seeing them merely as projections of their own personal theory of personality and maladaptive behavior. The influence of existential therapy on all other schools of counseling and psychotherapy has been apparent (May & Yalom, 1989).

Existential therapy regards every client as a unique individual existing in the center of his or her own world of experience. The fundamental concept in existential philosophy is that an individual cannot be objectively defined by others in the true sense of being or existing (May, 1961). The existential viewpoint is that meaning radiates from each person to the object world after the person has defined himself or herself relative to his or her unique circumstances at specific moments in time; thus Sartre's mantric statement: "existence precedes essence." This concept represents a precondition to existential therapy being successful—the client must choose *being* rather than *nonbeing* (i.e., nothingness) to be able to find solutions to his or her problems (May & Yalom, 1989). The existential therapy process is an ontologic "I-Am" experience in which the client recognizes "I am living and I am unique. I have the right to be and to choose the nature of my being."

The idea that one's existence is unique can lead to feelings of *existential isolation* or loneliness. In existential therapy the client is helped to experience his or her uniqueness as *freedom* and *responsibility*. Freedom and responsibility are related concepts in existential therapy; although individuals are free to control their life, they must take responsibility for confronting the limits of their destiny (May, 1981). May and Yalom (1989) note that individuals differ greatly in their desire to take such responsibility because of the anxiety it might entail.

Existential therapists are concerned about *anxiety* and *guilt* generally; they hold that everyone experiences both in either normal or neurotic forms (May, 1977). Normal anxiety is proportionate to the cause, is not repressed, and can be used to creative ends; neurotic anxiety is just the opposite. Normal guilt arises from violations of the laws and mores of society. Neurotic guilt develops from one's perception that he or she is responsible for events actually outside his or her control or for events that are fantasized. May and Yalom (1989) describe a third type of guilt, an existential guilt, which occurs when individuals believe that they have not developed or achieved up to their potential. Clients are helped in existential therapy to develop the ability to distinguish between normal and neurotic guilt and anxiety and to change the neurotic forms to normal ones.

*Death* is considered in existential therapy to be a primary source of anxiety as it is the ultimate concern of human beings. Individuals erect denial defenses against the inevitability of death, defenses which at times can manifest as maladaptive behavior. Related to the issue of death in existential therapy is the idea of *boundary situations*. Boundary situations occur when individuals are forced to confront existential situations, such as death. Boundary situations can involve death confrontation in a real or a symbolic sense; for instance, symbolic death might be experienced as the result of a career ending, a marriage dissolving, self-concept loss due to a communicative disorder, or the birth of a child with a communicative disorder. Boundary situations can be experienced in a manner that brings positive changes for the individual—heightened awareness of the joys of living, improved interpersonal relationships, savoring of each moment of the here-and-now. Or, they can result in an individual's becoming depressed about past events or excessively apprehensive about future ones.

Existential therapy does not emphasize clinical techniques as much as it does the therapy relationship. The client is helped by the clinician, in a more confrontational and direct manner than in person-centered therapy, to accept responsibility for his or her destiny, to use anxiety as an impetus to creativity, and to learn and grow from boundary situations. Frankl (1960, 1969, 1978) describes techniques used in his logotherapy that help clients achieve the goals of existential counseling and choose to be. Two basic techniques Frankl describes are: (a) *dereflection,* which involves helping clients become less self-absorbed and more interested and engaged in other persons and activities in order to resolve feelings of *meaninglessness* (Frankl, 1963)—another source of anxiety and existential despair and isolation—and (b) *paradoxical intention,* which involves encouraging clients to confront and defuse their anxiety by doing voluntarily and exaggeratedly what they are apprehensive about or regard as involuntary behavior, such as stuttering on purpose if they are fearful of being dysfluent.

## GESTALT THERAPY

Another well-documented and widely used experiential approach to counseling is *Gestalt therapy*. Gestalt therapy was founded in the 1940s by Frederick "Fritz" S. Perls (1883–1970) and is in part derived from the Gestalt psychology principles forwarded by Max Wertheimer, Wolfgang Koehler, and Kurt Koffka. The Gestalt approach to counseling (Perls 1969a, 1969b, 1973) is based in the *here-and-now* and relates anxiety to dwelling on the past or preoccupation with the future, much the same as in existential therapy. In Gestalt therapy, as in existential therapy, responsibility for behavior is placed with the client. As with person-centered therapy, Gestalt therapy is phenomenological in its view of human behavior and recognizes an innate human tendency to self-actualize. Gestalt therapy operates on the primary concept of Gestalt psychology: when individuals at any given moment encounter constellations of stimuli they organize them into patterns or *gestalten* and perceive them as a whole. The organization of stimuli into gestalten is determined by the perception principles of *similarity, proximity, closure,* and *direction;* by each individual's *integrative mechanism* or gestalt function; and by the whole constellation of stimuli encountered. The gestalt is a perceptual experience in which physiologic and psychological phenomena are so closely integrated that the whole is more than a sum of its parts. Thus, in the Gestalt therapy viewpoint, an individual's thoughts, emotions, and perceptions can be understood only by considering them in a "whole person" context.

The primary goal of Gestalt therapy is to help clients become *self-regulating* through *awareness,* regardless of their specific presenting problem. "Awareness includes knowledge of the environment, responsibility for choices, self-knowledge, self-acceptance, and the ability to contact" (Yontef & Simkin, 1989, p. 339). To help a client move from being dependent to being independent Gestalt therapists help the client achieve greater self-awareness through a process rather than a content approach to therapy. Owing to this orientation, Gestalt therapy focuses more on the counseling relationship than on specific clinical techniques. The Gestalt therapy client-clinician relationship emphasizes the same characteristics as in the person-centered therapy relationship—caring, acceptance, and warmth expressed toward the client by the clinician.

But the most essential aspect of the counseling relationship in Gestalt therapy is *dialogue.* Emphasis on dialogue in Gestalt therapy is an indication of its existential perspective (Yontef & Simkin, 1989). This is the *I-thou relation* concept of Gestalt therapy, which assumes the client has meaning only in relation to others. The client is an equal with the clinician who recognizes the client's experience but also observes experiences of which the client is not aware. In this relationship both the clinician and the client are self-responsible—for themselves and each other. Four characteristics represent Gestalt therapy dialogue:

1. *Inclusion* involves the client and clinician fully entering the therapy experience while maintaining their individual identities, without judgment or interpretation of the client's experience, which provides a safe environment for therapy and promotes the client developing self-awareness.
2. *Presence* involves a phenomenological sharing with the client by the clinician of his or her observations, thoughts, feelings, and personal opinions, not to manipulate the client but to encourage the client to become self-regulating.
3. *Commitment to dialogue* involves allowing interpersonal contact between client and clinician to take its course rather than manipulating it to predetermined outcomes.

4. *Dialogue is lived* means that dialogue is concerned with doing, which in addition to verbal expression, can involve any means of communication such as art, song, dance, music, or nonverbal expression.

Techniques have been described (Levinsky & Perls, 1970; Levinsky & Simkin, 1972; Passons, 1975; Perls, 1969a, 1969b) to facilitate dialogue in Gestalt therapy, to increase clients' self-awareness, and to reveal clients' avoidances and resistances to becoming independent and self-regulating. These techniques include:

1. *Use of personal pronouns,* which encourages clients to personalize dialogue and to indicate acceptance of responsibility—for instance, "I think" rather than "people think."
2. *Assuming responsibility,* which requests clients to end all of their expressed opinions, beliefs, or positions with "and I take responsibility for it," as well as changing all of their "I can't" statements to "I won't."
3. *Converting questions into statements,* which forces clients to change evasion questions (e.g., "So you think therapy might be helpful?") to statements that reveal their belief system (e.g., "I don't think you really believe therapy might be helpful."
4. *Empty chair technique,* which helps clients work through approach-avoidance conflicts and to center in the now, by arguing with an empty chair their reasons for avoiding and then occupying the chair and arguing back with reasons for not avoiding.
5. *Sharing hunches,* which helps clients recognize their tendency to project meaning by clinicians using "I see . . . I imagine" statements in response to clients' behaviors and verbalizations.
6. *Playing the projection,* in which clients are asked to play the part of others onto whom they project.
7. *Now I'm aware,* which helps clients become aware of their inner psychological and physiologic states by closing their eyes, relaxing, and prefacing statements such as "Now I'm aware," "Now I'm aware of the tension in my larynx," "Now I'm aware that I worry about what people think of my hearing loss."
8. *Game of dialogue,* which encourages clients to use dialogue to argue both roles in personality conflicts such as passive-aggressive, top dog-underdog, and so forth, in order to recognize and resolve the conflicts.
9. *Role rehearsal and reversal,* which facilitates playing the projection, wherein clients are asked to rehearse new roles and to play roles that are the opposite of their usual, conflicted ones to increase self-awareness.
10. *Expressing resentments and appreciations,* which gets clients to recognize both the positive and negative attributes of significant others in their lives, rather than expressing recognition of the negative attributes only, which improves interpersonal relationships.

CREATIVE ARTS THERAPY

An experiential approach to counseling that does not have a theoretic base in the sense or to the degree of other approaches is creative arts therapy (CAT). CAT involves using creative activity to foster the client's emotional and physical health. Used in this approach are art therapy, bibliotherapy, dance therapy, drama therapy, and music therapy (Fleshman & Fryrear, 1981). CAT has proved effective in enabling communication between clinicians and cognitively impaired and nonverbal clients (Robbins, 1985); Nystul (1993) describes a case in which he used art therapy to help a client who stuttered develop social interest by using the illustrations the client produced to identify his basic mistakes and self-defeating behavior.

## Person-Centered Therapy

Person-centered therapy was developed by Carl R. Rogers in the 1940s, although Meador and Rogers (1979) note that it is "a continually developing approach to human growth and change . . ." (p. 131). Part of the reason for its continuing development is that the hypotheses on which person-centered therapy is based have been and continue to be extensively researched in numerous counseling settings. That Rogers encouraged testing of his hypotheses and that person-centered therapy lends itself to scientific examination have led to its hypothesis being backed up with a considerably solid base of empirical data.

Person-centered therapy has been found to have application in many professional disciplines involved in helping and educational relationships intended to promote human growth to its potential. In its application to education (Rogers, 1969), person-centered therapy has been known as student-centered therapy. Other examples of its application are with encounter groups addressing various concerns such as terminal illness and drug abuse, minority populations, intercultural groups, marriage relationships, families, international relationships, and industry. The widespread popularity among professional disciplines of person-centered therapy is due, in part, to its historical link to psychology rather than to medicine; to the fact that it is relatively easy to learn and use and does not require clinicians to have expertise with personality development, personality dynamics, and diagnosis of personality disorders; and to the tendency of clients to achieve counseling goals in person-centered therapy in a relatively brief period of time (Hall & Lindzey, 1978).

### HISTORICAL PERSPECTIVE

Carl Rogers' background is discussed in Chapter 3 in the section on self-theory. Rogers developed the *nondirective* approach to counseling, which became a third major force in counseling and psychotherapy, the other two being psychoanalysis and behaviorism. His nondirective approach to counseling was introduced in his 1942 book *Counseling and Psychotherapy*. Rogers' ideas initially were roundly criticized as being heuristic and a direct challenge to the counseling approaches based on the assumption that the counselor knew best and should be in charge of change in the client's behavior. He expanded on his approach to counseling and introduced his theory of personality in *Client-Centered Therapy* (1951). Other works followed in which Rogers continued to refine the process of client-centered counseling: *A Theory of Therapy, Personality, and Interpersonal Relationships as Developed in the Client-Centered Framework* (1959), *On Becoming a Person* (1961), *Freedom to Learn* (1969), *Carl Rogers on Encounter Groups* (1970), and *On Becoming Partners: Marriage and Its Alternatives* (1972). The evolving character of Rogers' approach to counseling is reflected in the various titles he has termed his therapy, "nondirective to client-centered to relationship-centered to 'experiencing'" (Bischof, 1964, p. 425). In 1974, in order to describe more adequately the human values his approach to counseling addresses, Rogers changed the name of his therapy from "client-centered" to "person-centered" (Meador & Rogers, 1979).

### BASIC CONCEPTS

The basic concepts underlying self-theory and Rogers' theory of personality on which person-centered therapy is based are described in Chapter 3. Rogers' theory of personality and approach to counseling are based in part on Snygg and Combs' (1949) theory of phenomenology, on the holistic and organismic psychology of Angyal (1941) and Maslow (1943), on the interpersonal theory of Sullivan (1945), and on the self-theory interpretations of Lecky (1945) and Raimy (1943), among other influences.

Person-centered therapy is humanistic and, as with Gestalt therapy, is closely aligned with existential philosophy. In both humanistic and existential approaches to counseling there is respect for the client's subjective experiences; for the client's autonomy, choice, values, and purpose; and for the client's responsibility and capability to effect change and growth. Existentialists, however, view life as having no basic or universal meaning and see individuals as being continually faced with the anxiety of confronting life's meaninglessness and attempting to create personal identity in a meaningless existence. Humanists, on the other hand, hold that individuals can and will find meaning in life, if afforded the right conditions to do so, through their inherent drive to actualize. Ansbacher (1977), an Adlerian psychologist, lists six characteristics common to humanistic approaches to counseling:

1. The creative power of individuals, in addition to heredity and environment, is a crucial force in their growth and change.
2. An anthropomorphic model of human personality and behavior is superior to a mechanomorphic one.
3. The decisive dynamic in human behavior is purpose rather than cause.
4. A holistic approach to counseling is more effective than an elementaristic approach.
5. Clinicians should take clients' subjectivity, opinions, viewpoints, and their conscious and unconscious levels of awareness into full account.
6. Effective counseling and psychotherapy are dependent on a positive client-clinician relationship.

In addition to being in consonance with existential, humanistic, and Adlerian concepts, person-centered therapy shares some principles with rational emotive behavior therapy (REBT) (Ellis, 1977). These shared principles include an optimism that even seriously disturbed individuals can change; the idea that negative self-attitudes are born out of unnecessary self-criticism, but that negative attitudes can be changed to positive ones; willingness to go to extreme effort to improve the human condition; willingness to explicate fully and demonstrate publicly the technique of person-centered therapy and REBT; and respect for scientific validation. Person-centered therapy and REBT differ, however, in that REBT does not place the importance on the client-clinician relationship as does person-centered therapy; in REBT, clinicians provide the goals of therapy whereas in person-centered therapy clients determine therapy goals; counselors practicing REBT challenge "basic mistakes" in clients' thinking but person-centered therapists unconditionally accept clients' ways of thinking; in REBT, direct action strategies for effecting changes in behavior are prescribed by clinicians, whereas in person-centered therapy actions are determined by the clients; and in REBT clinicians act didactically and confrontationally when necessary, pointing out clients' irrational beliefs and self-defeating thinking, but person-centered therapists at all times maintain a respectful and accepting relationship with clients (Raskin & Rogers, 1989).

Assumptions

The assumptions basic to self-theory are listed in Chapter 3. The major assumptions on which the process-oriented approach (one of its distinguishing characteristics) to person-centered therapy is based are listed below (Rogers, 1951; Rogers, 1954; Rogers & Sanford, 1985; Rogers & Wood, 1974).

1. *Effective outcome of therapy is ensured if clinicians possess the appropriate attitudes.* This is the fundamental tenet of person-centered therapy—that clinician attitudes that create a clinical atmosphere of respect and trust are what is necessary for clients to change in positive, constructive directions. It is in diametric opposition to traditional psychoanalytic and directive approaches. In his nondirective orientation to counseling, Rogers es-

chews the techniques used in traditional psychoanalysis and directive approaches to therapy (e.g., teaching, evaluation, diagnosis, advising, persuasion, confronting, interpreting, and so forth).

2. *Clients, not clinicians, are best able to set therapy goals and to determine how to modify their behavior.* This idea is based on the belief that clients possess the inherent potential for positive growth and change and to self-actualize and they will change and self-actualize if given the proper conditions and adequate self-awareness.

3. *Individuals react to their phenomenal field as they perceive it.* As discussed in Chapter 3, the client's perceptions of reality, rather than external reality, has the greatest influence on their personality and behavior.

4. *Clients' behavior can best be understood from their internal frame of reference.* This is the idea that clinicians should have a phenomenological perspective of therapy, recognize that each client's perception of reality is unique, and understand that it is important and possible to comprehend the client's internal frame of reference.

5. *It is the responsibility of the clinician to be accessible to the client.* This enables clinicians and clients to experience together the moment-to-moment, here-and-now, experiential nature of the counseling relationship.

6. *Individuals tend to behave in ways consistent with their concept of self.* As described in Chapter 3 under self-theory, the self is a differentiated portion of the phenomenal field that consists of perceptions of "I" and "me." The organism demands consistency between the individual's behavior and perceptions of self.

7. *The same principles of counseling and psychotherapy apply to all clients.* This is considered in person-centered therapy to be the case regardless of whether the client is classified as normal, neurotic, or psychotic. It is held that all individuals possess the inherent desire to self-actualize and person-centered therapy is optimistic about their potential to do so.

COUNSELING TECHNIQUE

Person-centered therapy is not structured around an array of therapeutic techniques that are employed directly by the clinician to expose "mistakes" in a client's patterns of thinking and behaving and to modify those patterns. Rather, clinical technique in person-centered therapy involves interpersonal characteristics of the counseling relationship only, namely the attitudes and beliefs the clinician brings to the therapy encounter. By being genuine, caring, and empathic the clinician is able to share in the client's internal frame of reference and gain insight, along with the client, into the structure of self and experiences that have proved to be obstacles to the client's personal growth.

Change is accomplished by the client, not by the clinician manipulating the client. In the nonjudgmental setting of person-centered therapy, clients are able to take responsibility for their growth, explore their internal frame of reference, discover attitudes denied to conscious awareness, and make changes in their concept of self. The clinician does not instruct the client to do anything, does not set goals for the client, and does not evaluate or diagnostically label the client's behavior. Instead, the clinician intently listens to the client and displays that he or she hears and understands what the client is saying. The clinician is *reflective* in a therapy climate of *nonpossessive warmth*. Clients are thus indirectly encouraged to abandon defensive behaviors, examine their attitudes and behaviors, and develop for themselves goals and strategies to resolve any crisis and resume forward-moving personal growth.

TRUST

Raskin and Rogers (1989) note that "perhaps the most fundamental and pervasive concept in person-centered therapy is trust" (p. 155). *Trust* is the foundation for Rogers' theoretic position on general human development as well as the rationale for his person-centered approach to therapy. There are essentially three placements of trust, the first being in the inherent tendency for all individuals to self-actualize and to move forward in constructive, positive directions in attempting to achieve their full potential.

The second placement of trust is in the client's ability to set realistic goals for change and growth and to monitor progress toward achieving those goals. In this regard, trust is placed in the client's judgment to determine the need for, type, and amount of therapy; the desired outcome of therapy; and the strategies for achieving insight, growth, and change. The same trust is afforded groups as well as individual clients. A third application of trust, and one that is particularly fundamental to the philosophy of person-centered therapy is placement of trust by the client in the clinician. For person-centered therapy to be maximally effective, trust must not be unidirectional, the client must place as much trust in the clinician as the clinician does in the client.

CLINICIAN QUALITIES

Rogers (1957) recognizes three essential qualities in clinicians that foster the trust discussed above and that serve to create the clinical atmosphere that is conducive to clients embarking on an experience of self-discovery and self-enhancement.

1. *Congruence.* According to Rogers (1957), congruence is the most important of the three essential clinician characteristics. Congruity means that clinicians are genuine in the therapy experience; they do not operate under false pretense; there is correspondence between their inner perceptions of the therapy experience and their verbalizations of those perceptions; and they honestly convey their attitudes and opinions to their clients. Professional facades are avoided by person-centered clinicians; their thoughts and behaviors match. Clinicians who are congruent in the counseling relationship can express both their positive and negative perceptions, which serves to foster a trust between them and their clients.
2. *Unconditional positive regard.* Another important attitude that clinicians should possess and communicate to the client is an unconditional respect and acceptance of the client as a person. This acceptance carries no condition, judgments, or evaluations; the clinician simply conveys to the client that he or she is accepted regardless of what feelings or opinions are expressed in the therapy relationship. The clinician's acceptance should be nonpossessive; that is, it should not be displayed to meet needs of the clinician (e.g., to be respected or valued). Unconditional positive regard for their clients does not mean that the clinician accepts or approves of all of the attitudes and behaviors that clients exhibit; it means that regardless of how individual client behavior is judged, the clinician accepts the client as a person worthy of respect. The more the client perceives the nonpossessive warmth, caring, and acceptance of the clinician, the greater the likelihood that therapy goals will be accomplished (Rogers, 1977).

   On the other hand, clinicians who experience active dislike, disapproval, or distaste for clients most likely will not meet with success in therapy; clients will perceive their lack of positive regard and acceptance and respond defensively to attempts at meaningful interaction. Rogers recognizes that it is not likely that clinicians feel unconditional positive regard for their clients at all times. He suggests, however, that positive change in behavior is less likely to occur if the client does not perceive the full acceptance and caring of the clinician.
3. *Empathy.* Empathy is used by clinicians to convey genuineness, caring, and unconditional positive regard to the client. This is one of the most important "techniques" of the person-centered clinician. Empathy, however, is not actually a technique or device used

to effect change in a client's behavior. It is an attempt by clinicians to identify subjectively with the feelings and meanings they experience rather than attempting only to objectify a client's feelings and meanings. The empathic clinician conveys to clients an attitude of deep, genuine interest in their moment-to-moment, here-and-now world of subjective experience.

Empathy involves more than the clinician reflecting the content of the client's comments; for instance, by repeating the client's last words. It is the sincere attempt by clinicians to share in a client's inner feelings from within the client's internal frame of reference; clinicians experience both the inner feelings of clients and their own inner responses to the client's feelings. If clinicians respond with respect, understanding, and warmth to this sharing, clients are more encouraged, in a nondirective manner, to explore their feelings more deeply and to resolve any incongruity that exists between their subjective experiencing and objective reality. One caution is that empathic clinicians should be careful to maintain their own separateness while sharing in a client's subjective experiences. Progress in therapy is enhanced if clinicians are able to have a high degree of empathy yet preserve and express their own identity.

Rogers (1986) reports that research has indicated that client success in counseling is positively correlated with the three clinician attitudes discussed above—congruence, unconditional positive regard, and empathy. These are the three most critical conditions of the counseling relationship (Rogers, 1954) and by their presence, client change can be spontaneously precipitated. These are not separate feeling or being states that can be selectively manipulated by skilled clinicians. According to Meador and Rogers (1979) they are "interdependent and logically related" (p. 132). They also are not "all-or-none" conditions, but exist on a continuum. The higher the degree of clinician congruence to the counseling relationship and unconditional positive regard and empathy for the client, the more likely is a client to become increasingly aware of inner experiencing and to behave in more congruence with thoughts and feelings.

## CLIENT CHARACTERISTICS

In addition to the three clinician characteristics discussed, three characteristics on the client side of the counseling relationship serve to characterize the process of the person-centered approach (Raskin & Rogers, 1989). Brief descriptions of these client characteristics follow.

1. *Self-concept.* Person-centered therapy is concerned primarily with a client's perceptions about self and with how those perceptions affect self-esteem. Clients who have self-concepts in conflict are likely to experience a lowering of self-esteem or negative self-regard. If a client's perceptions of self can be enhanced, self-regard tends to become more positive as well and the prognosis for maximal success in therapy is improved. Success in therapy typically leads to clients experiencing more positive self-regard.
2. *Locus-of-evaluation.* At the outset of therapy a client is often found to be operating on conditions of worth. To maintain positive self-regard, the client lives according to the standards and values of others rather than in congruence with personal internal, organismic values. These clients, in effect, care too much about what others think of them and so develop a locus-of-evaluation of self that is external. With success in therapy, along with increase in self-esteem, clients tend to shift the evaluation of themselves from an external to an internal locus.
3. *Experiencing.* A third characteristic of person-centered therapy that relates to client progress is experiencing. Initially clients tend to some degree to be rigid in how they ex-

perience the self and the world. If therapy progresses successfully, clients become more flexible and open in their experiencing of inner feelings and external reality.

The above characteristics that are manifested by clients illustrate the process nature of person-centered therapy. As the counseling relationship progresses because of clinician congruity, positive regard, and empathy, progress is simultaneously made by the client along the dimensions of self-concept, locus-of-evaluation, and experiencing.

## GOALS OF THERAPY

The one general goal of the person-centered counselor is to establish the clinical conditions that are conducive to the central client goal of re-establishing progress toward self-actualization. As discussed in Chapter 3, the self-actualization process can be inhibited by the development of conditions of worth—imposed standards of others that individuals might use, rather than their organismic values, to maintain positive self-regard. This state, in turn, can lead to incongruity between the organismic drive to self-actualize and the ability to channel that drive into constructive, positive action.

The person-centered counselor is in effect only removing obstacles to change by providing an environment in which change is encouraged by clients gaining insight into their attitudes and experiences. Other than the general goal of reinstituting the self-actualization drive, the client sets both the individualized goals in person-centered therapy (Rogers, 1970) and the means to achieve them. In the person-centered framework, counseling basically is the "releasing of an already existing capacity in a potentially competent individual" (Rogers, 1959, p. 210).

## IF-THEN CONDITIONS

What are the conditions that promote change in a client's behavior and reactivate progress toward self-actualization? They can be stated in an *if-then* sequence—if certain conditions exist, then change in the client's behavior is likely to occur. According to Rogers (1951, 1959), the necessary and sufficient conditions for success in counseling are:

1. *Minimal psychological contact.* To establish a relationship, at least two people, in this case the client and clinician, have to be in at least a minimal state of psychological contact.
2. *Minimal state of anxiety.* The client must be anxious for change to occur for it to happen. The more anxious the client is about incongruity between his or her concept of self and behavior the better the prognosis that constructive change will occur in counseling.
3. *Clinician congruity.* The importance in therapy of this clinician characteristic was discussed above. Clinicians who are congruent can recognize and express their inner experiencing of the feelings displayed by the client in the clinical relationship. The more self-actualizing and fully functioning the clinician is, the more effective he or she will be in counseling.
4. *Unconditional positive regard.* As discussed above, if the clinician does not judge a client's behavior as positive or negative and has an unconditional positive regard for the client irrespective of his or her value system, then the client will perceive both self-worth and the potential for growth and change.
5. *Empathy.* This condition also was discussed above and is the essence of therapy being person-centered (Rogers, 1959). Although no clinician can ever fully comprehend a client's internal frame of reference, an attempt by the clinician to do so promotes trust in the therapy relationship which in turn fosters a sense of security for the client in exploring his or her inner feelings.
6. *Client awareness.* The client must perceive that the clinician is empathic and has unconditional positive regard for him or her for maximal change to occur for the client in ther-

apy; it is not merely enough for the clinician to possess these characteristics, they must be demonstrated to the client.

PROGRESS OF THERAPY

The progress of person-centered therapy is recognized by the client as a sequence of experiences. Rogers (1951) describes person-centered therapy as consisting of six distinct client experiences.

1. *Responsibility.* The first experience the client typically has is that of responsibility for himself or herself in the counseling relationship. After initial reactions of isolation and anger, the client should show signs of increasing independence and responsibility.
2. *Exploration.* The client begins, as a result of the warm, caring person-centered counseling relationship, to explore his or her inner feelings and attitudes. Incongruity between feelings and behaviors is discovered through verbalized exploration with the clinician and internalized, nonverbalized exploration outside the counseling relationship.
3. *Discovery of denied attitudes.* Attitudes that had been denied to conscious awareness, both positive and negative, are discovered by the client as a result of exploration. The client identifies attitudes that are inconsistent with the concept of self and symbolizes them in conscious awareness.
4. *Reorganizing the self.* Once denied attitudes are discovered and symbolized in awareness by the client, a reorganization of his or her concept of self occurs, which results in more positive perceptions of the self. It is at this stage in therapy that the client starts to become a fully functioning organism, experiencing congruence between internal awareness and external experience.
5. *Progress.* If the therapeutic relationship is founded on clinician congruity, positive regard, and empathy, the client begins to experience progress at the outset of therapy. Experiencing progress may come with an emotional price; the discovery and resolution of denied attitudes can cause consternation and depression for the client. But each time the client confronts his or her feelings and reorganizes a portion of the self in a positive, constructive direction, he or she is reinforced to continue taking risks in exploring, confronting, and reorganizing the self.
6. *Ending.* Just as a client determines whether or not to enroll in counseling, what are the goals of therapy, and what are the strategies to be used to achieve those goals, so too does the client determine when counseling will end. Ending of counseling may cause clients to experience a nonspecific sense of loss or fear. One way to minimize the negative client emotion occasioned by ending therapy is to set time limits. Time limits alert clients from the initial counseling session that there will be a specific and foreseeable ending date. Time limits also tacitly force progress in therapy, as clients know that they do not have the luxury of limitless time to achieve therapy goals.

OUTCOMES OF COUNSELING

The hoped for ultimate outcome of person-centered therapy is that the client overcomes the internalized restrictions of conditions of worth, establishes congruity between organismic values and need for self-regard, and resumes or initiates movement toward self-actualization. If complete congruence is established and self-actualizing movement is optimal, a client becomes what Rogers calls a *fully functioning* individual (Rogers, 1959). Becoming more fully functioning is a process that involves gradual change along several dimensions. Rogers (1961) describes four dimensions that characterize the changes typically observed in clients and which are regarded as successful outcomes of therapy.

1. *Openness to experience.* Clients who become more fully functioning permit more experiential data to enter conscious awareness and accurately symbolize it, rather than constructing defense mechanisms to deny, distort, and falsify reality. They do not operate on rigid belief systems, can tolerate ambiguity, and seek new ways to learn and grow.
2. *Self-trust.* As therapy progresses and clients become more open to experience, they tend to place more trust in their own judgments and decisions. By placing more trust in their organismic valuing system, clients can take responsibility for their decisions and take corrective action when unsatisfactory decisions are made.
3. *Internal locus of evaluation.* Increasing trust of self encourages clients to shift the evaluation of their behavior from external standards to internal ones. Clients increasingly look to themselves for life choices and for validation of the self.
4. *Willingness to continue growing.* Rogers eschewed the term "well-adjusted" as a client characteristic manifested as an outcome of successful therapy as it implies that an end-goal has been achieved and that the experiencing of that goal is static. Self-actualization is not an end-goal of therapy. Rather it is a process reclaimed in therapy by clients, a process that affords limitless opportunity for growth; in the person-centered view, no one ever becomes fully self-actualized. Fully functioning clients are in a continuing process of becoming and being open to new experiences. They challenge their internal beliefs and test their perceptions of external reality.

### Relevance to Speech-Language Pathology and Audiology

Of all approaches to counseling, perhaps person-centered therapy is most obviously relevant to speech-language pathology and audiology. It does not take specialized, extensive training in counseling or psychotherapy to apply its principles to working with persons with speech, language, and hearing disorders. It is a relatively safe approach to counseling compared with approaches that employ direct counseling technique. As Corey (1986) notes: "For a person with limited background in counseling psychology, personality dynamics, and psychopathology, the person-centered approach offers assurance that prospective clients will not be psychologically harmed" (p. 112).

The basic clinical skills used by person-centered therapists—active listening, reflecting, clarifying, and so forth—are applicable to all helping professions. If clinicians do not possess these skills and the characteristics of congruity, unconditional positive regard, and empathy, they might be less effective in modifying speech, language, and hearing disorders, whether or not their intent is holistic treatment of the client.

The emotions that persons with communicative disorders and their families and significant others might experience were discussed in Chapter 2. These emotions can be barriers to success in therapy and can diminish the quality of life and social effectiveness for individuals with speech, language, and hearing disorders. Clinicians can nondirectly help clients work through the grief or sense of crisis they experience when they, their child, or their significant other develops a communicative disorder.

Clients with communicative disorders oftentimes report for therapy in a state of incongruity between their perceptions of reality and reality itself. For instance, a client might see himself or herself as a completely ineffective communicator when in fact he or she possesses adequate interpersonal skills and the speech, language, and hearing ability to be quite effective as a communicator. Or, the reverse scenario might be observed at times— the client has an exaggerated, positive impression of the present status of his or her communicative functioning or has unrealistic expectations of what he or she will be able to achieve in therapy. A person-centered approach to counseling might prove effective in helping clients resolve such incongruity by accurately aligning their beliefs and attitudes about their communicative disorder with the external present and future reality the status of the disorder presents. By taking the time in therapy to explore with clients the question of congruence, speech-language pathologists and audiologists might find that the prognosis for successful therapy is enhanced. This counseling focus is important also to the philosophy of holistic therapy, which is a particularly meaningful consideration in cases where the therapy prognosis for a client is guarded.

The primary clinical objective in speech-language pathology and audiology is to help clients, regardless of age or type of disorder, become more fully functioning than they were at the outset of therapy. This is accomplished primarily by direct treatment of their speech, language, or hearing disorder. If improvement in their communicative behavior is not appreciable or at best minimal, after some duration of therapy, reality begins to set in for the client that his or her concept of self, in part, may always be that of one who has disordered speech, language, or hearing. Will that idea promote a decrease in the client's self-esteem and lead to him or her developing conditions of worth, subjugating organismic values and standards to the values and standards of others to maintain positive self-regard? Or, will it exacerbate conditions of worth that already exist chiefly because of their communicative disorder? Possibly so, is the answer to both questions. And not just for the clients themselves. Parents, spouses, and significant others of individuals with communicative disorders are at risk to be derailed in their self-actualization process by having to confront and cope with the challenges presented by the communicative disorder of their loved one.

Speech-language pathologists and audiologists can assist clients and their significant others in maintaining their self-actualization urge if they are committed to holistic treatment of clients—treatment of the person and the disorder, rather than treatment of the disorder only. If the anticipated outcome of therapy is a client who is more open to experience; who trusts in his or her own judgments and decisions; who evaluates personal values, standards, and behaviors within themselves; and who desires continuing growth even after therapy terminates, then behavioral therapy might be augmented with experiential counseling, possibly within a person-centered framework.

REFERENCES

Adler, A. (1917). *Study of organ inferiority and its physical compensation.* New York: Nervous and Mental Diseases Publishing Company (1917).

Adler, A. (1929). *The science of living.* New York: Greenburg.

Adler, A. (1930). Individual psychology. In C. Murchison (Ed.), *Psychologies of 1930.* Worcester, MA: Clark University Press.

Adler, A. (1931). *What life should mean to you.* Boston, MA: Little, Brown & Co.

Adler, A. (1935). The fundamental views of individual psychology. *International Journal of Individual Psychology, 1,* 5–8.

Adler, A. (1964). *Social interest: A challenge to mankind.* New York: Capricorn.

Adler, A. (1969). *The practice and theory of individual psychology.* Paterson, NJ: Littlefield, Adams.

Alexander, F., & French, T. M. (1946). *Psychoanalytic therapy.* New York: Ronald Press.

Allen, J. W. (1971). The individual psychology of Alfred Adler: An item of history and a promise of revolution. *Counseling Psychologist 3,* 3–24.

Angyal, A. (1941). *Foundations for a science of personality.* New York: Commonwealth Fund.

Ansbacher, H. L. (1959). A key to existence. *Journal of Individual Psychology 15,* 141–142.

Ansbacher, H. L. (1977). Individual psychology.In R. J. Corsini (Ed.), *Current psychotherapies.* Itasca, IL: FE Peacock.

Ansbacher, H. L., & Ansbacher, R. (Eds.), (1956). *The individual-psychology of Alfred Adler.* New York: Basic Books.

Ansbacher, H. L., & Ansbacher, R. (Eds.), (1964). *Superiority and social interest by Alfred Adler.* Evanston, IL: Northwestern University Press.

Arlow, J. A. (1989). Psychoanalysis. In R. J. Corsini & D. Wedding (Eds.), *Current psychotherapies* (4th ed.). Itasca, IL: FE Peacock.

Ayllon, T., & Azrin, N. (1968). *The token economy: A motivation system for therapy and rehabilitation.* New York: Appleton-Century-Crofts.

Bandura, A. (1974). Behavior theory and the models of man. *American Psychologist, 29,* 859–869.

Bandura, A. (1986). *Social foundations of thought and actions: A social cognitive theory.* Englewood Cliffs, NJ: Prentice-Hall.

Beck A. T. (1976). *Cognitive therapy and emotional disorders.* New York: International Universities Press.

Beck, A. T., & Emery, G. (1985). *Anxiety disorders and phobias: A cognitive perspective.* New York: Basic Books.

Beck, A. T., Rush, A. J., Shaw, B. F., & Emery, G. (1979). *Cognitive therapy of depression.* New York: Guilford Press.

Beck, A. T., & Weishaar, M. E. (1989). Cognitive therapy. In R. J. Corsini & D. Wedding (Eds.), *Current psychotherapies* (4th ed.). Itasca, IL: FE Peacock.

Berne, E. (1961). *Transactional analysis in psychotherapy.* New York: Grove Press.

Berne, E. (1964). *Games people play.* New York: Grove Press.

Berne, E. (1966). *Principles of group treatment.* New York: Oxford University Press.

Berne, E. (1972). *What do you say after you say hello?* New York: Grove Press.

Bischof, L. (1964). *Interpreting personality theories.* New York: Harper & Row.

Bordin, E. S. (1955). *Psychological counseling.* New York: Appleton-Century-Crofts.

Bottome, P. (1939). *Alfred Adler: A biography.* New York: Putnam.

Bugental, J. (1976). *The search for existential identity.* San Francisco: Jossey-Bass.

Corsini, R. J. (1953). The behind-the-back technique in group psychotherapy. *Group Psychotherapy, 6,* 102–109.

Corey, G. (1986). *Theory and practice of counseling and psychotherapy* (3rd ed.). Monterey, CA: Brooks/Cole.

Dinkmeyer, D., & Dinkmeyer, D. C., Jr. (1985). Adlerian psychology and counseling. In S. Lynn & J. Garske (Eds.), *Contemporary psychotherapies: Models and methods.* Columbus, OH: Merrill/Macmillan.

Dreikurs, R.(1957). *Psychology in the classroom: A manual for teachers.* New York: Harper & Row.

Dreikurs, R. (1960). *Group psychotherapy and group approaches: Collected papers.* Chicago: Alfred Adler Institute.

Dreikurs, R. (1971). *Social equality: The challenge of today.* Chicago: Henry Regnery.

Ellenberger, H. F. (1970). *The discovery of the unconscious.* New York: Basic Books.

Ellis, A. (1962). *Reason and emotion in psychotherapy.* New York: Lyle Stuart.

Ellis, A. (1970). Humanism, values,rationality. *Journal of Individual Psychology, 27,* 50–64.

Ellis, A. (1973). *Humanistic psychotherapy: The rational-emotive approach.* New York: Julian Press.

Ellis, A. (1977). The basic clinical theory of rational-emotive therapy. In A. Ellis & R. Greiger (Eds.), *RET handbook of rational-emotive therapy.* New York: Springer-Verlag.

Ellis A. (1979a). The practice of rational-emotive therapy. In A. Ellis & J. Whiteley (Eds.), *Theoretical and empirical foundations of rational-emotive therapy.* Monterey, CA: Brooks/Cole.

Ellis, A. (1979b). Rational-emotive therapy as a new theory of personality and therapy. In A. Ellis & J. Whiteley (Eds.), *Theoretical and empirical foundations of rationale-emotive therapy.* Monterey, CA: Brooks/Cole.

Ellis A. (1979c). The theory of rational-emotive therapy. In A. Ellis & J. Whiteley (Eds.), *Theoretical and empirical foundations of rational-emotive therapy.* Monterey, CA: Brooks/Cole.

Ellis, A. (1984). The essence of RET—1984. *Journal of Rational-Emotive Therapy, 2,* 19–25.

Ellis, A. (1989). Rational-emotive therapy. In R. J. Corsini & D. Wedding (Eds.), *Current psychotherapies* (4th ed.). Itasca, IL: FE Peacock.

Ellis, A. (1991). The revised ABC's of rational-emotive therapy (RET). *Journal of Rational-Emotive and Cognitive-Behavior Therapy, 9* (3), 139–172.

Ellis, A. (1993). Changing rational-emotive therapy (RET) to rational emotive behavior therapy (REBT). *Behavior Therapist, 16,* 257–258.

Ellis, A. (1994). *Reason and Emotion in Psychotherapy* (2nd ed.). New York: Birch Lane Press.

Ellis, A., & Harper, R. (1975). *A new guide to rational living* (revised ed.). Hollywood: Wilshire Books.

Erickson, E. H. (1963). *Childhood and society* (2nd ed.). New York: WW Norton.

Fleshman, B., & Fryrear, J. L. (1981). *The arts in therapy.* Chicago: Nelson-Hall.

Frankl, V. E. (1960). Paradoxical intention: A logotherapeutic technique. *American Journal of Psychotherapy, 14,* 520–535.

Frankl, V. E. (1963). *Man's search for meaning.* New York: Washington Square Press.

Frankl, V. E. (1967). *Psychotherapy and existentialism: Selected papers on logotherapy.* New York: Touchstone/Simon & Schuster.

Frankl, V. E. (1969). *Will to meaning.* New York: World Publishing.

Frankl, V. E. (1970). Forerunner of existential psychiatry. *Journal of Individual Psychology, 26,* 38.

Frankl, V. E. (1978). *The unheard cry for meaning.* New York: Touchstone/Simon & Schuster.

Frankl, V. E. (1984). *Man's search for meaning: An introduction to logotherapy* (3rd ed.). New York: Touchstone/Simon & Schuster.

Glasser, W. (1961). *Mental health or mental illness?* New York: Harper & Row.

Glasser, W. (1965). *Reality therapy: A new approach to psychiatry.* New York: Harper & Row.

Glasser, W. (1969). *Schools without failure.* New York: Harper & Row.

Glasser, W. (1976). *Positive addiction.* New York: Harper & Row.

Glasser, W. (1980). Reality therapy. An explanation of the steps of reality therapy. In N. Glasser (Ed.), *What are you doing? How people are helped through reality therapy.* New York: Harper & Row.

Glasser, W. (1984). *Take effective control of your life.* New York: Harper & Row.

Glasser, W.(1986). *Control therapy in the classroom.* New York: Harper & Row.

Glasser, W. (1990). *The quality school.* New York: Harper & Row.

Hall, C. S., & Lindzey, G. (1978). *Theories of personality* (3rd ed.). New York: John Wiley & Sons.

Hummel, R. C. (1962). Ego-counseling in guidance: Concept and method. *Harvard Education Review, 32,* 461–482.

Jones, E. (1955). *The life and work of Sigmund Freud* (Vol. 2). New York: Basic Books.

Jung, C. G. (1916). *Analytical psychology.* New York: Moffat, Yard.

Kaufer, F. H. (1975). Self-management methods. In F. H. Kaufer & A. P. Goldstein (Eds.), *Helping people change.* New York: Pergamon Press.

Kroeber, T. C. (1963). The coping functions of the ego-mechanisms. In R. W. White (Ed.), *The study of lives.* New York: Atherton Press.

Levinsky, A., & Perls, F. S. (1970). The rules and games of Gestalt therapy. In J. Fagan & I. Shepherd (Eds.), *Gestalt therapy now.* New York: Harper & Row.

Levinsky, A., & Simkin, J. S. (1972). Gestalt therapy. In L. N. Solomon & B. Berzon (Eds.), *New perspectives on encounter groups.* San Francisco: Jossey-Bass.

Lecky, P. (1945). *Self-consistency: A theory of personality.* New York: Island Press.

Manning, W. H. (1996). *Clinical decision making in the assessment and treatment of fluency disorders.* Albany, NY: Delmar.

Maslow, A. H. (1943). A theory of human motivation. *Psychology Review, 50,* 370–397.

Maslow, A. H. (1970). Holistic emphasis. *Journal of Individual Psychology, 18,* 125.

May, R. (1953). *Man's search for himself.* New York: WW Norton.

May, R. (Ed.) (1961). *Existential psychology.* New York: Random House.

May, R. (1970). Myth and guiding fiction. *Journal of Individual Psychology, 26,* 39.

May, R. (1977). *The meaning of anxiety* (revised ed.). New York: WW Norton.

May, R. (1981). *Freedom and destiny.* New York: WW Norton.

May, R., & Yalom, I. (1989). Existential psychotherapy. In R. J. Corsini & D. Wedding (Eds.), *Current psychotherapies* (4th ed.). Itasca, IL: FE Peacock.

Meador, B. D., & Rogers, C. R. (1979). Client-centered therapy. In R. J. Corsini (Ed.), *Current psychotherapies* (2nd ed.). Itasca, IL: FE Peacock.

Meichenbaum, D. (1977). *Cognitive-behavior modification: An integrative approach.* New York: Plenum.

Mosak, H. H. (1967). Subjective criteria of normality. *Psychotherapy, 4,* 159–161.

Mosak, H. H. (1989). Adlerian psychotherapy. In R. J. Corsini & D. Wedding (Eds.), *Current psychotherapies* (4th ed.). Itasca, IL: FE Peacock.

Munroe, R. (1955). *Schools of psychoanalytic thought.* New York: Holt, Rinehart & Winston.

Nystul, M. S. (1993). *The art and science of counseling and psychotherapy.* New York: Merrill/Macmillan.

Pavlov, I. P. (1906). The scientific investigation of the psychical faculties of processes in the higher animals. *Science, 24,* 613–619.

Passons, W. R. (1975). *Gestalt approaches in counseling.* New York: Holt, Rinehart & Winston.

Patterson, C. (1966). *Theories of counseling and psychotherapy.* New York: Harper & Row.

Perls, F. S. (1969a). *Gestalt therapy verbatim.* Moab, UT: Real People Press.

Perls, F. S. (1969b). *In and out of the garbage pail.* Moab, UT: Real People Press.

Perls, F. S. (1973). *The Gestalt approach.* Palo Alto, CA: Science and Behavior Books.

Rapaport, D. (1958). The theory of ego autonomy: A generalization. *Bulletin of the Menninger Clinic, 22,* 13–35.

Raimy, V. C. (1943). *The self-concept as a factor in counseling and personality organization.* Unpublished doctoral dissertation, Ohio State University, Athens, OH.

Raskin, N. J., & Rogers, C. R. (1989). Person-centered therapy. In R. J. Corsini & D. Wedding (Eds.), *Current psychotherapies* (4th ed.). Itasca, IL: FE Peacock.

Robbins, A.(1985). Working towards the establishment of creative arts therapies as an independent profession. *The Arts in Psychotherapy, 12,* 67–70.

Rogers, C. R. (1942). *Counseling and psychotherapy.* Boston: Houghton Mifflin.

Rogers, C. R. (1951). *Client-centered therapy; its current practice, implications, and theory.* Boston: Houghton Mifflin.

Rogers, C. R. (1954). *Psychotherapy and personality change.* Chicago: University of Chicago Press.

Rogers, C. R. (1957). The necessary and sufficient condition of therapeutic personality change. *Journal of Consulting Psychology, 21,* 95–103.

Rogers, C. R. (1959). A theory of therapy, personality, and interpersonal relationships, as developed in the client-centered framework. In S. Koch (Ed.), *Psychology: A study of a science, general systematic formulations, learning, and special processes.* New York: McGraw-Hill.

Rogers, C. R. (1961). *On becoming a person.* Boston: Houghton Mifflin.

Rogers, C. R. (1969). *Freedom to learn: A view of what education might become.* Columbus, OH: Charles E. Merrill.

Rogers, C. R. (1970). *Carl Rogers on encounter groups.* New York: Harper & Row.

Rogers, C. R. (1972). *On becoming partners: Marriage and its alternatives.* New York: Delacorte.

Rogers, C. R. (1977). *Carl Rogers on personal power: Inner strength and its revolutionary impact.* New York: Delacorte.

Rogers, C. R. (1986). Client-centered therapy. In I. L. Kutash & A. Wolf (Eds.), *Psychotherapist's casebook: Therapy and technique in practice.* San Francisco: Jossey-Bass.

Rogers, C. R., & Sanford, R. C. (1985). Client-centered psychotherapy. In H. I. Kaplan, B. J. Sadock, & A. M. Friedman (Eds.), *Comprehensive textbook of psychiatry* (4th ed.). Baltimore, MD: Williams & Wilkins.

Rogers, C. R., & Wood, J. (1974). Client-centered theory: Carl Rogers. In A. Burton (Ed.), *Operational theories of personality.* New York: Brunner/Mazel.

Skinner, B. F. (1938). *The behavior of organisms.* New York: Appleton-Century-Crofts.

Skinner, B. F. (1953). *Science and human behavior.* New York: Macmillan.

Standal, S. (1954). *The need for positive regard: A contribution to client-centered theory.* Unpublished doctoral dissertation, University of Chicago, Chicago, IL.

Sullivan, H. S. (1945). *Conceptions of modern psychiatry.* Washington, DC: W. A. White Foundation.

Snygg, D., & Combs, A. W. (1949). *Individual behavior: A new frame of reference for psychology.* New York: Harper & Brothers.

Vaihinger, H. (1925). *The philosophy of "as if."* New York: Harcourt, Brace, & World.

Wolpe, J. (1958). *Psychotherapy by reciprocal inhibition.* Stanford, CA: Stanford University Press.

Yontef, G. M., & Simkin, J. S. (1989). Gestalt therapy. In R. J. Corsini & D. Wedding (Eds.), *Current psychotherapies* (4th ed.). Itasca, IL: FE Peacock.

# 5. Multicultural Considerations in Counseling Communicatively Disordered Persons and Their Families

Dolores E. Battle

Counseling is an educative problem-centered experience occurring between people that allows the expression of feelings and permits and encourages growth in both parties (Luterman, 1991). It is a process designed to help persons work toward an understanding of themselves, reduce depression, anxiety, guilt, anger, and frustration and to learn new ways of coping with and adjusting to life situations (Rollin, 1987). Counseling by speech-language pathologists and audiologists is designed to provide information that allows clients to explore feelings related to communication disorders and their treatment, to help and support clients and their families as they change communication or communication-related behaviors, and to help them make use of the resources available (Stone & Olswang, 1989).

Although most speech-language pathologists and audiologists agree on the importance of counseling, many are uncertain about their role in the counseling process and their ability to incorporate counseling in their work. This uncertainty is increased when they are confronted with the need to provide counseling for culturally and linguistically diverse clients (Stone & Olswang, 1989). Because different cultures have different world views which affect counseling, it is important that speech-language pathologists and audiologists understand the role that culture plays in the counseling process.

According to the 1990 census, the minority population in the United States exceeds 60 million or nearly 25% of the entire population (U.S. Bureau of Census, 1991). Persons with European roots constitute 76.3% of the population and are usually considered the majority. African-Americans constitute nearly 12% of the population; Hispanics nearly 8.6%; Native Americans, including Aluets and Eskimos, 0.75%; and Asian/Pacific Islanders 2.78%.

There has been a rapid increase in the number of persons immigrating to the United States from Central and South American, the Caribbean Basin, Asia, and the Pacific Islands. If the current trends in immigration continue, by the end of the century population increases will be largely due to significant increases in immigrants from a variety of culturally and linguistically diverse countries. The Hispanic population will have increased by 21%, the Asian presence by about 22%, African-Americans by almost 12%, and whites by a little more than 2%. The result will be that the United States will reflect a mosaic of cultural and linguistic diversity, with considerably more diversity than has been present to date. Compounding the difficulty resulting from increased diversity are differences among variables (Wong, 1985; Cheng, 1993), such as:

- migration and relocation history
- degree of assimilation and of acculturation
- facility with the native language and with English as a second language
- family composition and intactness
- amount of education
- degree of adherence to religious and cultural beliefs

The Asian populations alone represent 29 different subgroups that differ in language, religion, and values. Until recently, Japanese-Americans represented the largest group of Asians in the United States. The Chinese and Filipino populations in the United States are rapidly increasing. At the present time over 60% of the Asian immigrants are Chinese. If current immigration trends continue, by 2020 the largest Asian group in the United States will be Filipino (U.S. Bureau of Census, 1991).

Using conservative estimates, 10% of the United States population have communication disorders. The National Health Interview Survey indicates that there is a greater prevalence of communication disorders among racial minorities and economically disadvantaged persons (Benson & Marano, 1994). These populations are more predisposed to disorders related to environmental, teratogenic, nutritional, and traumatic factors than other groups. In addition, although minority persons may have the same types of communication disorders found in the majority population, the causes and effects of the disorders may be different, may be understood differently by clients and families, and thus may indicate different approaches to treatment and different needs for counseling. As contact with persons from other cultures increases, the basic assumptions on which counseling is based will be challenged and techniques modified to reflect the cultural diversity among clients.

This chapter provides information to assist the speech-language pathologist and audiologist in understanding the counseling needs of persons from culturally and linguistically diverse groups and to provide suggestions to improve the delivery of counseling services to these persons and their families.

## MULTICULTURAL COUNSELING

### Race, Ethnicity, and Culture

Race refers to biologic differences and physical characteristics of genetic origin that differentiate one group of people from another. Ethnicity refers to the social or cultural heritage a particular group shares that relates to customs, language, religion, and habits passed from one generation to the next. It does not depend on a biologic or genetic foundation.

Culture refers to all those things that a people have learned to do, believe, value, and enjoy in their history. It is a framework that guides and binds life practices; a shared pattern of learned behavior that is transmitted to others in an ethnic group. These patterns of behavior, whether implicit or explicit, are transmitted by symbols that constitute the distinctive achievements of the historical group. It is the totality of implicit ideas, skills, values, and beliefs; explicit skills, tools, customs, and institutions; and sociopolitical histories that determines a person's cultural identity.

## Cultural Assumptions in Counseling

Multicultural counseling is an attempt to integrate and coordinate majority assumptions with contrasting assumptions of persons from different cultures (Pedersen, 1988). Most literature on counseling is based on cultural assumptions that are relevant to white middle class culture in the United States. Counselors by their training and life experiences generally base their perceptions of the client and the client's problems on assumptions that are relevant to the majority culture. Monocultural assumptions in counseling must be challenged for the following reasons:

1. We do not all share a single measure of "normal" social, cultural, economic, and political behavior. However, behavior described as pathologic in one culture may be viewed as adaptive in another (Wilson & Calhoun, 1974).
2. In European or Western cultures, individuals are the basic building blocks of society. However, in several cultures, such as Middle Eastern, Hispanic, and Asian/Pacific, the family is considered the basic building block of society.
3. Problems are defined by cultural values. Behavior that is considered abnormal or problematic in one culture may be considered acceptable in another. For example, in Japan, children are not considered to be late talkers if they are able to talk before entering kindergarten. In Western societies, parents become concerned if a child is not talking well by 3 years of age. Although African-American and west African cultures have a very high incidence of dysfluency by Western standards, dysfluency is not considered a problem for which one seeks professional services.
4. The meaning of abstract terms such as "good" and "bad" is not universal. Terms have different interpretations depending on the frame of reference of the culture. Behavior such as premarital sex that is considered "bad" in one culture, may be culturally accepted behavior in another. For example, modes of discipline that may be considered as abuse in one culture may be the accepted norm in another.
5. European cultures expect children to develop independence at an early age. However, some non-Western cultures value dependence on members of the family and do not expect or value independence in young children. Value is placed on dependence on the social group or family. For example, Japanese "*amae*" represents the relationship in which the eldest son is preparing for the time when the mother will be dependent on the eldest son. Efforts to develop independence in these cultures will not be readily accepted.
6. Although persons in Western cultures assume that clients are helped more by formal counseling, persons in non-Western cultures feel that the natural support provided by the family or community is sufficient for solving problems.
7. Western cultures assume that persons depend on linear thinking to understand the world. There is the belief that everything has a cause and every cause has an effect. In some non-Western cultures, however, cause and effect are seen as two aspects of the same undifferentiated reality with neither cause nor effect being separate from the other. This is evident in the Chinese concepts of ying/yang.
8. Western cultures assume that individuals need to change to fit the system. In other cultures, it is believed that the system can be changed to fit the individual.

9. Western approaches to counseling assume that sociopolitical history is not relevant for the proper understanding of personal contemporary events. However, cultural history both of the ethnic group and the client's personal life history are important to understanding the client's present behavior. This is especially true when one considers the sociopolitical history of racism related to African-Americans and recent relocation history of immigrants from Central and South America and Southeast Asia.

10. Counselors assume that they know all of their own assumptions. It is not expected that persons are able to express or recognize all personal and cultural assumptions. The cultural assumptions may be so institutionalized that despite the best intentions, counselors may be unaware of and be unable to confront their own personal assumptions, values, and biases that may affect counseling relationships.

## Multicultural Versus Cross-Cultural Counseling

Most literature on multicultural counseling refers to a situation in which the counselor is a member of the majority culture and the client is from any one of a number of minority cultures. More realistically, multicultural counseling is that in which the client and the counselor are from different cultures, regardless of whether one or both are from minority cultures. To that extent, most counseling is multicultural or cross-cultural. The counseling literature focuses on efforts to make the majority counselor familiar with the values of the minority client. However, in a more broad perspective, cross-cultural counseling occurs when the counselor and the client are members of different (*a*) cultures, (*b*) racial or ethnic groups, (*c*) genders, (*d*) sexual orientations, or (*e*) different socioeconomic strata. Using this view, cross-cultural counseling refers to situations in which the counselor is a member of one racial or ethnic group and the client is a member of another group regardless of whether either or both are members of the cultural minority or majority (Atkinson, Morten, & Sue, 1979).

Counseling literature through the 1970s and 1980s was concerned with the importance of same-culture counselor-client relationships. Co-membership in a culture was thought to enhance the counseling relationship because of shared interest, status, and characteristics. Terrell and Terrell (1981, 1984) report that African-Americans may mistrust white counselors and may lack confidence in "white" solutions to their problems. Zitzow and Estes (1981) also report that, dependent on the degree of assimilation, Native Americans may feel uncomfortable dealing with non-Native Americans because of lack of trust developed from the historical sociopolitical treatment of Native Americans in this country.

Culturally different clients often approach counseling with a great deal of suspicion as to the counselor's conscious or unconscious motives in a cross-cultural context. People of African descent are especially reluctant to reveal aspects of their personal lives in cross-cultural counseling because of mistrust brought about by racism in the U.S. society (Terrell & Terrell, 1981; 1984). Native Americans and Hispanics share intimate relationships only with close friends established through prolonged relationships.

Some minority clients resent minority counselors, are jealous of them, and view them as less than competent counselors (Hilliard, 1986). However, in a counterbalanced study (Carhuff & Pierce, 1967) to test the effects of white and African-American counselors on same and different culture clients, there were no significant differences in the perceived outcome of counseling sessions. The African-American clients stated that they would return to the African-American counselor, but none indicated that they would return to the white counselor. White clients made no distinction in preference in counselor or willingness to return to counseling. Preference in culture or race of counselor in this study may have been a preference for a particular style of communication. African-American counselors were described as using more active expressive skills, whereas white counselors were reported to have more genuine empathy with white clients. Mexican-American and white clients attributed more skill, understanding, and trust to white professionals (Carhuff & Pierce, 1967).

## BARRIERS TO EFFECTIVE COUNSELING

Counselors are often culturally encapsulated by measuring reality against their own monocultural assumptions and values and by demonstrating insensitivity or superficial acceptance of cultural variations in clients. Differences in class-bound values, culture-bound values, and language and communication differences between counselor and client are barriers to effective counseling.

## Class-Bound Values

Counseling is usually an activity involving middle class counselors and lower or upper class clients (Sue & Sue, 1990). Persons from lower socioeconomic groups are disproportionately represented among persons from non-Western cultures in the United States. The resulting class differences affect the counseling situation. The ethnic minority reality relates to racism and poverty that dominate the lives of many minorities. Clients who are concerned with the realities of daily existence and survival may not value counseling as a means of solving their problems.

Insight into the nature of problems is an important consideration in counseling. Counselors expect clients to develop insight into the underlying dynamics and causes of their problems. Individuals who are concerned with personal survival may not perceive the development of insight as important to their life situations. Their primary concerns may revolve around employment, child and family care, finances, and survival on a day-to-day basis. They may not feel that taking time to reflect on the nature or cause of problems, will solve their problems. They may prefer immediate tangible solutions to problems without concern for the cause or nature of the problem.

Asians are urged to keep busy and not to think about problems when encountering feelings of frustration, anger, depression, or anxiety. They believe that thinking too much about something can cause problems. Avoidance of morbid thoughts is the road to mental health. The role of insight is lessened when the avoidance of morbid thought is added to concern for survival among lower-class Asians (Lum, 1982).

Social class differences are factors in making and keeping appointments. Clients from lower socioeconomic groups concerned with survival may not keep appointments made weeks in advance. They also may not perceive 50- to 60-minute weekly sessions as consistent with their need to seek immediate solutions to problems.

The level of intervention intensity also varies with socioeconomic status. Hollingshead and Redlich (1968) report that middle class clients remain in treatment longer than lower class clients. Lower socioeconomic minority clients tend to terminate counseling at a rate of greater than 50% after only one contact with the counselor, whereas only 30% of white clients terminate services after only one contact. The higher termination rate of African-American clients is thought to be related to the perception that white counselors are antagonistic and inappropriate to their life experiences, that they lack sensitivity to the circumstances and hardship affecting their lives, and that they may lack an understanding of oppression and racial discrimination (Sue & Sue, 1990).

Sue and Sue (1990) cite a situation which is not uncommon in schools. JJ, a 12-

year-old African-American male was referred for special services because of apathy, indifference, inattentiveness, and inability to follow classroom instruction. Teachers reported that he did not pay attention and fell asleep in class. He was thought to have a problem with attention deficit disorder (ADD) and a language disability. After 6 months of speech therapy it was noted that he came from a home life of extreme poverty, where hunger, lack of sleep, and overcrowding served to diminish his energy and motivation. Behaviors observed were more a result of poverty than ADD or language disability. The goals established for therapy were not consistent with his immediate needs and did not consider the life circumstances that may have contributed to his school performance.

Counselors and clinicians need to consider life circumstances and socioeconomic class values in determining the nature of a disorder and the course of treatment including counseling.

## Culture-Bound Values

Attitudes, beliefs, customs, and cultural institutions affect the counseling relationship. When the cultural values of the client and counselor differ, the counseling relationship and specific techniques used may be affected. Counseling is influenced by the sociocultural framework from which it arises.

### HEALTH AND DISABILITY

Counseling theories are influenced by assumptions that theorists make regarding the goals for counseling, expectations of counselors, expectations of clients, the methodologies used to invoke change, and the culturally determined definitions of health and disability.

Different cultures assign different meanings to disability, health, and wellness. The cultural view of disability and wellness affects the nature of the counseling situation and the expectation of counseling results. For example, the Chamarro view the disabled child as everyone's child and a gift from God. The Chinese, on the other hand, regard a disabled child as a curse brought about by the wrong doings of their ancestors. Neither may be willing to participate in counseling as a part of treatment for a communication disorder.

Westerners or European-Americans seek formal counseling from psychiatrists, psychologists, social workers, ministers, or other professionals. Members of other cultures look to elders, family members, friends, or folk healers for assistance. African-Americans frequently seek assistance from ministers or co-workers. Hispanic-Americans more commonly seek assistance from *Curanderos* or healers, *Espiristas* or *Santerios.* Asian-Americans may seek assistance from herbalists, family and friends, or diviners (Randall-David, 1989).

Native Americans believe that there must be harmony with nature. Rather than seeking to control the environment, Native Americans accept things as they are. A child with a disability may be accepted as nature's intention. Events are a part of the nature of life and one must learn to live with and accept what comes. There may be reluctance to seek assistance, rehabilitation, or counseling that may alter the course of nature.

Cultural differences in perception of health and disability extends to the distinction between physical and mental well-being. Western cultures make a distinction between physical well-being and mental well-being. Medical personnel are sought for medical problems and counselors, psychiatrists, or psychologists are sought for assistance with psychosocial problems. Some non-Western cultures may not make this distinction. They view physical and psychosocial problems as one. They often locate psychological feelings in the physical body, such as headaches, lightheadedness, and other pains.

Asians have difficulty accepting disability. If there is no overt physical disability, as is often the case with communication disorders, the problem may be perceived as willful.

There may be denial that a problem exists. There will be no reason for the person to have intervention or rehabilitation. In some cases, the mother may have a deep sense of failure because she is perceived within the culture to have failed to train her child properly. Disability may be thought to bring shame on the family. The clinician may be in the position of identifying a disability that the parents or family do not understand or recognize and may recommend a treatment that they find unfamiliar or unacceptable.

Some Asians believe the cause of disability is spiritual or moral brought about by the wrong doings of the ancestors. Because the problem is thought to be spiritual, it cannot be cured or corrected by secular means. To the Filipino, for example, illness is due to imbalance in cosmic forces and a lack of will power. A disability is more acceptable if it is expressed as a physical complaint or given a naturalistic explanation such as the mother's failure to follow prescribed dietary practices during pregnancy (Lynch & Hanson, 1992). Such a disability is expected to be managed by physical or medical means that provide concrete, tangible forms of treatment such as medication. If a speech-language or hearing disorder is thought to be related to a physical disorder, a medical specialist will be sought, not a speech-language pathologist or audiologist. If the disorder is thought to be related to a spiritual cause, it will be treated by confession or other forms of consolation. The clients may have limited faith in the counseling process and in talking to a stranger about their disabilities. They may be concerned about the stigma attached to the need for counseling and be less confident that counseling will help. Help for the disabilities may be sought in support groups or from family and friends. Long-term counseling focusing on feelings, attitudes, and beliefs may not be consistent with the culture's view of treatment for disabilities.

## INDIVIDUALISM VERSUS COOPERATION

Counseling has traditionally been conceptualized in Western individualistic terms (Atkinson, Morten, & Sue, 1979; Ivey, 1981,1986). However, the cultural values held by members of different cultures can have a significant effect on their (a) willingness to engage in counseling, (b) expectations of counseling goals, and (c) expectations of their role and responsibility within the counseling relationship. Individualism and competition between individuals for status, recognition, and achievement form the bases of Western tradition. The individual is the building block of the culture. Problems are located within the individual and solutions are based on the individual.

In Asian-American, Hispanic, and African-American cultures, the psychosocial unit of operation is the family, group, or collective society (Sue & Morishima, 1982; Nobles, 1976; Mays, 1985). For example, the Filipino focuses on interdependence rather than personal choice and independence. Their goal in life is to preserve harmony and avoid stress and confrontation among individuals, family members, and groups. Achieving smooth interpersonal relationships may take precedence over clear communication and accomplishing a particular task. They are concerned with appearance before others and are thus intolerant of public criticism or critique of their actions (Gochenour, 1990).

The personal pronoun "I" does not exist in Japanese. The notion of "atman" in India is defined as participating in unity with all things and not being limited by the temporal world. Greetings such as, "How is your family today?" are more common than "How are you today?" In the Samoan language there is no word for "person" because the person is only a part of the whole group.

When the family or group is the basis of psychosocial identity, it is not culturally appropriate for persons to make decisions without consulting the group or family. Issues surrounding the care of a child or disabled family member are considered the responsibility of the family. Interference from persons outside the family or outside the culture may be interpreted as indicating that the family is guilty of severe neglect or mistreatment. Having a problem that requires outside assistance may bring shame on the group or family, rather than only creating guilt for the family member with the problem (Sue & Sue, 1990). If the family or group views the locus of the problem as within society, not within the individual, the development of personal insight will not be highly valued and will be inappropriate for use in counseling.

## TIME ORIENTATION

Western cultures are oriented toward the present and future. Long-term goals and preparation for the future are highly valued. The perception of lessened personal worth in old age or after retirement and an emphasis of youth reflects this value. Many non-Western cultures are focused on the past as shown in their respect for the elderly and ancestors. When persons are present and past oriented, they are less likely to accept the importance of establishing long-term goals or treatments that may produce results in the distant future. In these cases, short-term goals with tangible observable results are more likely to be understood.

## Language Usage and Communication Style Differences

Language usage and communication style are strongly correlated with race, culture, and ethnicity. All cultural groups have unique communication styles that have major implications for counseling. Language usage communication differences affect both nonverbal and verbal communication.

## NONVERBAL COMMUNICATION

Nonverbal communication is information that is transmitted by means other than words. Nonverbal communication conveys feelings, emotions, and intensity of emotions. It adds clarity to verbal communication by inflection, stress, voice tone and intensity, and gestures. Nonverbal communication reveals the general emotional state of the speaker and listener including the degree of comfort or tension in the communication situation. It also reveals specific feelings regarding topics under discussion and the intensity of those feelings (Lane & Molyneaux, 1992).

Nonverbal communication in counseling involves many behaviors including proxemics, kinesics, eye contact, paralanguage, silence, and directness. Nonverbal cues in communication (e.g., eye contact, physical contact, and body language) are rooted in cultural contexts. It is generally believed that 60 to 70% of human communication is nonverbal (Ramsey & Birk, 1983; Condon & Yousef, 1975). Nonverbal aspects of communication operate on an unconscious level of awareness and are therefore not under conscious control.

Nonverbal aspects of communication tend to be more spontaneous and are more difficult to censor and falsify; thus, they are more trusted than words (Wolfgang, 1985). Both Native Americans and African-Americans feel that nonverbal communication is a more accurate barometer of one's true feelings and beliefs than verbal communication (Hall, 1966; Kochman, 1981; Stanback & Pearce, 1985; Weber, 1985). The counselor who does not adequately deal with his or her own biases and attitudes may unwittingly communicate them to the client through nonverbal communication.

Nonverbal communication is used differently by different groups. Western men are usually low keyed, dispassionate, impersonal, and issue oriented in counseling sessions. Some African-American clients may be low-keyed or "play it cool" to hide their true feelings. Counselors unfamiliar with this communication style may interpret low-keyed demeanor as apathy or depression. Other African-Americans may be animated in their communication style. A counselor may misinterpret the client's raising of the voice and animated communication as anger, or irrational, out-of-control behavior when actually a culturally appropriate communication style that is high-keyed, animated, and rhythmic is being used (Hall, 1966; Weber, 1985).

Various nonverbal aspects of communication are classified into three general categories: proxemics, kinesics, and paralanguage. An additional category is chronemics, the use of time in interpersonal communication.

## Proxemics

Proxemics refers to the use and perception of an individual's personal space. Conversational distances are a function of racial and cultural background of the conversants (Susman & Rosenfeld, 1982; Wolfgang, 1985). Hall (1966) defines Western interpersonal distance zones as 0–18 inches for intimate interactions; 1.5–4 feet for general personal interactions; 4–12 feet for social contacts; and more than 12 feet for public interactions. Acceptable distances for various types of communication behavior vary in different cultures. Asians typically prefer to maintain greater conversational distance than Westerners. Hispanics, African-Americans, Indonesians, and Middle Easterners use a closer stance and may touch during conversations (Jensen, 1985). Arabs stand closer, touch each other more, are more likely to face head-on, use more eye contact, and speak louder than do people from Western cultures (Watson & Graves (1966). A counselor who backs away from a client because of a need for greater space may be perceived as aloof, cold, or lacking in the desire to communicate with the client.

Proxemics also applies to the relation between counselor and client in seating arrangements. Whereas Western professionals, particularly European-Americans, prefer a desk or table between them and the client, Latin Americans are not comfortable with this arrangement as they prefer more physical contact with the counselor. Eskimos prefer to sit side-by-side when talking about intimate aspects of their lives. Native Americans consider it rude and intimidating behavior for the counselor to sit directly facing the client (Sue & Sue, 1990).

Placing one's feet on the desk in a counseling setting is often used to indicate a relaxed and informal attitude to North Americans. However, Latin Americans and Asians consider such positioning to be rude and arrogant, especially if the bottoms of the feet are shown. Crossing or stretching one's legs in a group setting is unacceptable to Middle Easterners.

## Kinesics

Kinesics or the meaning of body movements includes such actions as facial expression, smiling, head movements, use of hands, and eye contact. Kinetic behavior is a rich source of information about internal emotive states. Counselors often rely on kinetic cues to assess emotive reactions of their clients to questions or to topics when the client is reluctant to share or acknowledge these reactions verbally.

### Facial Expression

Charles Darwin (1872) described facial expressions and body movements of persons suffering from excess grief. Faces express emotions and indicate the individual's degree of responsiveness to and involvement in counseling.

Kinesics is linked to biologic reaction and learned cultural responses. Ekman, Friesen, and Hess (1984) studied the recognition of emotional states by people from various cultures. They concluded that movements of specific facial muscles during primary emotions such as anger, sadness, happiness and disgust are universal. Schwartz, Fair, Salt, Mandel, and Klerman (1976) studied facial expression in depressed subjects and found that electromyographic patterns of facial muscles could differentiate when subjects were imagining happy versus sad scenes. The universality of expressions of emotion refers to the immediate reaction evidenced in emotion-arousing situations. How the person acts once the emotion has been triggered varies considerably among individuals and among cultures. Facial expressions are more controllable than hands, legs, and the rest of the body (Hansen, Stevic, & Warner, 1982). In Japanese and Chinese cultures, restraint of feeling is a sign of maturity and wisdom. Value placed on control of emotional expression contributes to a demeanor among some Asian groups that is often interpreted by Eurocentric individuals as stoic, flat, enigmatic, or even inscrutable. Koreans, for example, may present with a demeanor referred to as *myu-po-jung* or lack of facial expression. A particular person's way of expressing feelings is likely to be a combined product of cultural tradition and personal conditioning.

## Smiling

Smiling is also a culturally determined nonverbal behavior. Te (1989, p. 54) says that "not all people smile in the same language." In Western cultures, smiling indicates liking or a positive affect. Western counselors consider persons who smile to be intelligent and pleasant (Lau, 1982). In Japanese cultures, however, a smile is a sign of embarrassment, discomfort, and shyness. Outward expression such as smiling is discouraged except in extreme situations (Yamamoto & Kubota, 1983). This lack of smiling may be interpreted as a lack of feeling.

To some Asians, a smile is considered an expression of apology for minor offenses or an expression of deference to an authority figure who scolds a child or criticizes an adult. To others, a smile indicates sincere acknowledgment of fault or a mistake committed and indicates that the person is neither offended nor harbors any ill feeling or resentment toward the interlocutor. Still other Asians consider smiling to be a sign of weakness. Vietnamese often think that North Americans are superficial because they smile too much (Barna, 1985). The people of the Philippines smile when things go wrong and refrain from losing their temper or expressing anger (Guthrie, 1968).

## Head Positioning and Head Nodding

How the head is positioned in conversation also sends nonverbal messages. Lifting the chin while conversing is considered to be poised and polite to Englishmen; however, to North Americans, lifting the chin in conversation is considered a sign of arrogance and snobbery.

Argyle and Dean (1965) note that head nodding plays an important role in communication; nodding the head rapidly reinforces the speaker, gives permission to continue speaking, or requests permission to speak. Shaking the head from side-to-side indicates "no" to North Americans and head nodding indicates "yes." However, Asians generally use repeated head nodding during conversation to indicate deference toward an authority figure and not to indicate agreement or disagreement.

## Shaking Hands and Sticking Out the Tongue

The manner of shaking hands is also culturally rooted. Latin Americans frequently shake hands more vigorously and for longer periods than do North Americans. Offering to shake the left hand or offering something in the left hand is considered an insult to Middle Eastern Moslems. Placing a hand on an Egyptian woman's left shoulder has connotations regarding pregnancy. In the Laotian culture, it is acceptable for men to shake hands in greeting one another but women do not shake hands.

Sticking out the tongue also has different meaning across cultures. In the Sung dynasty in China sticking out the tongue was a mark of terror and ridicule. To the Ovimbundu of Africa, sticking out the tongue indicates that you are a fool; Mayan statues of the gods sticking out the tongue indicates wisdom. However, in North America sticking out the tongue indicates a quasi-obscene gesture of defiance, mockery or contempt (Sue & Sue, 1990).

### Eye Contact

Among the more important aspects of kinesics is eye gaze or eye contact. Much has been written about the importance of eye contact in interpersonal communication in Western cultures. There is considerable cultural variation in the use of eye contact. Although North Americans make eye contact 80% of the time when listening, they tend to look away about 50% of the time when speaking to others. African-Americans, on the other hand, make infrequent eye contact when listening and make greater eye contact when speaking. Argyle and Dean (1965) report that the amount of looking is a signal for intimacy in Western cultures. Averting the eyes or looking away can signal lack of interest. Prolonged looking between sexes can be described as harassment or leering.

In Asian/Pacific Island cultures nonverbal "reading the eyes" takes precedence over verbal communication. The Chinese examine the face and observe the overall expression (Cheng, 1993). They feel that the eyes are windows to the person's emotional state and are private; eye contact is avoided.

Among Asian/Pacific Islanders, direct or sustained eye contact with relative strangers is interpreted as a sign of hostility and is considered impolite or shameful. Similarly, direct eye contact with an elder, an authority figure, or a family member of higher status is considered disrespectful. Asians consider direct eye contact rude and an invasion of privacy. Asians generally use repeated head nodding, avoidance of direct eye contact, and minimal verbalization as a way of showing deference toward an authority figure.

Respect is highly valued among Native Americans. Eye contact between Native American children and elders indicates a lack of respect, defiance, or rudeness. To signify respect for another person, especially an elder, Native Americans avoid eye contact by looking down. They are taught to "see" without looking directly at someone (Clarke & Kelly, 1992).

Among persons from the Middle East, lack of eye contact between men and women during conversations is expected to maintain respect and proper distance between genders (Sasson, 1992). Eye contact between a man and woman is believed to have sexual connotations.

### Paralanguage

Paralanguage refers to all things that can be done with speech and voice to communicate meaning, other than making words, such as pitch changes, inflections, varying rate, silence or pauses, loudness, and inflection. Paralinguistic factors can provide clues to personality characteristics, mental illness, group membership, and status within a group. Paralinguistic factors can provide information about a speaker's emotive state. There is a wide variation in the use of paralinguistic features across cultures.

### Silence

Silence, pause, and hesitation are important components of any therapeutic relationship. Silence is more than just the absence of speech. It is a culturally rooted practice that can indicate respect, or thoughtful consideration of or agreement with what was just spoken. North Americans feel uncomfortable with pauses or silent stretches in communication. They believe that long pauses or periods of silence in conversations indicate tension or reluctance to respond. To Middle Easterners, silence during conversations allows individuals periods of personal privacy. "Tuning out" in conversations is quite accepted and valued. Filling in the silence is not desired or expected. To the Russians, French, and Spanish, silent periods during conversation indicate agreement among the parties (Hall, 1976).

To Asians silence indicates respect for elders and is a sign of politeness. The relative importance of silence in Asian cultures is shown in proverbs such as, "Keep your mouth shut and your eyes open," and "He who knows, talks not; he who talks, knows not." Silence is a primary control strategy among some Chinese. A typical practice is to refuse to speak any further when unable to accept the speaker's attitude, opinion, or way of thinking about particular issues or subjects.

Native Americans also use silence as an indicator of respect for elders. Silence is used to prevent discord and disharmony and to indicate agreement with suggestions of elders, even though the young listeners may not follow through with those suggestions.

Generally speaking, silence can serve as an expression of interest and respect, but if silence follows consistent verbal responses and verbal acknowledgment it may indicate disagreement or negative emotional reactions such as anger (i.e., the silent treatment). This can greatly affect the client-clinician interaction in the counseling situation.

### Loudness

As with silence, speaking voice volume is a cultural phenomenon. Asians tend to speak more softly than do persons from other cultures. Use of lower volume is not a sign of weakness, shyness, or depression. On the other hand, persons in Middle Eastern, African-American, and Hispanic cultures prefer to be bathed in sound, preferring louder volume in both speaking and music (Lynch & Hansen, 1992).

### Inflection or Vocal Stress

Vocal inflection or stress that accompanies a speaker's words often gives clues to how the words are to be interpreted. The speaker indicates feelings by saying, "It was very upsetting," with emphasis on the word "very." The same utterance pronounced with a rising inflection, "It was very upsetting?," indicates that a question about someone else's feelings has been asked. As with facial expression, personal circumstances or cultural variables can affect the use of inflection in verbal language. Persons who are having difficulty with verbal expression may not stress words that reflect their feelings. Also, interpreters or translators may not include subtle changes in stress that reveal the emotive state of the speaker.

### Chronemics or Time Orientation

Time or the amount of time a person is willing to commit to a situation sends a nonverbal message. Cultural differences in orientation to time concepts can affect counseling. Western cultures are oriented to the future with a focus on the youth as hope for a better future. There is an understanding that the hope for the future lies in the youth so an emphasis is placed on development of the youth and equipping them for their lives as adults. There is a devaluing of personal worth in old age or following retirement. On the other hand, Asians value the past with focus on ancestors and the wisdom of the elderly.

Native Americans and African-Americans have a present time orientation with a focus on the here-and-now. They seek immediate concrete solutions to problems rather than abstract goals to be reached sometime in the future. They may not understand the importance of activities undertaken in the immediate or short-term that do not have an immediate, observable result.

Punctuality or planning for the future may not be important and long-term planning is not valued among many Native Americans. Things get done according to a rational order or rhythmic or circular pattern marking time with the months, seasons, or years not according to deadlines (Ho, 1987). It may be difficult for Native Americans to develop long-term goals and to understand the importance of developing skills that will be useful in the future. Developmental milestones may not be marked by motor development, but by when the child has tribal rituals such as the naming ceremony, the "first laugh," or the puberty ceremony (Joe & Malach, 1992).

Cultural differences in time orientation are also reflected when clinicians attempt to establish timeliness for appointments. Hispanics, who are more present oriented, mark time by events rather than by the clock. They are more likely to agree to appointment times that are related to important family events, such as "after I pick up the children," rather than a strict time (e.g., at 2:30). Vocabulary can also reflect the relative values of time in a culture. For example, in English "a clock runs," but in Spanish, "a clock walks."

## VERBAL COMMUNICATION

Verbal communication is accomplished by what we know as language with words. The components of verbal communication can influence the counseling interaction with culturally and linguistically diverse persons with communication disorders. Verbal communication can be reduced both by the nature of the communication disorder or by the influence of limited English or bilingualism.

If a client's phonology is influenced by a nonstandard English dialect or by the influence of a second language such that the client's speech is less intelligible, the level of comfort in the communication environment is reduced.

If use of syntax or sentences is difficult, the client may use short sentences. If the client has difficulty using complex sentences with dependent clauses, the relative meaning of clauses may be confused. For example, the client may not use "because," "since," or "however" to express or understand causal relationships. The counselor may use sentences of such length and complexity that the client may be unable to process them appropriately.

Difficulty with meanings of words or semantics, limited vocabulary, and cultural variation in subtle word meanings may lead to difficulty in expression and understanding. The client's vocabulary may be such that the words used by the counselor do not convey the intended meaning to the client. For example, the counselor may use the term "mother" to refer to a specific female biologic parent. The client may understand the term to refer to a foster parent or the current caretaker. One client may use the term "mother" to refer to a gentle, loving elder whereas another may use the term to refer to a tired, overworked, shrew. Meanings of synonyms and double meaning words such as "hot" and "bad," and figurative language including idioms and metaphors can also be misinterpreted in cross-cultural verbal interactions. Failure to understand imagery, analogies, and nuances of cultural sayings may render the counselor ineffective in establishing relationships and building credibility.

Pragmatics concerns how language is used in different environments to serve the user's purpose. It involves those aspects of communication that are larger than linguistic word and sentence units. Pragmatic variables vary across cultures. Differences in the use of language have significant impact on the counseling relationship. They may render the client and counselor unable to understand the nuances and subtleties of each others' language and to express and describe feelings and problems, making rapport building difficult. Differences in the use of the more ritualized sociolinguistic rules, such as accepting compliments and greeting and taking leave phrases, may lead to communication barriers and may affect the counseling relationship. The ways in which clients acknowledge agreement or disagreement, role status in who may initiate or start a conversation, and how one responds to others are culturally determined. Every culture has conversational topics that are acceptable and others that are taboo in certain circumstances. For example, in Saudi Arabian culture, it is inappropriate to ask questions about the women of a family. In the U. S. culture is considered polite to ask about the well-being of a person's spouse.

Social Status or Roles in Communication Patterns

Counselors expect clients to exhibit openness, verbalize emotions, and express insight into their personal problems. Understanding cultural variation in communication styles and patterns is indispensable for speech-language pathologists and audiologists who work with culturally and linguistically different clients.

Verbal behavior patterns are culturally determined. Western patterns of verbal behavior are horizontal with persons having equal responsibility and freedom within the communication exchange regardless of status. Role status lines are not clearly defined. Children are encouraged to speak freely to elders as well as to their social peers. In non-Western cultures patterns of communication tend to be vertical, flowing from those of higher prestige and status to those of lower (Sue & Sue, 1990). For example, Native Americans, Asian-Americans, and Hispanic children are taught not to speak until spoken to by their elders and to respond minimally.

Non-Western clients respect the counselor as wiser and as occupying a higher status than they and they expect the counselor to be authoritarian, direct, and active in the relationship (Henkin, 1985; Mau & Jepson, 1988). They may respond to inquiry with short phrases or statements. For example, when African-American clients are expected to communicate their feelings in standard English, they may use shorter, incomplete sentences with less grammatical elaboration and a heavier reliance on nonverbal cues (Mays, 1985). A client's brief or limited verbal expression may lead counselors to impute inaccurate characteristics or motives to the client. A client may be seen as uncooperative, sullen, negative, nonverbal, repressed, or having limited verbal ability on the basis of limited language expression alone. If clients are encouraged to express themselves in their native language or to use their cultural communication style, they may be more open to counseling.

Direct Versus Indirect Communication Style

Cultural values can affect particular aspects of communication in the counseling situation. The use of direct versus indirect communication style is an important factor in counseling interactions. Direct statements and direct suggestions for changing behavior may not be accepted by persons who prefer to use an indirect style. The preference for indirect expression may have an impact on the counselor's interpretation of the client's intent.

Western families prefer to express themselves and to deal with problems directly. Asians and other non-Western cultures often prefer to use an indirect communication style to deal with problems, accommodate the will of others, create harmony, and avoid conflict. For example, a Western client may make a statement such as, "Why don't you turn off the television," or the less direct, "You'll be grounded unless you turn off that television." An Asian client may use an indirect expression to accomplish the same task, "Looks like a boring program," or "I think your friend must be doing his homework now."

Persons in Western and European cultures are very direct in their response to questions. However, persons in other cultures communicate their preferences very indirectly and rely on the listener to understand the intended meaning. For example, to persons with

Middle Eastern roots, a direct "no" is considered impolite and may lead to confrontation. To avoid conflict with professional recommendations and give the impression of agreement, the client may use a weak "yes" instead of saying "no" or "that won't work." A weak "yes," "maybe," or "perhaps" either takes the place of "no" or may mean agreement (Sharifzadeh, 1992). Middle Easterners may use "thank you" or "it's fine" to mean "yes."

Asians usually do not say "no" directly. Direct disagreement is considered confrontational and a threat to the harmony of the group. To the Japanese, a direct "no" is considered offensive and insulting. The Vietnamese use "yes" as polite acknowledgment of a question, rather than as agreement. It may be used because the client believes that this is the desired response or because the client does not wish to appear rude or confrontational.

Asian, Native American, and Hispanic clients consider directness in communication to be immature, rude, and lacking in finesse. The Japanese are baffled by Western attitudes toward formalities, insensitivity to status, embarrassing critical remarks, prying questions, unnatural physical intimacy, predilection for premature decisions, and endless conversations. On the other hand, Westerners consider indirect, evasive statements to be baffling (Barlund, 1975). The confusion that direct communicators may experience as they try to sort out what is actually intended by indirect communication may require a cultural mediator's skill until they are familiar enough with a client's communication style.

Verbal self-disclosure, the willingness to express feelings both verbally and behaviorally, is considered necessary for effective counseling. In some Chinese and Japanese cultures emotional restraint is highly valued. Hispanic and Asian cultures emphasize that maturity and wisdom are associated with one's ability to control emotion and feeling. Persons in cultures that value emotional restraint may be reluctant to engage in self-disclosure. Also, Native Americans or clients from lower socioeconomic groups often resist attempts at self-disclosure, preferring to ascribe their problems to forces beyond their control. If, because of cultural values, the client is reluctant to verbally self-disclose, the counselor may deem the counseling ineffective.

## COUNSELING BILINGUALS AND LIMITED ENGLISH PROFICIENT CLIENTS

Persons participating in counseling may have limited verbal ability because of a communication disorder. The communication disorder itself may limit the client's ability to understand and express abstract concepts and feelings. When difficulties in language coexist with bilingualism, the problems incumbent in multicultural counseling are multiplied.

Counseling techniques that heavily rely on verbal interaction to build rapport and express ideas presuppose that the participants are capable of expressing their ideas and understanding each other. In counseling, abstract concepts and values are often discussed. If the client has difficulty understanding or expressing complex abstract ideas and feelings in the language of the counselor, the counseling relationship will be affected.

Communication disorders or limited English proficiency may have significant impact on the counseling relationship. Reliance on verbal interaction to build rapport presupposes that the participants in the counseling dialogue are capable of understanding each other. A client who has difficulty with English, either because of limited English proficiency, bilingualism, or a communication disorder, is less able to express abstract feelings and concerns and less able to understand the counselor's advice.

According to the 1990 Census (U.S. Bureau of Census, 1991), 32 million or 13% of the people in the United States speak a language other than English at home. There are many more who do not speak English well. At minimal estimates, 10% of these persons have a communication disorder and may need to be involved in counseling to help them understand or treat the disorder.

Bilingualism refers to language proficiency in two languages. Balanced bilingualism is exemplified by a speaker who has attained an equal level of proficiency in one or more languages. The true balanced bilingual is equally able to express abstract concepts in both formal and informal settings. Nonbalanced bilingualism is far more usual. Nonbalanced bilingualism exists when the person has a higher level of proficiency in one language than in another across the areas of speaking, listening, reading, and writing. What is more usual is that the bilingual person has mixed dominance in that he or she is dominant in one particular skill or language in one setting and dominant in another skill in another setting. Speaking ability may be better in one language, but listening ability equal in both.

Cummins (1984) refers to differences between basic interpersonal communication skills (BICS) and cognitive academic language proficiency (CALP). Persons who have basic interpersonal communication skills communicate adequately during informal communication interactions where there is a high level of sensory-motor images and weaker cognitive demands. They do not necessarily have the language proficiency to function in de-contextualized situations or situations that require expression of more abstract reasoning as may be required in counseling. For example, although there are 87 mutually intelligible languages and dialects in the Philippines, including Tagalog, Ilicano, Cebuano, Visayan, and Pampango, English is the official unifying language. English is the language of education, commerce, law, government, and entertainment. However, many Filipinos do not speak English at home and have little daily experience with the English language. Philippine-English is a mixture of indigenous language elements, and various dialects, intonations, vocabulary items, and syntax (Santos, 1983). Often because of perceived basic conversational fluency in English, it is assumed that Filipino comprehension of more abstract English is extensive. Although it may appear that Filipinos understand and express themselves in English, the influence of various dialects often renders questionable their level of comprehension of more abstract concepts necessary for counseling in English.

Most speech-language pathologists and audiologists are monolingual. Fewer than 1% of the members of the American Speech-Language Hearing Association are able to provide speech-language or hearing services in a language other than English. This implies that most speech-language pathologists and audiologists providing counseling to culturally and linguistically diverse persons with communication disorders are monolingual. These clinicians may have difficulty understanding the language of their clients or have difficulty expressing concepts in ways that are comprehensible to them. This may lead to misunderstanding of a client's feelings and attitudes and in turn lead to inappropriate suggestions for solutions to problems.

The bilingual or limited English proficient client may have difficulty expressing abstract concepts or feelings in the language of the counselor and thus may not be able to fully describe or express feelings. These clients may have difficulty distinguishing between literal and figurative meaning or intent in communicative acts. The subtleties of language may lead to misunderstandings in expressing concepts in the language of the client versus the language of the counselor in the counseling relationship. These subtleties may force the client to assume ways of thinking about personal behavior that are contrary to cultural values. For example, the client may use "can't" when the intended meaning is "I chose not to" (i.e., "I can't change my speech"). "Should" or "ought to" may be used instead of "want to" ("I should use my new voice"); "have to" may be used instead of "choose to" ("I have to stay home").

Differences in the use of language may mislead the counselor as to the client's intent or vice versa. The client may not understand the ideas expressed by the counselor and thus may respond in a way that does not match the intent of the counselor. Questions such as, "Do you have any ideas about how to encourage more communication?" may be answered literally with "no" rather than by responding to the intent of the message, which may be to provide some suggestions.

## Using Interpreters in Counseling

Differences in language and culture between counselor and client may be addressed by using a cultural mediator, translator, or interpreter. Translators provide literal translation of words. However, translation may lead to miscommunication in counseling. For example, in some Native American languages the term for hearing loss is translated "without ears" because there is no equivalent word for hearing loss.

Interpreters provide a communication of the message rather than a literal translation of the words alone. The use of interpreters with persons who have limited English proficiency in counseling has many potential problems. The client may not be willing to express personal information to a member of his or her community who serves as the interpreter. Unless the interpreter is properly trained, there may be omissions or distortions in the intended message of the counselor. The interpreter who may have some limitations in the language of the counselor or that of the client may not accurately express the meaning of words and abstract concepts being expressed and may omit significant detail because of not perceiving the detail to be important. The interpreter may elaborate or editorialize the comments or fail to explain a concept accurately. Because the interpreter may not fully understand the concepts being expressed he or she may make an error or misunderstand the intent of the client or counselor. There may be confusion about words or terms and incorrect references, which lead to inappropriate responses and comments. In addition, many interpreters have unequal skill in both languages and may fail to interpret nonverbal messages from facial expression, gestures, and other factors in paralanguage.

In some cases, in spite of the many limitations, it may be necessary to work with an interpreter. In these cases there are three basic steps—briefing, interaction, and debriefing—that should be taken to minimize difficulties (Medina, 1982). The counselor and the interpreter should meet prior to the counseling session to (a) learn proper protocols and forms of address, (b) review the general purpose of the session, (c) describe respective roles, (d) discuss the areas that are likely to be covered, and (e) remind the interpreter to interpret accurately both verbal and nonverbal messages. Special terminology that may be used should be explained so that it can be used accurately during the exchanges. During the actual session, the counselor should speak clearly and somewhat more slowly in a calm and unhurried manner addressing remarks and questions directly to the client or family. The counselor should look at and listen to family members and observe their nonverbal communication while they are speaking. The counselor should avoid using nonverbal communication that may be misunderstood by the client and should use a positive tone of voice and facial expression that sincerely conveys respect and interest in the client. The counselor should limit remarks and questions to a few sentences between translations, avoid giving too much information or discussing too many complex or abstract topics in a single session, and avoid technical jargon, colloquialism, idioms, slang, and abstractions. However, oversimplifying and condensing important explanations should also be avoided. Time should be allowed for the interpreter to interpret as immediately and accurately as possible. If it is not possible to interpret the intent of the message accurately, the interpreter should explain this to the counselor. There should be periodic checks on the family's understanding and accuracy of the translation by asking the client or family to repeat in their own words instructions or explanations of whatever has been communicated, with the interpreter facilitating. When possible, verbal information should be reinforced with materials written in the family's language and with visual aids or behavior modeling, if appropriate. Following the session, the counselor and the interpreter should discuss general observations and review the pertinent aspects of the session to be certain that both counselor and client have a mutual understanding of what has occurred (Lynch & Hanson, 1992).

## CROSS-CULTURAL FAMILY COUNSELING

### Nature of Families

There are conflicting value systems about the nature of families across cultures. The nuclear family, which is common among Western cultures, involves the parents and siblings in one family unit. However, definitions of the Western family are changing. Blended families from second and third marriages and living units of unmarried adults, same-gender adults, single-parent families, grandparent custodians, stepparents, foster parents, and guardian relationships have re-defined the meaning of family in today's Western societies. The extended family, which is more common among non-Western cultures, may include relatives, friends, preachers, boyfriends, and other persons. Counselors must be aware of the various configurations of families and accept the unit that is presented without value judgment.

Western families place greater value on the individual and on individual achievement. Almost all non-Western families place greater value on families' historical lineages, ancestors, interdependence among family members, and submergence of self for the good of the family (Kim, 1985; Yamamoto & Kubota, 1983). The Native American family is structurally open and assumes villagelike characteristics (Red Horse, 1983). In Middle Eastern families, the extended family is most important with as many as three generations living in the same household (Scharifzadeh, 1992).

The roles of members within the family vary across cultures. In Hispanic families there is the extended family with attendant sex roles. *Machismo* exists in Mexican and Puerto Rican families in which the oldest male is head of the family, is dominant in the household, and has greater authority than any female. Male children are given independence at younger ages than females. There is unwavering love for the mother who serves as a unifying factor in the family. Formalized kinship relationships such as *compadrazgo* or "godfathers" exist in which loyalty to the family takes precedence over other social systems (Kayser, 1993).

In Asian families there is strict adherence to hierarchal role status with unquestionable obedience to the authority of the elders and males. In African-American and Filipino families obedience is highly valued; however, the roles of males and females are more egalitarian with each parent using compromise and mutual respect to maintain smooth interpersonal relationships with the children.

Customs, language, and type of family structure vary across the 530 heterogeneous Native American nations, 478 of which are recognized by the U. S. government. This includes the 200 Alaskan native villages and the 280 tribes that have a land base or reservation. Approximately 50% of Native Americans live on reservations with the remainder living in urban areas with varying degrees of acculturation. Although there is great variation among Native Americans, it is generally held that for most, family and group have precedence over the individual (Everett, Proctor, & Cortmell, 1983; Wise & Miller, 1983).

Among Native Americans, the tribe is the most important social unit. This extended family is the basic unit, with individuals being extensions of the tribe and having strong respect for the wisdom and knowledge of their elders. All children belong to the tribal family and cannot be reared or adopted by nontribal members without the permission of the tribal leaders. Children are often raised by relatives (e.g., aunts, uncles, cousins, and grandparents) who may live in separate households. Nearly 90% of Native American grandparents are involved with their grandchildren on a daily basis, although they may live in separate homes. It is not uncommon for children to move frequently between the homes of relatives, depending on who is best equipped to care for the child at a given time. Differences in family structure and relationships can significantly affect the role and expectations of the family in counseling.

## Goals of Family Counseling

The goal of family counseling is to modify relationships within the family to achieve harmony (Foley, 1984). Application of family counseling to speech-language pathology and audiology is based on the assumptions that (*a*) it is logical to involve in counseling all persons in the family who operate within the communication system of the client; (*b*) that the communication problems of a client affect communication within the family (i.e., the family is the client); and (*c*) that the task of the speech-language pathologist or audiologist is to modify and improve relationships within the family to facilitate the development of communication for the client.

Depending on their cultural value system, families differ in their understanding of the goals of family counseling. Some culturally and linguistically diverse families enter into counseling to address problems of the client—not problems in the family. Attempts to focus directly on family dynamics as contributing to the client's problem may be met with negativism and possible termination. For many culturally and linguistically diverse families, counseling and parent conferences are unfamiliar experiences for which they have no frame of reference. Their previous experience with counseling may have been negative. They may have been made to feel that they are at fault for any problems that the child has or they may have mistrusted the motivation of the counselor.

Counselors often expect clients to discuss intimate aspects of lives or relationships within the family. Intimate evaluations of personal or social problems reflect on the entire family. Asians (Sue & Sue, 1990), Hispanics (Laval, Gomez & Ruiz, 1983) and Native-American clients, therefore do not reveal personal matters to persons outside the family (Everett, Proctor, & Cortmell., 1983). Counselors should take care not to violate the family's understanding of counseling and their expected role in the treatment of the communication disorder of the client. Any discussion of problems and intrafamily dynamics should directly relate to the communication disorder and the role that the family can directly play in helping the client to develop appropriate communication.

## Roles of Members Within Families

In some cultures the seat of problems is often thought to lie within the family rather than within the individual. Because internal relationships within families differ across cultures, the internal structure of family counseling differs cross-culturally. The roles of family members, the person's ability to make decisions independent of the family, and the willingness of persons to express feelings or reveal information about the family vary across cultures and play important roles in family counseling with culturally and linguistically diverse clients. For example, in some Native American tribes families may seek the advice of elders and participate in tribal ceremony to protect the child and family before seeking professional assistance (Joe & Malach, 1992). If the elders do not see the need, intervention will not be supported by the extended tribal family even when the mother wants it and does not agree with the elders' decision. Decisions for intervention need to be supported by the extended family with the blessing of the tribal healer or elders before professional intervention can be obtained.

It is extremely difficult to be specific about applying cross-cultural strategies and techniques in minority families because of the great variation not only among Asian-Americans,

African-Americans, Hispanics, and Native Americans and white North Americans, there are large variations within the groups themselves. Asian-Pacific cultures include at least 32 distinct subgroups. In addition, many families are bicultural or multicultural in their cultural value systems. For example, Filipinos with a Western orientation may have many traditional Asian beliefs, values, and practices, as well as many Western religious and Euro-Christian ethics. Native Hawaiians may have an Asian view of the extended family, both traditional and Christian religious beliefs; and may use both traditional and Western medicine and both English and traditional language.

Counselors need to understand differences among various cultural groups including differences in family structure, parent-child relationships, and spousal relationships. They need to understand the help-giving structures in the community that may be more acceptable to the family as sources of counseling. Regardless of cultural background, the family can be best engaged in counseling and therapy in supportive roles by (a) asserting that the client's problem is indeed a problem not only for the individual, but also for the family; (b) recognizing and reinforcing the family's concern to help change the client's behavior; and (c) emphasizing that each family member's contribution is needed to resolve the problem and, without it, the problem either will remain or get worse bringing on further difficulty within the family (Kim, 1985).

The ability to enter into a counseling relationship with family members goes well beyond the use of interviewing skills, to both education and the creation of communication-enhancing relationships. Family-centered counseling may focus on improving communication and relationships among family members or it may focus on the interlocking roles of family members, in the process of structuring and restructuring the family communication systems.

## STRATEGIES FOR COUNSELING CULTURALLY AND LINGUISTICALLY DIVERSE CLIENTS WITH COMMUNICATION DISORDERS

1. Be formal and status conscious by adopting the role of an authority figure. Use formal introductions made with correct titles. Do not encourage the use of first names as this confuses many clients about status and reduces the status of the counselor in the eyes of the client. Greet clients as soon as they arrive, extending your hand and introducing yourself by your full name and title.
2. Learn the correct pronunciation of the client's name and the appropriate honorific title and use them. Do not attempt to use nicknames or to shorten the name used by the client. Many cultures address persons by their honorific title long after personalized and informal relationships have been established.
3. Allow the development of rapport and a trusting working relationship at the beginning of counseling as culturally appropriate. Many families may be reluctant to participate in counseling as they feel uncomfortable and inadequate in an environment in which they may already feel disenfranchised. This feeling may be increased if there is a language barrier in addition to cultural differences. Allowing the client time to finish statements and thoughts, speaking slowly and clearly to the client, and not interrupting the client facilitate the development of rapport and help to reduce cultural and linguistic barriers.
4. Identify the client's expectations in the counseling situation. Remember, the expectations of the client may be different from those of the counselor.
5. Explain the counseling process—how it will be useful to the client and how it will be useful in addressing the client's immediate needs. Explain the roles and responsibilities of each person in the counseling relationship.
6. Assure the client of confidentiality. Explain the limits of the information that will be shared with others, with the client's permission, and why it is necessary to share the in-

formation with specific others. Be aware that there may be a stigma or cultural taboo against sharing personal information outside the immediate family.

7. Acknowledge the concern that the client may have in dealing with a person who does not share his or her culture or language. Assure clients that every effort will be made to understand the problem as it relates to them and ask their assistance in helping to understand areas that may result in cultural conflict.

8. Obtain information on the family and household and on the roles of individuals within the family and household in relation to the client. Use restraint in gathering information being careful not to ask questions that are not directly related to the perceived problem. Asking for childhood or other histories should be done judiciously and only if a direct connection can be made to the perceived problem.

9. Use indirect approaches to taking the histories rather than by asking direct questions. Using indirect approaches does not require the client to reveal embarrassing or personal information. If the counselor is interested in possible emotional trauma that may be contributing to the problem, a general inquiry about the family's immigration and resettlement may be appropriate, allowing the client to reveal only that information with which he or she is comfortable revealing.

10. Expect differences in the client's willingness and ability to express concerns verbally. Many clients are not socialized to express inner thoughts and feelings. Emotional inhibition and lower verbal participation may indicate the need for a more direct active approach on the part of the counselor. However, person-centered counseling combined with behavioral techniques may be effective depending on the individual client. Clinician qualities and behaviors, such as respect and acceptance of the client and his or her values, unconditional positive regard for the client, allowing the client to explore personal feelings, and helping the client arrive at his or her solution are core counseling attributes that transcend culture.

11. Identify strengths within the family and resources within the community that may provide support for the client with the problem. For example, Native American clients may be unfamiliar with resources in a non–Native-American community and may be reluctant to seek services from non–Native Americans (Sue & Sue, 1990).

12. Determine the client's view both of the problem and its possible outcome in therapy or counseling.

13. Establish mutually agreed-on specific short-term goals that will make an observable, tangible difference in the immediate future. Reaching consensus on the expectations of counseling should be viewed as the first step toward acceptance of recommendations.

14. Make initial appointments immediately and schedule follow-up appointments as soon as possible. Discuss the approximate number of sessions and establish a mutually agreed-on timetable for reaching the goals. The number of sessions should be limited and scheduled within a short time period. The client may not understand the importance of sessions that are scheduled once a week for 3–60 minutes. In addition, individual sessions should be short, allowing sufficient time for the development of rapport but not permitting long sedentary discussions which may not be tolerated by the client.

15. Establish mutually agreed-on active means to reach the goals and solve specific problems. The counselor may have to take a more active directive role in counseling rather than to expect the client to participate in nondirective introspective techniques.

16. Recommendation decisions should take into account the financial needs and resources of the families as well as being relevant to their "real life" situation.

17. Because of the involvement of the family, counseling may be more effective and more productive in the home or with group or family counseling. Ask the parents or client

who they want to be included in the counseling sessions, especially during home visits. If doing home or family counseling, address comments to the entire group, not just to the client or parent, thus showing respect to the entire family.

## BECOMING A CULTURALLY COMPETENT COUNSELOR

When there is a cultural difference between the client and the counselor, there is significant potential for cultural conflict in the clinic or counseling situation. The sources of this conflict are cultural values, class values, and communication barriers. Given an awareness of these sources of potential conflict, counselors should be proactive in their attempts to become culturally competent. They should develop an understanding and awareness of multicultural beliefs and attitudes, a knowledge and comprehension of cultures, and skill in interaction with persons from other cultures. A culturally competent counselor seeks continuous self-assessment regarding cultural differences, knowledge, and resources to be competent to practice in a multicultural world.

### Develop an Awareness of Beliefs and Attitudes

Multicultural awareness is not an end in itself, but rather it is a means of increasing a person's power, energy, and freedom of choice in a multicultural world (Pedersen, 1988). Counselors should move from being culturally unaware to being aware and sensitive to their own cultural heritage; they need to understand how their own values and biases affect others before they can adjust to the value systems of others. They should understand and value the differences that may exist among clients and should develop an awareness of topics, techniques, questions, and responses which can be changed and modified to be correct for each culture. In developing an awareness of beliefs and attitudes, the counselor should recognize the need to deliver quality services and seek to improve them. The counselor should ask, "What can I do to serve this client in a culturally appropriate manner?" This approach applies both to multicultural clinicians who have been trained in the dominant society's frame of reference and to mainstream clinicians.

### Develop Knowledge of the Particular Culture

Counselors should develop an understanding of the sociopolitical systems operating in the United States with respect to the treatment of the culturally and linguistically diverse, as well as specific knowledge and information about the particular group with which they are working. This knowledge should include clear and explicit understanding of the institutional barriers that operate on the particular group so that there can be an understanding of the client's interaction in the counseling situation.

### Develop Skill in Interacting with Persons from the Particular Culture

Skill in interacting with a client from a different culture includes having the ability to generate a wide variety of verbal and nonverbal responses that are appropriate to a specific culture. Counselors should be able to send and receive both verbal and nonverbal messages accurately and appropriately in each culturally different context. They should be able to use institutional intervention skills on behalf of the clients as appropriate to each cultural context.

REFERENCES

Argyle, M., & Dean, J. (1965). Eye contact, distance and affiliation. *Sociometry, 28,* 32–49.
Atkinson D. R., Morten, G., & Sue D. W. (1979). *Counseling American minorities.* Dubuque, Iowa: Wm. Brown & Co, Publishers.
Barlund, D. C. (1975). *Public and private self in Japan and the United States.* Tokyo: Simul Press.

Barna, L. M. (1985). Stumbling blocks in intercultural communication. In Samovar, L. A., & Porter, B. E. (Eds.), *Intercultural communication: A reader* (4th ed). Belmont, CA: Wadsworth Publishing.

Benson, V., & Marano, M. A. (1995). Current estimates from the National Health Interview Survey, 1993. *Vital and Health Statistics Series 10*(190). Hyattsville, MD: National Center for Health Statistics.

Boyd-Franklin, N. (1989). *Black families in therapy: A multisystems approach.* New York: Guilford Press.

Carhuff, R. R., & Pierce, R. (1967). Differential effects of therapist race and social class upon patient depth of self-exploration in the initial clinical interview. *Journal of Consulting Psychology, 32,* 632–634.

Cheng, L. L. (1993). Asian-American cultures. In Battle, D. E. (Ed.), *Communication disorders in multicultural populations* (pp. 38–77). Stoneham, MA: Butterworth-Heinemann.

Clarke, S., & Kelly, S. D. (1992). Traditional Native American values: Conflict or concordance in rehabilitation. *Journal of Rehabilitation, 58* (2), 23–27.

Condon, J. C., & Yousef, F. (1975). *An introduction to intercultural communication.* New York: Bobbs-Merrill Co.

Cummins, J. (1984). *Bilingualism and special education.* San Diego: College Hill Press.

Darwin, C. (1965; originally published in 1872). *The expression of emotions in man and animals.* Chicago: University of Chicago Press.

Ekman, P., Friesen W. V., & Hess, P. (1984). The international language of gestures. *Psychology Today* (May) 64–69.

Everett, F., Proctor, N., & Cortmell, B. (1983). Providing psychological services to American Indian children and families. *Professional Psychology, 14,* 588–603.

Foley, C. D. (1984). Family therapy. In Corsini R. J. (Ed.), *Current psychotherapies.* Itasca, Il: F. F. Peacock Publishers.

Gochenour, T. (1990). *Counseling Filipinos.* Yarmouth, ME: Intercultural Press.

Guthrie, G. M. (1968). *The Philippine temperament: Six perspectives on the Philippines.* University Park: Pennsylvania State University Press.

Hall, E.T. (1966). *Beyond culture.* New York: Anchor Press.

Hansen, J. C., Stevic, R. R., & Warner, R. W. (1982). *Counseling: Theory and process.* Toronto: Allyn-Bacon.

Henkin, W. A. (1985). Toward counseling the Japanese in America: A cross-cultural primer. *Journal of Counseling & Development, 63,* 500–503.

Hilliard, A. (1986). Keynote address. Presented at the First National Symposium on Multicultural Counseling, Atlanta, GA.

Ho, M. K. (1987). *Family therapy with ethnic minorities.* Newbury Park, CA: Sage.

Hollingshead, A., & Redlich, F. C. (1968). *Social class and mental illness.* New York: John Wiley & Sons.

Ivey, A. E. (1981). Counseling and psychotherapy: Toward a new perspective. In Marsella A. J., & Pederson, P. B. (Eds.), *Cross-cultural counseling and psychotherapy.* Elmsford, NY: Pergamon Press.

Ivey, A. E. (1986). *Developmental therapy.* San Francisco: Jossey-Bass.

Jensen, J. V. (1985). Perspective on nonverbal intercultural communication. In Samovar, L. A., & Porter, R. E. (Eds.), *Intercultural communication: A reader.* Belmont, CA: Wadsworth.

Joe, J. R., & Malach, R. S. (1992). Families with Native American roots. In Lynch, E. W., & Hanson, M. J. (Eds.), *Developing cross-cultural competence: A guide for working with young children and their families* (pp. 89–120). Baltimore, MD: Brookes Publishing Co.

Kayser, H. (1993). Hispanic cultures. In Battle, D. E. (Ed.), *Communication disorders in multicultural populations* (pp. 114–157). Stoneham, MA: Butterworth-Heinemann.

Kim, S. C. (1985). Family therapy for Asian Americans: A strategic structural framework. *Psychotherapy, 22,* 342–356.

Kochman, T. (1981). *Black and white styles in conflict.* Chicago: University of Chicago Press.

Lane, V. W., & Molyneaux, D. (1992). *The dynamics of communicative development.* Englewood Cliffs, NJ: Prentice Hall.

Lau, S. (1982). The effect of smiling on person perception. *Journal of Social Psychology, 117,* 63–67.

Laval, R. A., Gomez, E. A., & Ruiz, P. (1983). A language minority: Hispanics and mental health care. *The American Journal of Social Psychiatry, 3,* 42–49.

Lum, R. G. (1982). Mental health attitudes and opinions of Chinese. In Jones, E. E., & Korchin, S. J. (Eds.), *Minority mental health.* New York: Praeger.

Luterman, D. (1991). *Counseling to communicatively disordered and their families* (2nd ed.). Boston, MA: Little, Brown & Co.

Lynch, E. W, & Hanson, M. J. (1992). *Developing cross-cultural competence: A guide for working with young children and their families.* Baltimore, MD: Brookes Publishing.

Matsuda, M. (1989). Working with Asian parents: Some communication strategies. *Topics in Language Disorders, 9*(3), 45–53.

Mau, W. C., & Jepson, D. A. (1988). Attitudes toward counselors and counseling processes: A comparison of Chinese and American graduate students. *Journal of Social Issues. 29,* 167–185.

Mays, V. M. (1985). The Black American and psychotherapy: The dilemma. *Psychotherapy, 22,* 167–185.

McAdoo, H. P. (1993). *Family ethnicity: Strength in diversity.* Newbury Park, CA: Sage.

Medina, V. (1982). *Interpretation and translation in bilingual B.A.S.A.* Superintendent of Schools, Department of Education, San Diego, CA.

Nobles, W. W. (1976). Black people in white insanity: An issue for Black community mental health. *The Journal of Afro-American Issues, 4,* 21–27.

Pedersen, P. (1988). *A Handbook for developing multicultural awareness.* Alexandria, VA: American Association for Counseling and Development.

Ramsey, S., & Birk, J. (1983). Preparation of North Americans for interaction with Japanese: Considerations of language and communication style. In Landic, D. & Buslin, R. W. (Eds.), *Handbook of intercultural training: Vol. III.* New York: Pergamon Press.

Randall-David, E. (1989). *Strategies for working with culturally diverse communities and clients.* Washington, DC: Association for the Care of Children's Health.

Red Horse, J. (1983). Indian family values and experiences. In Powell, G. J., et al.(Eds.), *The psychosocial development of minority group children* (pp. 258–272). New York: Brunner/Mazel.

Rollin, W. J. (1987). *The psychology of communication disorders in individuals and their families.* San Diego: College-Hill Press.

Santos, R. A. (1983). The social and emotional development of Filipino-American children. In Powell, G. J. (Ed.), *The psychosocial development of minority group children* (pp. 131–146). New York: Brunner/Mazel.

Sasson, J. (1992). *Princess.* New York: William Mollor & Co.

Schwartz, G., et al. (1976). Facial expression and imagery in depression: An electromyographic study. *Psychosomatic Medicine, 38,* 337–347.

Sharifzadeh, V. (1992). Families with Middle Eastern roots. In Lynch, E. W., & Hanson, M. J. (Eds.), *Developing cross-cultural competence: A guide for working with young children and their families* (pp. 319–354). Baltimore: Brookes Publishing.

Stanback, M. H., & Pearce, W. B. (1985). Talking to "the man": Some communication strategies used by members of "subordinate" social groups. In Samovar, L. A., & Porter, R. E. (Eds.), *Intercultural communication: A reader.* Belmont, CA: Wadsworth.

Stone, J. E., & Olswang, L. B. (1989, June-July). The hidden challenge in counseling. *ASHA,* 27–31.

Sue, D. W., & Morishima, J. K. (1982). Mental health of Asian Americans. San Francisco: Jossey-Bass.

Sue, D. W., & Sue, D. (1990). *Counseling the culturally different.* New York: John Wiley & Sons.

Susman, N. M., & Rosenfeld, H. M. (1982). Influence of culture, language and sex on conversation distance. *Journal of Personality and Social Psychology, 42,* 66–74.

Te, H. D. (1989). *The Indo-Chinese and their culture.* San Diego: San Diego State University Multifunctional Resource Center.

Terrell, F., & Terrell, S. L. (1993). African-American cultures. In Battle, D. E. (Ed.), *Communication disorders in multicultural populations* (pp. 3–37). Stoneham, MA: Butterworth-Heineman.

Terrell, F., & Terrell, S. L. (1981). An inventory to measure cultural mistrust among blacks. *Western Journal of Black Studies, 5,* 180–185.

Terrell, F., & Terrell, S. L. (1984). Race of counselor, client, sex, cultural mistrust level, and premature termination of counseling among black clients. *Journal of Counseling Psychology, 31,* 371–375.

U.S. Bureau of the Census. (1991, June 12). *Census on specific racial groups.* U.S. Department of Commerce News (not paginated).

Watson, O. M., & Graves, T. D. (1966). Quantitative research in proxemic behavior. *American Anthropologist, 68,* 971–985.

Weber, S. N. (1985). The need to be: The social significance of Black language. In Samovar, L. A. & Porter, R. E. (Eds.), *Intercultural communication: A reader.* Belmont, CA: Wadsworth.

Wilson, W., & Calhoun, J. F. (1974). Behavior therapy and the minority client. *Psychotherapy; Theory, Research and Practice, 11,* 317–325.

Wise F., & Miller, N. B. (1983). The mental health of American Indian children. In Powell, G. J., et al. (Eds.), *The psychosocial development of minority group children* (pp. 344–361). New York: Brunner/Mazel.

Wolfgang, A. (1985). The function and importance of nonverbal behavior in intercultural counseling. In Pedersen, P.B. (Ed.), *Handbook of cross-cultural counseling and therapy.* Westport, CT: Greenwood Press.

Wong, H. Z. (1985). Training for mental health service providers to Southeast Asian refugees: Models, strategies and curricula. In Owan, T. C. (Ed.), *Southeast Asian mental health treatment, prevention services, training and research.* Washington, DC: National Institute of Mental Health.

Yamamoto, J., & Kubota, M. (1983). The Japanese American family. In Yamamoto, J, Romero, A. & Morales, A. (Eds.), *The psychological development of minority group children.* New York: Brunner/Mazel.

Zitzow, D., & Estes, G. (1981). The heritage consistency continuum in counseling Native American children. In Spring conference on Contemporary American Issues, *American Indian issues in higher education* (pp. 133–139).

Zuniga, M. E. (1992). Families with Latino roots. In Lynch, E. W., & Hanson, M. J. (Eds.), *Developing cross-cultural competence: A guide for working with young children and their families* (pp. 151–180). Baltimore, MD: Brookes Publishing.

Section 2.

# Counseling Process

# 6. **Fluency Disorders**

Eugene B. Cooper

---

---

This chapter focuses on defining and describing a counseling process for adolescents and adults experiencing those kinds of fluency disorders that warrant the label "stuttering." For the purposes of this discussion, the term *stuttering* is used as a diagnostic label referring to a clinical syndrome characterized most frequently by abnormal and persistent dysfluencies in speech accompanied by characteristic affective, behavioral, and cognitive patterns. When viewed as a syndrome involving characteristic affective, behavioral, and cognitive components, it follows that counseling is the foundation on which most, if not all, successful stuttering intervention programs are based.

Counseling processes consist of the mutual exploration and exchange of thoughts, attitudes, and feelings between a counselor and a client. Counselors encourage clients to explore and to clarify their attitudes and feelings about their concerns through thinking aloud. A primary goal of counseling individuals experiencing a stuttering syndrome is to enable the client to choose, from the many strategies available for altering the disabling features of stuttering, those strategies most compatible with the client's productive coping patterns. The key to successful counseling is the establishment of client-clinician relationships in which clients come to feel free in expressing their thoughts and feelings openly and honestly. The successful counseling process concludes when a client thinks, acts, and feels in a manner that indicates he or she is capable of applying productive coping patterns in real life situations to gain and maintain a feeling of fluency control. Because most, if not all, fluency disorders are characterized as having affective, behavioral, and cognitive components, it is apparent that speech-language pathologists need to be skilled in creating counseling-type helping relationships in which clients address their feelings, behaviors, and attitudes.

Unfortunately, with the popularization of behaviorally oriented fluency therapy programs beginning in the 1960s and 1970s and continuing into the 1990s, too many clinicians focus primarily on the behavioral aspects of stuttering syndromes, rather than on the generally more significant affective and cognitive components for which a counseling-type relationship is more appropriate. With the popularity of exclusively behaviorally oriented intervention programs, clinicians choose to establish instructional-type helping relationships with their dysfluent clients rather than a counseling-type helping relationship in which they address the client's feelings and attitudes.

Cooper (1965) and Cooper and Cooper (1966, 1985, 1991, 1995), noting the need for setting more appropriate fluency therapy goals than those included in behavioral intervention programs, described the "frequency fallacy" and its deleterious effects to the understanding and treatment of those persons experiencing a fluency disorder. The frequency fallacy is the erroneous assumption that the frequency of dysfluencies is the single most significant factor in determining the severity of stuttering and in measuring progress in therapy. By focusing on the dysfluencies, clinicians too frequently neglect the far more significant affective and cognitive aspects of the disorder. In addition, such myopia on the part of clinicians leads many individuals who are receiving therapy by behaviorally oriented clinicians to criticize speech-language pathologists in general for being more interested in their stuttering than in them.

The development in recent years of self-help support groups for persons who stutter is resulting in the widespread dissemination of such well-deserved and perceptive criticisms. Fortunately, the significance of the affective and cognitive characteristics of stuttering syndromes with respect to both their etiology and their maintenance is being studied and reported by an increasing number of investigators (Cooper, 1993a). These investigators conclude that whatever central neurologic factors may underlie or affect the syndrome of stuttering, they are complex and interactive and vary in relation to changes in an individual's cognitive and affective states. Such observations, based on both research and clinical experience, are fostering an awareness that the feelings and attitudes of individuals experiencing a stuttering syndrome are significant factors needing to be addressed in attempts to ameliorate the syndrome.

## DEFINING FLUENCY DISORDERS

"Fluency disorders" is popularly used as an umbrella term to refer to speech rate, rhythm, and prosodic abnormalities of any origin. Fluency disorders are observed in the speech of individuals having experienced cerebral vascular accidents, those with the Tourette's syndrome, and individuals experiencing such conditions as dysarthria, dyspraxia, cluttering, spasmodic dysphonia, palilalia, and, of course, the most commonly thought-of disorder when fluency disorders are mentioned, stuttering. Although the principles and procedures for counseling presented in this chapter are described specifically as they relate to those persons experiencing a stuttering syndrome, they are applicable to assisting those coping with fluency disorders of any origin.

### Defining Stuttering and Stuttering Syndromes

In recent years more circumspection appears to be justified in using the single term "stuttering" in writing or discussing clinical intervention strategies for those who stutter. In addition to there being no universally accepted definition of stuttering, researchers are still unable to distinguish between isolated fluency failures of normally fluent speakers and the isolated dysfluencies of chronic stutterers. There is also an increasing understanding of the relationships between dysfluencies and a host of diagnosable diseases, syndromes, and disorders. For these reasons, in place of the term stuttering, the terms *fluency, dysfluency, fluency failures,* and *fluency disorders* are suggested as appropriate semantically unburdened and descriptive umbrella terms. For the purposes of this discussion, stuttering is used as a diagnostic label referring to a clinical syndrome characterized most frequently by abnormal and persistent dysfluencies in speech accompanied by characteristic affective, behavioral, and cognitive patterns.

Three major stuttering syndromes have been identified: developmental, remediable, and chronic perseverative (Cooper & Cooper, 1991, 1995; Cooper, 1993a,b).

## DEVELOPMENTAL STUTTERING

Two of every five children under the age of seven, exhibiting dysfluencies beyond what could be judged as being normal, experience the developmental stuttering syndrome. Typically, without significant professional help, but with knowledgeable and supportive parental assistance, these children achieve normal fluency control by the age of seven. Few of these children in subsequent years can recall early difficulty with fluency; virtually none of them as adults remember having stuttered. Also, these children do not experience a feeling of loss of control when being dysfluent or are unable to verbalize such a feeling. They may indicate awareness of their dysfluencies but give little evidence that they think or feel the dysfluencies are problematic for them.

## REMEDIABLE STUTTERING

Two of every three individuals who stutter *after* the age of seven experience the remediable stuttering syndrome. Typically these individuals, with professional assistance and a supportive home environment, are able to make the necessary adjustments in the way they feel (the affective component), behave (the behavioral component), and think (the cognitive component) to achieve normal fluency. In adulthood, most frequently they can recall their struggle with stuttering but generally do not think of themselves as still stuttering. Although these individuals experience a feeling of loss of control during moments of dysfluency, their periods of dysfluency are generally episodic and, more frequently than not, can be related to changes in the individual's physical or mental condition, or environmental situation.

## CHRONIC PERSEVERATIVE STUTTERING

One of every five children before the age of 7 who is said to stutter because of fluency problems beyond the normal developmental dysfluencies experiences the chronic perseverative stuttering syndrome. For these individuals, maintaining an acceptable level of fluency may require a lifetime of coping. Because the chronic perseverative stuttering syndrome consists of multiple coexisting and interactive affective, behavioral, and cognitive components coalescing over a period of years, the hope for a complete cure or remission of symptoms appears remote. However, the outlook for these individuals is not bleak. With assistance, they are typically able to develop and maintain a feeling of fluency control that enables them to communicate successfully in even the most challenging speech situations. The abundant number of successful individuals who are chronically dysfluent testifies most tellingly to an optimistic outlook for those experiencing the chronic perseverative stuttering syndrome.

## CHARACTERISTIC AFFECTIVE, BEHAVIORAL, AND COGNITIVE COMPONENTS OF STUTTERING SYNDROMES

Although it is evident that individuals experiencing the remediable and chronic perseverative stuttering syndromes frequently share several common feelings, behaviors, and attitudes particularly pertaining to their speech, it is equally evident that these individuals cannot be described as having characteristic personality traits (Bloodstein, 1995). Unfortunately, as with most minority groups, popular stereotypes have been developed about individuals who stutter, which are not only inaccurate when applied to the vast majority of those who stutter but are negative in nature (e.g., most individuals who stutter are shy). The characteristic affective, behavioral, and cognitive components of the stuttering syndromes noted in this discussion refer specifically to feelings, behaviors, and attitudes related to the communicative process (e.g., the feeling of loss of control during moments of stuttering, avoiding answering the telephone, and thinking that most people believe stuttering is an indication of an emotional disorder). Although many feelings, behaviors, and attitudes can be identified as being common among those who stutter, feeling a loss of control during moments of stuttering and the dysfluencies themselves are examples of what may be only a few components that can be universally noted in those who stutter and, to make matters even more complex, in some instances they may not be present either. Thus, any helping relationship with individuals experiencing a stuttering syndrome should include a continuing assessment of the individual's characteristic fluency-related feelings, behaviors, and attitudes.

## HELPING RELATIONSHIPS AND COUNSELING

Helping relationships may be viewed as ranging from the straightforward instructional relationship, appropriate for the well-adjusted and functioning individual, to the complex psychotherapeutic relationship for the nonfunctioning psychotic (Cooper, 1982, Cooper & Cooper, 1985). In such a conceptualization, the continuum's underlying variable could be described as being the degree of complexity of the interpersonal relationship between the individual being helped and the individual helping. The counseling relationship, viewed on this continuum of complexity of interpersonal interchange, is placed in the center. Such a placement indicates that the relationship is more complex than the instructional relationship between a student and a teacher, but less complex than the psychotherapeutic relationship between patient and therapist. It is the counseling relationship that appears to be most appropriate for most stuttering therapy relationships.

At the instructional end of the continuum, the interchange between student and teacher is limited to the material being taught because the maximally adjusted and functioning student is capable of focusing exclusively on the subject at hand. A maximally adjusted student's learning is not impaired by impeding feelings, behaviors, and attitudes resulting from distorted perceptions of self or the environment. Obviously, the ideal situation just described rarely exists. Experienced instructors recognize the need to attend to those individual factors that impede the learning process in even the most "all-together" students. The instructional type of relationship, however, is characterized by the teacher focusing primarily on the concepts to be transmitted rather than on the feelings and attitudes of the student.

What is involved in the psychotherapeutic relationship at the other end of the continuum, by necessity, is more complex. To help the patient achieve the goals of the relationship, which, in contrast to the goal of most instructional relationships, may not be understood by the patient at the onset of therapy, the clinician deals with the client's perceptions that result in the feelings, behaviors, and attitudes necessitating the need for the helping relationship. In contrast to the teacher in an instructional relationship, the psychotherapist involved in a psychodynamically involved relationship initially focuses on the client's attitudes and feelings rather than on the transmittal of a predetermined body of information. When viewed in this manner, the type of relationship most appropriate for assisting an individual is dependent on the extent to which the individual's cognitive and affective responses, with or without the individual's awareness, preclude the attainment of the goals for which the helping relationship was initiated.

Cognitive (thinking) and affective (feeling) factors, which determine the type of helping relationship an individual might need, can be described as consisting primarily of three variables: extent of (*a*) misperceptions, (*b*) affective overlay, and (*c*) affective-cognitive disparity.

## Extent of Misperceptions

An individual's misperceptions can range from a simple distorted perception of an object peripheral to the individual's self-concept that can be altered easily by instruction to multiple and complex self-misperceptions that can be altered typically only through intense and prolonged self-study in a psychotherapeutic environment.

## Extent of Affective Overlay

Perceptions pertaining to an individual's self-concept are imbued with more affective significance than are perceptions of events, persons, and objects peripheral to the individual's self-concept. The closer a perception is to the individual's self-concept, the more that perception is accompanied by feelings. The affective significance attached to a perception and subsequently to behavior based on the perception, can be an impeding or a facilitating factor in modifying both the perception and the behavior resulting from the perception. Misperceptions with little or no emotional significance can typically be altered through instruction. However, the modification of affect-laden misperceptions usually requires establishing helping relationships characterized by emotionally significant interchanges such as those found in counseling and psychotherapeutic relationships.

## Extent of Cognitive-Affective Disparity

The lack of congruity between the ways an individual thinks and feels indicates the type of helping relationship the individual needs. Clients may know they are bright, but may not feel they are bright. Clients may be intellectually committed to modifying their speech, but may not be *emotionally* committed to doing so. Clients experiencing a significant lack of affective-cognitive congruence, particularly with respect to the issues with which the helping relationship must deal, are best served in a counseling relationship or, if the disparity is extreme, in a psychotherapeutic relationship.

Individuals ranking high on all of any one the three factors (misperceptions, affective overlay, or affective-cognitive disparity) are most effectively served in helping relationships that are more psychotherapeutically than instructionally oriented. Conversely, individuals ranking low on the three factors are excellent candidates for an instructional relationship. Thus, something more than an instructional relationship appears appropriate when clients (*a*) hold significant misperceptions not only of the problem itself, but also about the ramifications of the problem; (*b*) hold feelings about their problems or themselves that significantly impede successful use of speech and language modification procedures; and (*c*) experience significant discrepancies between the way they think and the way they feel about their problem and about themselves.

## ROLE OF COUNSELING IN TREATING ADOLESCENTS AND ADULTS EXPERIENCING A STUTTERING SYNDROME

Just as researchers have demonstrated that individuals who stutter do not possess characteristic personality patterns, they also have demonstrated that individuals who stutter *cannot* be judged as being more in need of psychotherapy than the general population. Researchers have demonstrated that those who stutter and who wish to alter the affective, behavioral, and cognitive components of their stuttering warrant a helping relationship best described as being a counseling-type relationship (Cooper & Cooper, 1985).

Altering an individual's feelings and attitudes concerning something as close to a personal sense of emotional and physical well-being as a fluency disorder might be difficult, if not impossible through an instructional-type helping relationship. Such attitudes and feelings are usually developed in one's early years through repeated and frequently emotion-laden interchanges with parents. In later years, self-perceptions continue to be modified primarily through interchanges with those with whom one becomes emotionally involved. One can adopt the attitudes of persons loved, respected, or admired more readily than the attitudes of those with whom there is no emotional involvement or for whom negative feelings exist. Clinicians also know that abrupt or significant changes in one's self-concept can be related to emotionally charged responses accompanying a single interaction or series of interactions with significant others. Helping relationships in which the goal is to develop, identify, or modify feelings and attitudes are viewed similarly. The clinician's task is to develop a relationship characterized by significant *affective* verbal interchanges (verbalizations accompanied by feelings) as well as significant cognitively based verbal interactions (verbalizations of an intellectual nature). Through significant interchanges of feelings and attitudes with the clinician, the client is provided the opportunity to identify, evaluate, and adopt therapy-facilitating feelings and attitudes.

It is unfortunate that terms such as *warm, personal, supportive, nurturing,* and *friendly* are often used to describe the type of helping relationship that facilitates changes in a client's feelings and attitudes. Clinical process studies indicate that although these terms are useful as an overall characterization of a relationship designed to alter feelings and attitudes, they are not helpful in describing how critical affective interchanges between client and clinician are engineered by the clinician. If terms such as warm and nurturing are used to describe the clinical relationship, the critical role that affective interchanges (positive and negative) play in altering attitudes and feelings in the therapy relationship may be neglected. In addition, such terms fail to remind clinicians that the ideal clinical relationship is a process and not a state.

During the course of helping relationships, a client's feeling toward the clinician follows a typical pattern of change independent of the type of therapy being employed (Cooper, 1966; Cooper & Cooper, 1966; Manning & Cooper, 1969). Clients typically become increasingly less positive toward clinicians soon after therapy begins. Subsequently, however, in successful therapeutic relationships they become even more positive than they were at the beginning of therapy. Toward the end of therapy, the client's feelings, although tending to become more positive, stabilize in comparison to the shifts noted in earlier stages of therapy. Such a pattern in client affect change is not surprising. Clients generally enter helping relationships with positive feelings about the clinical process. These positive feelings are primarily based on the client's expectation of symptom relief and faith in the clinician's ability to bring about that relief. Clients become less positive as they learn that the clinician has no instant cure and improvement comes only after the expenditure of significant energies. The increase in positive feelings following the initial decline is attributed to the client's sense of well-being as he or she experiences success in obtaining goals. The stabilization of client feelings noted as the therapy process nears termination is also to be expected. By this time in the therapy process clients are adjusted to the clinician and the number of affective, behavioral, and cognitive changes decreases. Being aware of these typical shifts in client feelings, clinicians, regardless of their therapeutic orientation, may avoid needless therapeutic failures and may even expedite the process.

## COUNSELING GOALS

The end goal of the treatment program described herein is the establishment and the maintenance of the feeling of fluency control rather than the attainment of an arbitrarily determined level of fluency. As noted, by focusing on the dysfluencies, a clinician may neglect the far more significant affective and cognitive aspects of the disorder. The significance of these stuttering features with respect to both etiology and maintenance has been observed in recent studies of the central neurologic processing systems of stuttering. As noted, whatever central neurologic factors may underlie or affect the syndrome of stuttering, they are complex and vary in relation to changes in the individual's cognitive and affective states.

The feeling of control appears to be the key variable in determining whether a person who experiences a fluency disorder will maintain an acceptable level of fluency after treatment terminates. Individuals are not asked to evaluate their success in terms of how fluent they are in various situations. They are asked whether they did or did not experience a feeling of fluency control as a result of applying any one of their affective, behavioral, or cognitive coping strategies. If a client reports feeling able to modify speech during a speech situation, the speaking experience is judged successful, although the client was dysfluent. The focus remains on the feeling of control and not on fluency.

Focusing on developing the feeling of control rather than on arbitrarily predetermined and generally meaningless fluency rates, assists clients, parents, and clinicians in maintaining the necessary perspective to the relative significance of the affective, behavioral, and cognitive components of the disorder. From the beginning of therapy, the focus should be on the development of feelings, attitudes, and motor skills that enhance the feeling of control. Behaviorally focused fluency programs not addressing the affective and cognitive features of oral language fluency control may be the single major factor leading to the needless guilt and shame experienced by an individual with the chronic perseverative stuttering syndrome who has been unable to attain or maintain normal fluency. By focusing on developing the feeling of fluency control, such issues as whether a client should be taught to accept the fluency disorder rather than to cope with it become academic, if not irrelevant.

Goals of a counseling-type helping relationship for individuals experiencing a stuttering syndrome with the end goal being that of establishing and maintaining a feeling of fluency control are:

1. To create client-clinician relationships that assist clients in identifying and exploring their feelings, behaviors, and attitudes regarding themselves and their stuttering.
2. To assist clients in identifying the feelings, behaviors, and attitudes that constitute the stuttering problem.
3. To assist clients in developing a reality-based perspective of the significance of their stuttering disorder as it relates to their sense of well-being and their personal and vocational goals.
4. To assist clients in identifying their typical affective, behavioral, and cognitive coping patterns and the relative success of those coping patterns.
5. To assist clients in applying their successful affective, behavioral, and cognitive coping patterns to their stuttering syndrome.
6. To assist clients in becoming more effective self-reinforcers.
7. To assist clients in the identification, development, and use of fluency initiating gestures.
8. To assist clients in obtaining and maintaining the end goal of stuttering syndrome treatment programs—the feeling of fluency control.

## COUNSELING PROCESS FOR ADOLESCENTS AND ADULTS EXPERIENCING A STUTTERING SYNDROME

The counseling process described herein consists of four stages: orientation, relationship, adjustment, and action.

## Orientation Stage

During this initial stage, the clinician assists the client in identifying feelings, behaviors, and attitudes that constitute the stuttering syndrome. The clinician informs the client of the procedures to be followed in the therapeutic process and the rationale for focusing on the client-clinician relationship as the key to the success of the therapy. The clinician explains that a basic interest, particularly in the beginning of therapy, is on how that relationship is developing. The clinician notes the success of the therapy process depends to a large extent on the development of an open, honest, and mutually respectful relationship. The clinician also advises the client that in the process of developing and maintaining such a relationship, the client will undoubtedly feel uncomfortable at times and have negative feelings toward the clinician. Although these clinician verbalizations may not be meaningful to the client at this point in the counseling process, they provide an orientation to which the clinician may refer as therapy progresses. Initially, clients are usually positive in their feelings regarding the clinician as he or she assists them in visualizing and defining their stuttering problem. In addition, the clinician has yet to suggest anything about what the client should or should not do that might cause clients to react negatively. The clinician describes a variety of therapeutic activities that might be undertaken by the client pending identification of the client's successful coping patterns, should they both agree on what is appropriate for the client. Clients typically feel a sense of optimism and are eager to begin. It is important that clients experience positive feelings toward the clinician in the initial interactions. Those positive feelings facilitate the clinician's elicitation of client feelings and attitudes early in the relationship.

Clients entering therapy for the first time typically are unable to conceptualize or objectively view their stuttering problem. They may describe their problem in terms that indicate a vague and generalized anxiety. Their situation appears analogous to individuals who know they are ill but do not know what is wrong; they live in fear, dreading the worst, until the illness is diagnosed. Even if the diagnosis is a threatening one, individuals generally experience an immediate reduction of anxiety as they begin to face the problem. The same is true for many individuals experiencing a stuttering syndrome. They are aware something is wrong, but are unable to grasp the exact nature of the problem and avoid seeking a diagnosis for fear of learning something even more fearful. Clinicians typically assist clients in bringing order to their thinking about stuttering as they engage clients in assessment activities that identify the feelings, behaviors, and attitudes that constitute their stuttering syndrome.

The Stuttering Apple, a therapy guide used in the Cooper Personalized Fluency Control Therapy program (Cooper & Cooper, 1985), is used to assist both children and adults in organizing their thinking about their stuttering and the therapeutic process. Although seemingly simplistic and at first glance of questionable use with adults, this therapy tool has been found useful in assisting clients of all ages to begin organizing their thinking about the problem. The Stuttering Apple consists of an outline of an apple with a circle in the center labeled "Core: Getting Stuck on Words." Surrounding the core within the outline of the apple are several empty circles. The directions on the form indicate that clients and clinicians should write in a circle things clients do when and because they stutter. As the client, assisted as necessary, notes such things as "I blink my eyes when I stutter," "My hand jerks when I get stuck," "I don't answer in class because I stutter," the clinician or the client makes a note of it on one of the circles. This procedure is continued until the client, with the aid of the clinician, puts all those behaviors associated with the moment of stuttering in the graphic display. As therapy progresses, clinicians and clients may identify additional stuttering-related behaviors and add them to the graphic display. The completed

Stuttering Apple represents the client's stuttering and stuttering-related feelings, behaviors, and attitudes in a graphic form.

The Stuttering Apple provides clients and clinicians with a similar conceptualization of the stuttering problem and facilitates communication between them. Because the Apple focuses on the "whens" and "becauses" of the stuttering problem, clients are not threatened by the clinician immediately directing their attention to feelings and attitudes before the client is comfortable enough in the relationship to address such issues. Although clinicians may successfully approach some adults with a direct question of how they feel about an issue, most clinicians have experienced the problem of having younger clients reply, "I don't know." By defining the problem in terms of "whens" and "because," clients are not being coerced at this early stage in therapy into introspecting to how they feel. Another important advantage in using a graphic display as a means of conceptualizing and identifying the client's problem is that the use of meaningless labels is avoided. Such terms as "secondary symptoms" and "avoidance devices" may be meaningless to the client. The Stuttering Apple provides a concrete description of the problem in the client's own words.

Clinicians may use the graphic representation to structure the therapy process. The clinician suggests that the Apple represents things the client wants to alter. Therapy become a matter of "eating the Apple to its core." Clinicians discuss which "bite" to take out first. Clients are led to choose a relatively uncomplicated behavior to eliminate, such as "I blink my eyes when I stutter." It is useful to suggest that after the Apple is eaten to its core, the remaining dysfluencies will be brought under control with the use of fluency-initiating gestures. Clients can see where they are going in therapy. Therapy procedures and materials for use in orienting clients to a counseling process for individuals experiencing a stuttering syndrome are described in more detail in the manual for the Cooper Personalized Fluency Control Therapy program (Cooper & Cooper, 1985).

## Relationship Stage

The second stage of the counseling process for adolescents and adults who stutter commences when clinicians direct clients to begin modifying some aspect of the stuttering syndrome. For example, clinicians might have clients practice maintaining eye contact in front of a mirror during the therapy session. In addition, the clinician might give clients a list of speaking situations in which they are to practice maintaining eye contact during moments of stuttering outside the therapy session. The primary goal of such assignments is to provide clinicians with opportunities to begin observing typical patterns of affective, behavioral, and cognitive responses of clients to suggestions that they alter any aspect of their stuttering syndrome. A secondary goal of such assignments, of course, is to begin modifying the stuttering syndrome itself. However, the key focus early in the relationship stage is on providing clients with maximal opportunities to express their typical patterns of coping. The clinician observes a client's affective, behavioral, and cognitive responses to these assignments and then directs the client's attention to those responses. In the process of making clients aware of responses to the assignments, clients and clinicians evaluate responses as being either facilitative or impeding with respect to attaining the goals of therapy.

Clinicians should not be surprised when clients knowingly or unknowingly resist doing their assignments. In some cases, the clinician may be asking a client to do something he or she has been trying hard not to do. Rather than viewing such resistance as a hindrance to therapy, the clinician can use it to expedite therapy by responding appropriately to the client's resistance. When, in the course of the therapy process the clinician identifies client coping patterns, whether they are therapy-facilitating or therapy-impeding, they should be pointed out to the client and the client should be encouraged to express them openly. This therapeutic strategy is termed "confrontation." Confrontation is defined as the clinician's verbalization of affective, behavioral, or cognitive client patterns that either facilitate or impede client progress in obtaining goals agreed on in establishing the helping relationship. Confrontation is different from the targeting of feelings, behaviors, and attitudes in the initial stage of therapy. In the orienting stage of therapy clinicians assist clients in describing and defining the stuttering problem. Confrontation helps clients accurately perceive their response patterns to their clinician's instructions for making changes.

How the confrontation is handled by clinicians is, of course, critical to the successful establishment of a productive counseling relationship. It is hoped that the clinician is aware of the distinction between accepting a person and accepting the person's behavior. What is accepted by the clinician is the person, not necessarily the person's behavior. Clinicians can be permissive on the feeling level but not necessarily on the behavioral level unless they are willing to work for an indefinite period in a dubiously supportive role.

Clinicians cite their clients patterns of affective, behavioral, and cognitive responses, as they become evident, but avoid labeling the patterns as being "good" or "bad." Most, if not all of the coping patterns identified as being detrimental to fluency change may be productive responses in other areas of the individual's life. For example, intellectualizing is a necessary cognitive skill for the college student and most appropriate in many situations. However, when a clinician comments on a client's use of intellectualizing with respect to the stuttering problem, the client typically assumes the clinician is disapproving. Clinicians may actually be admiring their client's creativity in the matter. Generally, it is only after the relationship matures that a client is able to sense that the clinician is understanding and accepting of the feelings and attitudes underlying the patterns being cited.

As clinicians continue to confront clients early in the relationship stage of therapy by citing their response patterns to the therapy assignments, clients typically respond in a defensive manner. They may deny the accuracy of the clinician's observations or they may indicate an intellectual acceptance of the observation even if they are angered by it. With continued confrontation, indications of client negativism (perhaps the first sign of client emotional involvement in the process) begin to be observed. For example, clients may become nonverbal, appear late for therapy, or subtly indicate they feel therapy is a waste of time. Such responses indicate clients are experiencing an *affective* response to the therapeutic relationship. The clinician's task is to motivate the client to express such feelings verbally.

Clinicians vary in their approaches to confrontation depending on their own needs and their perceptions of each client. One technique that many clinicians find useful is that of consistently requesting clients to define terms the clients use in reporting their reactions to fluency-related experiences. For example, clients might report they are embarrassed when explaining their failure to carry out the clinician's assignment to control eye blinks while shopping in a drug store. The clinician's response might be, "I'm not sure what you mean by 'embarrassed.' I know what I mean by that word, but what do you mean?" By continuing to seek an operational definition of terms used by the client, the clinician is confronting the client. Such a semantic approach has proved useful in provoking feeling responses from clients. Typically, the client's initial reaction to this type of clinician behavior is negative. The following statements reflect how clients often feel following such client-clinician interchanges: "My clinician doesn't believe anything I say," or "My clinician must be playing games with me." Again, the clinician's tasks are to motivate clients to express feelings verbally and to reinforce their expressions of feelings.

Clinicians confront clients with honest positive feelings in response to the client's affective, behavioral, and cognitive patterns perceived by the clinician as indicators of client worth. Such expressions of clinician positive affect toward clients are based on specific references to a client's behavior. Expressions of positive affect by the clinician without identifying an eliciting stimulus may be misinterpreted by a client as condescension or pandering. Clients might feel the clinician is being patronizing or might reject the expression of positive affect as the clinician's method of building them up. "Sweet talk" is not acceptable. The expression of positive affect is made contingent on a specific coping pattern. For example, perhaps the clinician admires the client for pursuing some form of continuing education while holding down a full-time job. The clinician expresses admiration with a specific reference to that coping strategy. At the same time, clinicians undoubtedly experience negative feelings in response to clients whose resistance to therapy persists. In such cases, the clinician is encouraged to express those feelings to the client. As with the expression of positive affect, this expression of feelings must be accompanied by a detailed description of the client's feelings, behaviors, or attitudes that elicited the negative response. Clinicians, of course, need to refrain from generalizing their negative feelings (e.g., you are *always* late for therapy; *all* you do is intellectualize). Skilled clinicians do not transfer their frustrations with other interpersonal relationships to their clients. To be therapeutically useful, the clinician's expression of feelings needs to be related to a specific client response of which the client is well aware.

The clinician's expression of feelings regarding the immediate interpersonal interaction serves a distinct purpose in this confrontational phase of the relationship stage of therapy. By such expressions of feelings, clinicians reassure clients that they are also involved in the relationship and that they also care about what happens. Frequently this expression of feelings can serve as an eliciting stimuli for client verbalizations of feelings. Again, to be successful in this stage of therapy, clinicians need to understand and be in control of their own feelings regarding the client-clinician relationship. If they are in control, their expressions of feelings toward clients will be warranted by the interaction taking place in the immediate relationship. It is not atypical to hear a beginning clinician state: "I get so frustrated with my clients; all they do is intellectualize!" The supervisor might reply, "Well, did you tell them so?" Clinician effectiveness, in such relationships, has been found to be related to the extent to which they openly express feelings (Cooper, Eggerston, & Galbraith, 1971). As noted, successful counseling is dependent on the interchange of feelings and attitudes between client and clinician. By expressing feelings as well as attitudes, the clinician provides a role model for clients to follow.

Clients are encouraged to verbalize both positive and negative feelings about their clinician as well as what is taking place in therapy. When clinicians encourage clients to express both negative and positive feelings about their clinician and their therapy, clients may question what the clinician is attempting to do. Clinicians reply they are working to establish the kind of therapeutic relationship in which clients feel comfortable enough to openly and honestly express feelings. The clinician suggests that the client may have feelings about the clinician and what is taking place in therapy. If the relationship is to proceed productively, such feelings need to be addressed. Initially, clients may deny such feelings or glibly agree to their existence. In any case, clinicians may need to pressure clients for several sessions before they can verbalize their feelings. At the beginning of this process, the client may express tentative indications of distress by observing that therapy has become a waste of time, or that they cannot understand how such feelings have anything to do with their stuttering. Clinicians may take the lead in suggesting to their clients that they feel their clinician is probably well-meaning, but "off base." The clinician's persistence in seeking expressions of both negative and positive feelings infrequently leads to what might be described as being an emotional outburst on the part of the client. During such an outburst, a client who had previously been noncommunicative with respect to feelings suddenly may openly express the negative feelings that have been "building up." If successful, the clinician leads clients to express their feelings about what has been taking place in therapy, their clinician, or feelings of frustration with their problem. These are the kinds of feelings that clients may not have been aware of possessing or have been hesitant to express.

Such expressions of negative feelings on the part of a client provide the clinician with an ideal opportunity. By communicating understanding and acceptance of the client's negative feelings, the clinician may make significant progress in establishing a helping relationships in which the client feels free to express openly both positive and negative feelings. Clinicians might respond to such expressions of negativism by telling the client, "Thank you for sharing these feelings with me. It makes me feel good that you can be honest with me. Of course, I am sorry for the negative feelings you have expressed, but I am delighted you could express such feelings to me. Now that I know how you feel, we can be open with one another and can deal with those feelings." Obviously, how such feelings of acceptance are expressed to clients varies markedly from clinician to clinician and from client to client.

Clinicians able to acknowledge a commonality with their clients are capable of conveying a basic feeling of respect and acceptance to them even while confronting them. As Murphy and FitzSimons noted long ago:

> One of the most valuable decisions which clinicians can make is to admit their commonality with the persons whom they are trying to help. . . . The principle of being different in degree and not in kind applies to all clinicians, all stutterers, all people. (1960, p.104)

If clinicians communicate understanding and acceptance of the client's feelings at this critical time, they will likely succeed in leading that client into an emotionally significant helping relationship characteristic of a counseling-type relationship. In such relationships, clients can evaluate their feelings and attitudes regarding themselves and their stuttering. Again, clinicians reinforce client verbalizations of both positive and negative feelings. Although clinicians may not share the negative feelings, they should be delighted that a client feels free to express them. Clients perceiving acceptance and honesty in a relationship express themselves more openly. They "check-out" their perceptions with those of their clinicians. In such a successful counseling relationship, a client tends to adopt the presumably more accurate perceptions of the clinicians.

Clinicians do not express psychodynamic interpretations of client behavior to their clients or provide clients with interpretations of abstract concepts such as anger, fear, and embarrassment. In addition to being inappropriate activities for speech-language pathologists, such interpretations may lead to a superficial intellectually based therapeutic relationship. Successful clinicians maintain a dynamic clinical relationship characterized by recurring feeling-based interchanges rather than emotionally sterile intellectual exchanges. Clinicians need to avoid client-clinician relationships that could be described as a forum for intellectual discussions and debates. When encouraging client involvement, successful counseling clinicians restrict themselves to citing affective, behavioral, and cognitive response patterns and avoid making psychodynamic interpretations to clients of the patterns observed.

Clinicians generally report that the use of confrontation strategies to elicit client feelings is one of the more difficult procedures in the counseling process. As they draw attention to a client's coping patterns, clinicians frequently are fearful that the client will misinterpret their observations as being critical evaluations of the client's feelings, behaviors, and attitudes. Unfortunately, inexperienced clinicians may refrain from using this potentially powerful strategy to expedite the development of a productive counseling relationship because they find the expression of negative feelings discomforting. Experienced clinicians perceive the expression of negative feelings as an ideal opportunity for them to re-assure clients that they value the expression of both positive and negative feelings. Confrontation, when used appropriately, communicates to clients that the clinician "cares." As therapy progresses, clients learn that clinicians "call it as they see it" and begin to value the clinician's perceptions. In such an atmosphere, clients find it difficult to accuse the clinician of playing games and of reporting only those events the clinician feels will make the client feel good. In summary, confrontation is an effective technique for expediting the development of the clinical relationship process.

The successful conclusion of the relationship stage of the counseling process finds clients expressing openly and honestly their feelings and attitudes regarding the clinician, the client-clinician relationship, and their stuttering-related feelings, behaviors, and attitudes. In addition, clients will have begun to identify and perhaps modify feelings, behaviors, and attitudes perceived as impeding progress toward developing the feeling of fluency control.

## Adjustment Stage

During the adjustment stage of the counseling process for adolescents and adults who stutter, the focus of therapy is on:

- altering misperceptions a client might have regarding the stuttering syndrome

- developing a reality-based perspective on the part of the client as to the affective, behavioral, and cognitive ramifications of the stuttering syndrome

- identifying the client's existing affective, behavioral, and cognitive coping patterns

- enhancing the client's self-reinforcement skills

- determining which strategies for achieving the feeling of fluency control are most appropriate in light of the client's typical coping patterns

As noted, a significant factor in facilitating changes in a client's affective, behavioral, and cognitive patterns is the extent to which the client values the feelings and attitudes of the clinician. These feelings and attitudes become known to the client through the verbal interchanges taking place in the therapy sessions. In the adjustment stage of counseling, clients are encouraged to "think-out-loud" regarding their feelings and attitudes about their stuttering and their coping strategies. Clinician responses to these verbalizations are limited primarily to statements reflecting and clarifying the client's verbalizations. It is during this time that clients may be discovering and expressing to another human being for the first time feelings and attitudes of which they had previously been unaware. During this phase in the counseling process the clinician's major responsibility is to reinforce the client's verbalizations of such introspective activity. At the same time, successful clinicians can assist clients in adopting more accurate perceptions of their stuttering and themselves. They do this, without valuing client perceptions on a good-bad continuum, by indicating the extent to which they perceive the client's verbalized attitudes to be reality-based. Verbalizations of feelings by the client, on the other hand, continue to be reinforced with the client being encouraged to explore the sources of such feelings.

Clinicians might experience difficulty in shifting their behavior from the relationship to the adjustment stage of counseling. Whereas in the relationship stage clinicians are directive with respect to confronting clients to elicit affectively significant responses, in the adjustment stage they are supportive of client self-evaluations and less overtly directive in leading the clients to "insights." If the clinician continues to be directive, the client may not feel comfortable in introspecting freely. Frequently the clinician observes significant affective, behavioral, or attitudinal coping patterns on the part of a client before the client becomes aware of them. Clinicians may want to expedite the process by conveying their insights to the client. Unfortunately, such verbalizations may cause a client to develop an intellectual understanding of the pattern being observed without any accompanying affective acceptance. Ideally, clients, through introspection facilitated by the clinician's encouragement of their thinking-out-loud, will come to a realization on their own of the significance of the issue being addressed.

In this stage of therapy, the clinician is called on to make the difficult discrimination between intellectualization and meaningful introspection. In an attempt to control intellectualization, the clinician may press a client to provide concrete examples of the feelings, behaviors, and attitudes being discussed. If the client is unable to relate the concept being discussed to a specific situation within his or her own experience, it may be assumed the client is intellectualizing. Perhaps one of the most common problems encountered in reinforcing introspection is that of clients substituting rumination for introspection. Too frequently clients engage in nondirectional and nonproductive "stewing" that characterizes rumination rather than in goal-directed analyses and problem-solving that characterize introspection. Clinicians frequently make this distinction for clients and then strive to reinforce introspective activities while punishing ruminative responses.

Disruptive cognitive processing takes many other forms. The following questions suggest examples of disruptive cognitive processing.

- Do the clients consistently evaluate themselves from a negative point of view?
- Are they unrealistically negative or positive thinkers?
- Do they view listener reactions to their stuttering unrealistically?
- Do they intellectualize inappropriately?
- Do they misinterpret affect-laden messages directed toward them?
- Do they misperceive the significance of their stuttering problem in relation to their productivity?

Throughout the period of self-evaluation, clinicians reinforce client verbalizations of feelings and attitudes which they judge to be accurate and indicative of client self-appreciation. Verbalizations indicating disruptive cognitive processing are punished. To do this, clinicians assist clients in identifying specific affective and cognitive patterns to be increased or decreased (e.g., "I feel dumb because I stutter; I think those who stutter should never take a leadership position.") Reinforcing or punishing responses to those patterns are then identified for both the client's and the clinician's use. Clinicians cannot assume that a simple nod of the head is a reinforcer or that a frown necessarily serves as a punishment. Typically, several sessions are required before the clinician and the client can begin to judge the effectiveness of the reinforcers and punishments chosen.

SHORT-TERM GOAL SETTING

Assuming a productive client-clinician relationship has been initiated, the major focus of the therapy discussions at this point in the counseling process shift to establishing mutually agreed-on short-term goals whose completion will result in the successful attainment of the end goal of therapy—the feeling of fluency control. The nature of these short-term goals varies significantly from client to client and is dependent on the extent to which each of the three components of the stuttering syndrome (affective, behavioral, or cognitive) are to be addressed. For example, clients with significant negative feelings regarding their self-worth because of their stuttering or with feelings of hopelessness with respect to their stuttering may wish to set a goal of increasing their feelings of self-worth or their feelings of hope. Other clients may wish to focus on increasing the accuracy of their perceptions regarding the nature of stuttering and the realities of the perceptions of others with respect to their stuttering. Others may elect, at this point in therapy, to focus on the behavioral aspects of the syndrome. Client-clinician discussions leading to the selection of appropriate short-term goals are invariably influenced by the continued identification of the client's successful and unsuccessful affective, behavioral, and cognitive coping strategies. Obviously, if the clinician and the client agree that one of the client's unsuccessful coping strategies is refusing to acknowledge negative feelings arising from stuttering-related experiences, they might select as a short-term goal the exploration of negative feelings as they relate to stuttering.

The success or failure of the counseling process is often determined during therapy's short-term goal-setting phase. If the client and the clinician are unable to agree on the client's patterns of coping strategies, the successes and failures of those patterns, the realities of the stuttering syndrome itself, and the short-term goals, the counseling process has stalled. In situations in which the clinician concludes the client is denying reality or does not accept the clinician's judgment to appropriate short-term goals, the clinician is well advised to consider referring the client to another professional. In addition, if the clinician perceives any of the client's coping patterns to be indicative of the client's need for psychological counseling, the clinician has the responsibility of bringing that to the client's attention. The continuation of the therapeutic relationship is, of course, dependent on the mutual agreement between client and clinician, both to the end goal of therapy and to the short-term goals that lead to the end goal. Short-term goals may need to be modified as additional client coping patterns are identified as facilitating or impeding the attainment of the feeling of fluency control.

## SELF-REINFORCEMENT

The ability of clients to self-reinforce has been found to be one of the most significant factors in predicting long-term success in obtaining and maintaining the feeling of fluency control. Clients must develop self-reinforcing behavioral as well as attitudinal patterns. They must not only *think* about reinforcing themselves on a continuing basis, but they must *do* something behaviorally to demonstrate and to foster attitudes conducive to self-reinforcement. New attitudinal and behavioral patterns are subject to extinction unless the individual is an effective self-reinforcer. Thus, as soon as a functional therapeutic relationship has been established, the clinician begins identifying and enhancing the client's self-reinforcement behavioral and attitudinal patterns. Just as with children, adolescents and adults are asked to give the clinician visible or audible signs each time they reinforce themselves for some thought or action. For example, if done without violating the client's sense of decorum, clients might be asked to do such things as pat their own shoulder or give a thumbs-up to indicate self-reinforcement. A client simply making a mental note of an act warranting self-reinforcement typically is not sufficient to foster the development and maintenance of self-reinforcement patterns. Clients need to *show* clinicians they are reinforcing themselves. Such signals enable clinicians to determine whether or not clients are in fact applying self-reinforcement strategies. Clinicians frequently need to assist clients in identifying and in rehearsing the actual internal thought processes and the overt behaviors they are to use to reinforce themselves.

## IDENTIFYING CLIENT AFFECTIVE, BEHAVIORAL, AND COGNITIVE COPING PATTERNS

Just as the client-clinician relationship process is critical to successful counseling, so is identifying the client's typical coping patterns. The psychology literature is replete with systems for identifying and categorizing "personality types." Popular self-help books are equally replete with procedures for determining how individuals organize themselves and how, by being aware of how they typically feel, act, and think, they use those existing patterns to their best advantage.

Fluency clinicians, in assisting their clients in selecting strategies to earn the feeling of control, can likewise enhance their clients' chances of success in obtaining their fluency goals by tailoring the therapeutic strategies to capitalize on their clients' successful coping strategies. For example, a client whose "specialty" and "joy" is performing detailed analyses of the frequency and complexity of behavioral patterns can be instructed in the anatomic, physiologic, and acoustic variables underlying alterations in the processes of phonation, articulation, and fluency. Such knowledge for these individuals appears critical to the development of their feeling of fluency control. For clients who are conceptually oriented and who thrive on developing personal hypothetic constructs to assist them in dealing with problems, the clinician can foster their feeling of fluency control by focusing on the development of cognitive strategies to cope with fluency failures. Some individuals who stutter develop and maintain, for significant periods of time, a "feeling of fluency control" that results in significant improvement in fluency, by focusing on feelings of well-being and power. They "psych themselves up," and successfully so, to *feeling* in control by self-talk, relaxation procedures, or other affect-inducing activities that have worked for them. Others focus on cognitive approaches to developing the feeling of fluency control. Such individuals might have discovered that various forms of imaging or meditation facilitate their development of the feeling of control, whether it is in regard to fluency or to other aspects of their lives.

For clients whose coping patterns include reliance on behavioral adjustments when it comes to addressing a problem, clinicians may instruct them in the use of such relatively simple behavioral strategies as the Coopers' FIGs—Fluency Initiating Gestures (Cooper & Cooper, 1985). The clinician's primary responsibility at this stage in the counseling process is to match the client's successful affective, behavioral, and cognitive coping patterns with therapy strategies dependent for their success on those very same coping patterns. Asking a feeling-oriented client to achieve the feeling of control through bibliotherapy does not appear an appropriate therapy strategy. Similarly, asking a cognitively oriented individual to focus on changing affricates and plosives to fricatives to gain the feeling of control may not be using the client's coping strategies effectively.

Identifying patterns of client coping strategies and then identifying fluency-facilitating strategies to capitalize on those patterns is challenging. However, our culture is filled with attempts at identifying various successful coping patterns common among the citizenry. Popular women's and men's magazines found on most newsstands typically contain one or two quick "checklists" to assist readers in identifying their affective, behavioral, or cognitive coping patterns in response to common life situations (e.g., screaming children, abusive relationships, eating patterns, and domineering bosses). The psychological literature is equally replete with more formal protocols for identifying coping patterns. Perhaps one of the most frequently applied systems for identifying psychological types is the Myers-Brigg Type Indicator (Myers, 1962, 1976). The most recent attempt at identifying and applying fluency-facilitating affective, behavioral, and cognitive coping patterns for adolescents and adults who stutter is Blood's (1995) *The POWERR Game: Dealing with Stuttering.* Clinicians can use such therapy tools effectively with clients in identifying and utilizing client coping patterns to facilitate gaining and maintaining fluency control. To provide lighthearted, humorous assistance to clinicians in identifying common affective, behavioral, and cognitive patterns observed in group therapy situations, Cooper and Cooper (1985) labeled and described the following patterns (presented here simply as examples of coping patterns):

- The *Oiler:* consistently "pours oil on troubled waters" by trying to smooth over any unpleasantness or discomfort in the group.

- The *Sunbeam:* interprets anything and everything that occurs in the group and is acknowledged by group members as being the harbinger of goodness, sweetness, and light.

- The *Moralist:* interprets almost everything in terms of being good or bad.

- The *Challenger:* consistently questions the accuracy of what is said whether or not the accuracy of any particular statement is relevant to the issue being discussed.

- The *Fountain:* constantly weeps real tears at any expression of feelings, positive or negative.

- The *Prosecutor:* questions in such a rapid-fire manner that the questioning suggests that the intent is to confuse rather than to learn.

- The *Sexist:* consistently interprets behavior and expressions of feelings as being related to gender.

- The *Doormat:* encourages others in the group to "tromp on me."

- The *Judge:* feels compelled to make pronouncements regarding the rightness or wrongness of the observations of others.

- The *Quipper:* is compelled to verbalize "one-liners" in response to any and all expressions of feelings, particularly when they are discomforting.

- The *Dreamer:* prefers to think and talk about what might have been, and what might be, rather than what is.

- The *Fog:* relates events as though seen through a heavy mist, never clearly and always devoid of detail.

- The *Sponge:* takes and adopts, as his or her own, the cares and worries of every member of the group.

- The *Interpreter:* is compelled to explain why other members of the group feel, act, and think as they do.

- The *Intellectualizer:* knows that everything (feelings included) can be rationalized to comfortableness.

- The *Defender:* jumps to the aid of others even when they are not being attacked.

- The *Amoeba:* is careful never to take a position on anything, just ebbs and flows with the tide.

- The *Reinforcer:* feels compelled to provide positive feedback whether appropriate or not.

- The *Denier:* sees, hears, and can think of no problems.

- The *Cloud:* casts a pall over any event, happy or sad.

- The *Cynic:* sees no value in anything anyone is doing.

- The *Doomsayer:* manages to utter "it'll never work" to almost any group suggestion.

- The *Procrastinator:* somehow manages to rationalize the postponement of initiating any behavioral or attitudinal changes at least until next time.

- The *Spacer:* seems to be mentally placed in outer space although physically present.

- The *Dogmatist:* specializes in making pronouncements about the way things are, and ought to be, in such a manner as to abruptly halt any further discussion.

Such labels for coping patterns should, of course, be used with caution particularly if they convey a negative valuing. More importantly, clients are encouraged to develop the ability to describe accurately and with precision their typical coping strategies. In fact, clients are encouraged to take joy and pride in coping patterns they identify as characteristic of themselves. Having identified the coping patterns, clients can begin to determine how they can use them to their advantage in altering those things about themselves they might wish to change. The clinician's role then becomes one of assisting the client in identifying the change agents most compatible with their coping patterns.

## TEACHING BEHAVIORAL STRATEGIES TO GAIN THE FEELING OF FLUENCY CONTROL

It is during the third stage (adjustment) of the fluency counseling relationship that the clinician begins instructing the client in the use of behavioral techniques, as well as affective and cognitive strategies, to alter fluency patterns to attain the feeling of fluency control. The extent to which clients rely on such behavioral techniques to earn the feeling of control is dependent, of course, on the coping strategies they ultimately wish to apply to their fluency disorder. Cooper and Cooper (1985, 1991) describe six speech techniques (FIGs—Fluency Initiating Gestures) that have been widely and successfully used in altering fluency in those who stutter:

> *Slow FIG* is a reduction in the rate of speech, typically involving equalized prolongations of syllables. The rate of speech is altered systematically, with the client prolonging each syllable or a word, phrase, or sentence.
> *Easy FIG* is a gentle superimposition of phonation on a gentle exhalation. It is most useful for those whose dysfluencies are characterized by laryngeal spasms. The client slowly exhales air before superimposing voice on the airflow. The client begins with a relaxed yawn and then gently initiates the process of articulation for speech.
> *Deep FIG* is a consciously controlled inhalation of air prior to the initiation of phonation.
> *Loud FIG* is a conscious and sustained increase or decrease in vocal intensity.
> *Beat FIG* is a change in the prosody (melody) and rhythm (beat) of speech accomplished by altering loudness, pitch, rate, and/or stress features during speech.
> *Smooth FIG* is a reduction of phonatory adjustments and use of light articulatory contacts, with plosives and affricative sounds being modified to resemble fricative sounds. It is characterized by continuous phonation or airflow combined with light articulatory contacts. (Cooper & Cooper, 1991, p. 30.)

Cooper and Cooper (1985, 1991, 1995) maintain that the use of such behavioral techniques are of value only in so far as they continue to assist clients in maintaining the feeling of control. To sustain the feeling of fluency control obtained through the use of FIGs, clients are instructed in "FIG switching" in which, within the same speech situation, they use a variety of combinations of the FIGs. It is apparent that unless a client experiencing a stuttering syndrome is capable of maintaining a *feeling* of fluency control, dysfluent episodes increase in both frequency and severity.

The fluency counseling third stage concludes when clients demonstrate the following:

1. Accurate perceptions of the affective, behavioral, and cognitive components of their stuttering syndrome.
2. An awareness of their affective, behavioral, and cognitive coping patterns and an ability to apply those coping strategies to earning and maintaining the feeling of fluency control.
3. An ability to develop and maintain positive self-reinforcement activities.
4. An understanding of and an ability to use fluency initiating gestures to assist in earning and maintaining the feeling of fluency control.

Although clinicians will have a significant amount of data with which to determine if a client meets the criteria noted above, the decision whether the client is ready for the action stage of the counseling process requires thoughtful analyses. Simply put, clients may or may not be ready to undertake "going for" the feeling of fluency control. For those clients who are not prepared to commit themselves to attaining the feeling of control, therapy might better be put on hold for an agreed-on period of time or even terminated if that appears to be the best course of action as far as a client's well-being is concerned. Unquestionably, to proceed to the final stage of therapy before the client is ready is not in the best interests of the client.

## Action Stage

To attain and maintain the feeling of fluency control, clinicians assist clients in maximizing the effectiveness of their affective, behavioral, and cognitive coping patterns that were identified, enhanced, or developed in the initial stages of therapy. Again, the primary goal in this final stage of therapy is the development of the feeling of fluency control.

The fourth and final stage of counseling dysfluent adolescents and adults is initiated when the clinician begins instructing the client in the use of coping strategies, including adjustments in speech production, outside of the clinical situation. Prior to this point in therapy, clinicians advise the client of their hesitancy to prescribe the use of specific strategies to earn the feeling of fluency control until they are convinced the client has attained the goals of the first three stages of therapy.

Initiating the final stage of therapy appears premature if clients:

- are not effective self-reinforcers
- do not view accurately their stuttering and its ramifications
- do not have a realistic emotional and intellectual appreciation of self
- do not understand their typical affective, behavioral, and cognitive coping patterns
- do not have a repertoire of fluency-enhancing affective, behavioral, and cognitive strategies
- do not believe the end goal of fluency therapy is the feeling of fluency control
- are unwilling or unable to expend a significant amount of psychic energy in the pursuit of the feeling of fluency control.

To avoid clients experiencing the frustrations that accompany failure with a therapy process, clinicians need to be confident clients are ready to commit themselves to earning and maintaining the feeling of fluency control before asking them to do so.

Frequently, as clients develop a more accurate self-concept, their perspectives of the significance of their fluency disorder to their sense of well-being changes markedly. Such changes in their perspectives may lead to alterations in their priorities with respect to what they want to do with their lives. They may conclude their fluency problem is not nearly as significant as they had perceived it to be and, further, the amount of energy they would need to spend in earning the feeling of control is not warranted at this period in their lives. Clients arriving at such a conclusion, based on a realistic assessment of their life situation, may be considered as successful in therapy as those who successfully commit significant amounts of energy to pursue the feeling of control. Adolescents and young adults typically find themselves committed to so many other productive and fulfilling activities that, in view of their more realistic perceptions of their stuttering, they cease to view stuttering as a major concern. Such clients can be dismissed from therapy with a real sense of accomplishment by both the client and the clinician. Clients can also be reassured that, if or when the control of their stuttering syndrome becomes a top priority in their lives, they can re-enter therapy with a real sense of hope in increasing their feeling of fluency control.

Clients begin to withdraw from the therapy relationship when they experience and maintain the feeling of fluency control outside of the clinic situation without the clinician's assistance. As clients begin attaining the feeling of control, therapy appointments are spaced with ever-increasing periods of time between appointments until clients indicate that they wish to terminate the formal therapeutic relationship. In this manner, the initial phase of follow-up procedures can be considered as part of the therapeutic process. Ideally, as the client-clinician relationship approaches termination, clients begin to develop a fluency-support system outside of the therapy situation. They might enroll themselves in a local self-help group for those who stutter. The National Stuttering Project, the National Council on Stuttering, and Speakeasy International all sponsor self-help groups. Toastmaster Clubs are found in many cities throughout the nation and historically have provided individuals who stutter with ideal opportunities to enhance and maintain their feeling of fluency control.

Just as fine artists can always see something they would like to add even to their finest paintings, clinicians, as they terminate a successful helping relationship, rarely feel a sense of completion. Clinicians invariably feel there is more that they might have done for the client. Similarly, clients typically feel there is more they might do to enhance their feeling of control. Thus, the termination of therapy is seldom achieved without clinician and client feeling incompleteness. However, assuming the goals of therapy were achieved, both client and clinician can look back on the therapy process with a sense of accomplishment, knowing they were able to modify, if not conquer, one of humankind's most tenacious and enigmatic disorders.

## THE EFFECTIVE COUNSELING CLINICIAN

The success of any therapy process involving the identification and modification of feeling, behavior, and thinking is dependent to a great extent on the clinician's ability to establish the kind of helping relationship that facilitates client introspection and self-evaluation. Murphy and FitzSimons (1960), in describing a counseling-type therapy for those who stutter, observed that: "The most important single variable affecting success in the treatment of stuttering is—the clinician" (p. 27). After reviewing what research was available at the time concerning the characteristics of the effective clinician, Cooper and Cooper (1985) concluded that effective clinicians could be described as follows:

> Affectively Verbal—Viscerally Vocal
> Affectively Honest
> Primarily Reflective—Not Affectively Directive
> Devoid of Dogma
> Noninterpretive
> Perseverative
> Informative
> Detail Disciplined (p. 27)

In a brochure distributed by the National Stuttering Project (1994) entitled *How to Get the Most Out of Stuttering Therapy*, Eugene B. Cooper advised those who stutter:

> If, from the very start, you don't like and respect your clinician, find another one. You need and deserve a clinician with whom you feel comfortable and with whom you can be open and honest about how you feel, think, and behave. If from the very first time you meet, your clinician doesn't make you feel good about being in therapy, find another.
>
> I am not saying everything should be sweetness and light in therapy. In fact, if it is, probably nothing is happening. But I am saying your clinician should make you feel good about being there. Research reveals that effective clinicians:
>
> - Express feelings openly—they let you know how they feel;
> - Are honest—they tell it like it is;

- Are positive in their attitudes—they see the good where many do not;
- Reflect feelings rather than direct feeling—they don't presume to tell others how they should feel;
- Are open minded—they are not judgmental;
- Are informative—they are perfectly clear about the purpose for each therapeutic activity;
- Are perseverative in their pursuit of goals—they hang in there;
- Are detail disciplined—they don't miss a thing.

Manning (1996) concludes his chapter on clinician characteristics in a recent text by noting:

> The best clinicians know that clients have much to teach us and can often benefit really as much from the treatment process as they do. Although we have been down this path before, the territory and timing of the steps will be new for our companion, to whom we must attend closely and with both determination and esteem. (p. 21)

An effective counseling clinician for those experiencing a stuttering syndrome is far more than an efficient technician. Technicians can implement well-defined, behaviorally oriented techniques, but the skills of a clinician are needed to assist clients in identifying, developing, and enhancing fluency-facilitating affective, behavioral, and cognitive coping patterns.

## SUMMARY

This chapter began by defining terms concerning fluency disorders and stuttering syndromes and describing a stuttering syndrome's characteristic affective, behavioral, and cognitive components. A brief discussion defining a continuum of helping relationships and counseling's place on that continuum followed as did a discussion of the goals for a counseling relationship for adolescents and adults experiencing a stuttering syndrome. A counseling process consisting of four stages (orientation, relationship, adjustment, and action) was then described. The chapter concluded with a brief description of an effective counseling clinician for adolescents and adults who stutter.

## REFERENCES

Blood, G. W. (1995). *The POWERR game: Dealing with stuttering.* Tucson, AZ: Communication Skill Builders.

Bloodstein, O. (1995). *A handbook on stuttering* (5th ed.). San Diego, CA: Singular Publishing Group.

Cooper, C. S., & Cooper, E. B. (1966). Variations in adult stutterer attitudes towards clinicians during therapy. *Journal of Communications Disorders, 2,* 141–153.

Cooper, E. B. (1965). An inquiry into the use of interpersonal communications as a source for therapy for stutterers. In D. Barbara (Ed.), *New directions in stuttering.* Springfield, IL: Charles C Thomas.

Cooper, E. B. (1966). Client-clinician relationships and concomitant factors in stuttering therapy. *Journal of Speech and Hearing Research, 9,* 194–297.

Cooper, E. B. (1982). Understanding the process. In S. Ainsworth (Ed.), *Counseling stutterers.* Memphis, TN: Stuttering Foundation of America.

Cooper, E. B. (1993a). Chronic perseverative stuttering syndrome: A harmful or helpful construct? *American Journal of Speech-Language Pathology, 3,* 11–22.

Cooper, E. B. (1993b). Red herrings, dead horses, straw men, and blind alleys: Escaping the stuttering conundrum. *Journal of Fluency Disorders, 18,* 375–387.

Cooper, E. B., & Cooper, C. S. (1985). *Cooper personalized fluency control therapy* (Revised). Austin, TX: Pro-ed.

Cooper, E. B., & Cooper, C. S. (1991). A fluency disorders prevention program for preschoolers and children in the primary grades. *American Journal of Speech-Language Pathology, 1,* 28–31.

Cooper, E. B., & Cooper, C. S. (1995). Treating fluency disordered adolescents. *Journal of Communications Disorders, 28,* 125–142.

Cooper, E. B., Eggerston, S. A., & Galbraith, S. A. (1971). Clinician personality factors and effectiveness. *Journal of Communications Disorders, 4,* 40–43.

Cooper E. B., & Gregory, H. (1994). *How to get the most out of stuttering therapy.* San Francisco, CA: National Stuttering Project.

Manning, W. H. (1996). *Clinical decision making in the diagnosis and treatment of fluency disorders.* New York, NY: Delmar Publishers.

Manning, W. H., & Cooper, E. B. (1969). Variations in attitudes of the adult stutterer toward his clinician related to progress in therapy. *Journal of Communications Disorders, 2,* 154–162.

Murphy, A., & FitzSimons, R. (1969). *Stuttering and personality dynamics.* New York, NY: The Ronald Press.

Myers, I. B. (1962). *The Myers-Briggs type indicator.* Palo Alto, CA: Consulting Psychologist Press.

Myers, I. B. (1976). *Introduction to type* (2nd ed.). Gainesville, FL: Center for Applications of Psychological Type.

# 7. Behavioral Counseling in Voice Disorders

R. E. (Ed) Stone, Jr.

> Where no counsel is, the people fall: but in the multitude of counselors there is safety.
>
> Proverbs 11:14

Anticipation of writing this chapter on counseling in voice disorders raised questions to what theories and what content could be addressed without repeating the contributions from Clark (1990), Lavorato and McFarlane (1988), and Stone and Olswang (1989). Of further consideration was how the practice of counseling could be taught by the written word and apart from the personal interaction of teacher and student or clinician and client (patient).

Help might come from referring to the dictionary for elaboration of the term counsel. There, one finds that the term can be a noun, as in the act of exchanging ideas and also in carefully considered advice. Additionally, counsel can be used as a verb, advise, as to give a person advice. Further explanations of this term used as a verb were: to exchange ideas; consult together; deliberate. The bottom line appears to be that counseling is a part of teaching, principally by verbal instruction.

## FOCUS OF BEHAVIORAL CONSULTATION

In considering that "behavioral" is a key idea in this chapter, we can exclude many of the medical, surgical, and psychological topics that are often important in the interventions in dysphonia. Behavioral narrows consideration to the things that *clinicians do* to foster and give focus to what *people do* with associated undesired and desired vocal and laryngeal consequences.

## Behavioral Counseling to Instate and Maintain Desirable Physiologic Events

Interestingly, most dictionary explanations of behavior, behaviorism, behavioristic, or behavior therapy address the issue of acting and reacting, but do little to emphasize that such action is based on physiologic events. In spite of the fact that behavior must be viewed as motor (neuromuscular) acts, behavior as *personal physiologic doing* is often not recognized by either clinician or client. For example, people often talk in terms of things happening (consequences, outcomes) to them rather than in terms of what they do that ends in consequences that are the "happenings." As further illustration, clinicians often talk to clients about "too much mucus in the throat" rather than what the client does that results in the laryngeal sicca. To illustrate the confusion of having a consequence instead of "doing" behaviors is viewing persistent mutational falsetto as a condition. Regrettably, clinicians often talk about a patient having a high pitch rather than indicating the client is elevating the larynx and increasing muscle activity during phonation.

## Behavioral Counseling to Eliminate Vocal Abuse Is Different Than to Correct Vocal Misuse

Clinicians often consider vocal abuse and vocal misuse as very closely related (if not synonymous) terms (Johnson, 1985; Stemple, Glaze & Gerdeman, 1995; Wilson, 1987). In this chapter, the terms "vocal abuse" and "vocal misuse" are used to designate different clinical entities. Here, vocal abuse refers to behaviors associated with a relatively normal sounding voice but which have a high risk for inducing vocal fold pathology (e.g., normal physiologic function resulting in shouting or screaming). The dysphonia subsequent to abuse is organically based. On the other hand, vocal misuse, refers to voice problems that arise out of behavioral manifestations of abnormal physiologic functioning of anatomic structures (Perkins & Curlee, 1969). Thus, functional dysphonia or vocal misuse refers to behaviors, not pathologic structures, that account for vocal aberrancy. Dysphonia from misuse is nonorganic based.

The content of consultation to prevent and correct vocal abuse assumes a set of considerations that differ from those in the intervention in vocal misuse. Consultation in vocal abuse reduction typically involves avoiding or eliminating risky actions of the client. Generally two aspects of intervention are involved in minimizing dysphonias in the absence of vocal fold pathology and which result directly from inappropriate behaviors brought to the task of voice production (muscular incoordination, vocal misuse). One aspect involves eliciting behaviors that result in different and closer to normal voice and then shaping the behavior to normal use. The other involves guiding the client to assume responsibility for applying newly learned coordinated muscular acts in speaking situations outside the clinical environment.

## CONSULTATION IN VOCAL ABUSE

### Definition of Vocal Abuse

Vocal abuse involves those behaviors that usually are first associated with relatively normal sounding voice but which make the vocal folds vulnerable to injury, subsequent tissue reaction, and associated dysphonia. Such pathologies typically present in the forms of vascular-based lesions (Chen, 1989; Remacle, Lagneau, Marbaix, Doyen, & Van den Eeckhaut, 1992); contact granulomas (Block, Gould, & Hirano, 1981; Sieron & Johannsen, 1992); polyps (Harma, Sonninen, Vartiainen, Haveri, & Vaisanen, 1975); nodules (Toohill, 1975); or cysts (Ford, 1994). In the clinical setting, differential diagnosis of the latter three pathologies often cannot be determined with certainty and, therefore, they generically might be referred to as *podulcysts*. Pulling, pressing, bending, twisting, and friction have been suggested as mechanisms of injury (Sonninen, Damste, Jol, & Fokkens, 1972). Shearing forces between tissues within the lamina propria or between the cover and body of the vocal folds may be another source of injury.

The term vocal abuse refers principally to the production of voice (for propositional as well as non-propositional purposes) in which pitch and loudness are elevated or there is excessive duration of production. Added to these concepts of voice production that is too high, too loud, or too long, vocal abuse also seems to imply voice production associated with excessive muscular effort. When techniques for study of phonation aerodynamics become more user friendly, increased subglottal pressure and high flow rates eventually may be added to a vocal abuse formula.

There is meager current evidence from scientific investigation that such factors contribute to the development of dysphonia and laryngeal pathology. While studying cricoid cartilage movement in canines resulting from stimulation of the superior laryngeal nerves, Stone and Nuttal (1974), induced phonation through controlled air flow and electrical stimulation of the recurrent nerves. They found the vocal folds occasionally developed inflammation and edema. In one animal, a vocal fold polyp was induced with high flow rates and supra-maximal stimulation when repeated for more than an hour. Gray and Titze (1988) described tissue changes in canine vocal fold epithelium resulting from hyperphonation over 2 to 4 hours of stimulation. Thus, there is indirect evidence that increased muscular activity and high flow rates may be associated with vocal abuse. Phonation at increased fundamental frequencies and at relatively great vocal intensity seems associated with voice quality changes according to Stone and Sharf (1973). They were not able, however, to document the vocal folds of their subjects before and after participation in the experimental procedures. Masuda, Ikeda, Manako, and Komiyama (1993) studied the speaking habits of 29 subjects for 131 days. Their results showed that office workers exhibited a phonation time of 33.6 ± 13.6 minutes over 8 hours of assessment. This is three times shorter than that of teachers and also of patients with vocal fold nodules (102.1 ± 22.9 minutes for 8 hours). For the teachers and patients with a long phonation time, half of the total time was at high intensity. Buekers, Bierens, Kingma, and Marres (1995) also studied the accumulated phonation times of various voice users. Figure 7.1 illustrates that nurses and speech-language pathologists yielded the greatest amount of voice use, at about 50% of a 12-hour day. Yet, their vocal intensities are relatively low in contrast to sports instructors who use voice less than 40% of the day. But, when sports instructors phonate, 60% of the time is in excess of 66 dBa.

From the meager experimental literature and a plethora of clinical experience represented in various textbooks on voice (e.g., Boone & McFarlane, 1993; Colton & Casper, 1990; Stemple, 1993; Greene, 1980), the definition of vocal abuse might be summarized by a statement such as, "Voice produced too long, too often, too high, too loud, with too much effort (or too much air) that leads to changes in the tissue cover overlying the body of the vocal folds."

An inventory of patients' vocal uses, therefore, becomes a significant feature of the counseling process. As early clinical procedures to reduce vocal abuse, Johnson (1985) recommends pinpointing specific vocal uses and identifying the times abuse is likely to occur.

## Gaining a Vocal Use Inventory

### PICTORIAL ASSAYS

Children seem to identify their vocal uses from pictures better than from verbal labels. Thus, Wilson (1987) employed line drawings of probable abuses. With the popularity of

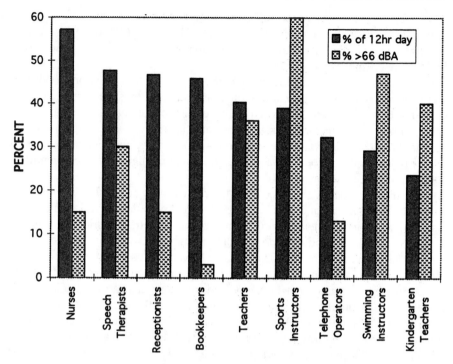

**Figure 7.1.** Voice duration and intensity loads. (From Buekers R., Bierens E., Kingma H., Marres, E. H. M. A. (1995). Vocal load as measured by the voice accumulator. *Folia Phoniatrica, 47*, 252–261.)

more recent activities for youth such as Little League baseball and football, soccer, competitive swimming, karate, Star Search for child performers, and so forth, his illustrations might benefit from expansion.

VERBAL ASSAYS

For the older person, a checklist rather than photos of possible vocal abuse behaviors is probably sufficient to indicate vocal abuse. Incorporating a graphic display may more poignantly illustrate risky behaviors to a patient and could be used as an adjunct to lists. Figure 7.2 illustrates a self-inventory of a rock singer/song writer who developed a unilateral excrescence on the lower lip of the left vocal fold. Unusual vocal noises, screaming, and alcohol and tobacco intake typically are included in an inventory; however, in this case these were null factors. This client indicated that most of her talking involved long telephone use (fone). An inventory usually might have the generic term "irritants." This person was more specific and indicated she was in an environment of stage smoke and bus fumes a lot.

## Consultation in Vocal Abuse Reduction in Children

Nearly every author dealing with the topic of vocal abuse indicates that abuses should be stopped. Yet, few are explicit in how to attempt cessation. Most consultants merely provide verbal admonitions. In contrast, Johnson (1985), in his book, *Vocal Abuse Reduction Program* (VARP), specifically describes how to assist children in the cessation process. He includes information on both content and methods of consultation; the nature of vocal

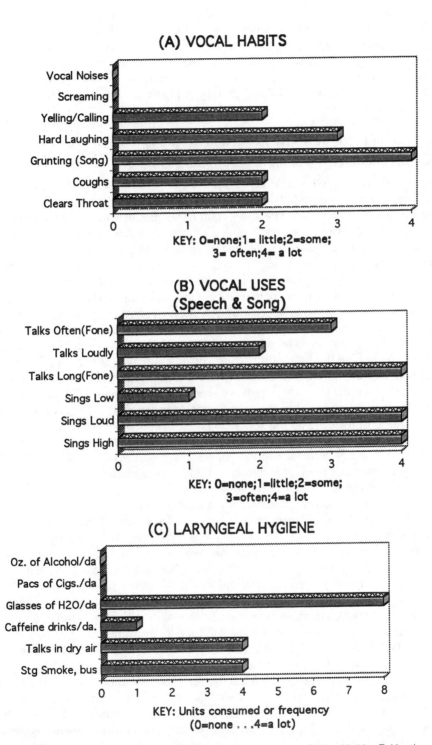

**Figure 7.2.** Self-inventory for determining possible factors of vocal abuse: **A.** Vocal habits. **B.** Vocal uses. **C.** Laryngeal hygiene.

abuse and its consequences; how to elicit parental and client participation in the program; and how to make telephone contacts for patient follow-up and counseling. This may be of particular interest in light of recent third-party payer surveillance on number of therapy sessions. Although this program has been summarized elsewhere (Stone, 1981), referral to the original work is strongly suggested. When the program is modified, there is a risk of success rates lower than the 80% and therapy going beyond the 2- to 15-week commitment Johnson describes.

## Consultation in Vocal Abuse Reduction in Adults

CONSIDERATIONS FOR THE GENERAL POPULATION

In contrast to working with children who usually are motivated by someone else to seek clinical intervention, most adults are self-motivated and generally require less convincing about the need to change vocal behaviors and habits. Because adults bring a broad range of knowledge and experiences to the clinical setting, consultation about the vocal mechanism and the effects of abuse is usually accomplished within a part of the first session. This session also may include beginning the voice inventory. Thus, an adult may use the period between the first and second session for a validity check of the inventory and bring suggestions for revising the inventory to be more personally appropriate to the next session.

In addition to eliminating specific abuses, the clinician also might teach principles of effective voice production. This involves assisting the client in selecting pitch and loudness levels and phonation styles that (a) yield the best sound, (b) allow the greatest durability, and (c) require the least effort. Thus, consultation against unnecessary muscle effort in both degree and location is appropriate. Excessive degree of laryngeal tension can be assumed when the false vocal folds are seen under laryngoscopy to move medially or when the epiglottis approaches the arytenoids. Unnecessary degrees of effort frequently are recognized by focusing on the abdominal area. People often extensively tense the abdominal muscles too much when talking. For one-on-one conversations, it is not necessary to use strong abdominal support. Instead, a person's effort for voice production should be comparable to quiet respiration. (This changes when teaching voice with increased vocal loudness.)

Unnecessary location of muscle activity is easily recognized in the person who stutters and has been called "secondary manifestations." In dysphonic individuals, such secondary manifestations usually are less blatant, but often can be seen when the clinician looks for them. For example, it is not necessary for one to show evidence of activity in the strap muscles when phonating. Yet, these muscles (jumpers, because they so readily come into view with the onset of voice) often are involved in the phonatory processes of vocal abusers. Also, laryngeal elevation reveals unnecessary activity of the supralaryngeal muscles that do not have to be involved in most phonations. Other sites may include forehead wrinkling, excessive lip pursing as a prephonation activity, and leg and arm movements. Unnecessary activity sets the stage for heightened levels of muscle activity in the larynx that approach or contribute to hyperkinetic phonation.

As part of the consultation for relaxed voice production, the clinician may consider guiding the client to implement voice production on the beginning of exhaled air, without breath holding at the transition of inspiration to expiration. Some clients require training via relaxation techniques (Jacobson, 1978) before they can produce steady voiceless exhalation. If production of intended sustained vowels shows quick waxing and waning in vocal intensity with concomitant jerky motions of the thorax and abdomen, preliminary relaxation and air flow training seems in order. When the client can produce even, sustained vowels without tension, vocalizations may be shaped into propositional speech following clinician counseling to implement technique in a hierarchy of speaking situations from vowels to dialogue. The counseling process may also include several sessions to pursue the extent to which the client succeeds in implementing good technique in the everyday world and in problem-solving any failures.

Effective maintenance of behaviors can be correlated with the clinician's skill in designing activities whereby the client learns to be responsible for the behaviors he or she brings to the task of speaking. It is the task of the behavioral counselor to develop strategies of approximation in using skills learned in the clinic to implement activities of daily living. This is an individualized strategy and, thus, programmed audio and video tapes and other productions for the general public often fall short of the mark.

## SPECIAL CONSIDERATIONS FOR PROFESSIONAL VOICE USERS

In addition to the foibles of vocal suicide experienced by the general public, professional voice users experience greater vocal abuse. Many such individuals in the past have been relatively disinterested in voice care but now there is a trend toward becoming more attuned to voice problems and to seek help. This possibly is due to recent media coverage of highly visible individuals such as Bill Clinton, Luciano Pavarotti, Sammy Davis, Jr., Jack Klugman, Kathy Mattea, and Larry Gatlin, who have had laryngeal and vocal disorders. Thus, with increasing frequency, a clinician may be asked about professional uses of voice, vocal hygiene, prevention of abuse, and preservation of vocal function. Consultation content might include some of the following ideas. Vocologists at the Vanderbilt Voice Center who have contributed to this topic include, specifically, Kimberly Chachere, Melissa Portell, Cheryl Rainey, Jackie Gartner, and Dr. Tom Cleveland.

Voice Use Program

*Outside the Venue*

When in a professional mode of voice use (e.g., on a performance or lecture tour, during days of rehearsals, recording sessions, cutting commercials, or song writing) a person should employ alternatives to oral communication as much as possible. This may involve relegating business negotiations to the an agent or manager. During heavy vocal demands professionals might well follow a basic rule: Avoid talking unless being paid for it. Another rule for survival might be: Minimize the duration of necessary conversations. Unnecessary and extended verbal intercourse that merely falls under the rubric of social niceties should be deferred until the professional demands are no longer present.

Another potential rule might be: Intersperse periods of vocal use with silence. Frequently, individuals may find that following an 80/20 or 90/10 minute rule to be helpful under which the larger numeral represents duration of voice use and the smaller numeral the duration of silence. Also, employ strategies that favor quiet rather than loud vocalizations. This can be done when a person emulates the voice used in a confidential sharing of thoughts. Using a "Ma Bell" voice suggests talking only when the speaker can reach out and touch someone (the listener); that is, when interpersonal distances favor using a quiet voice. Following such a guideline, the client avoids calling from one room to another, from one end of a tour bus to the other, from inside to outside, and so forth.

*At the Venue*

The counselor might also choose to review a singer's program of numbers to place the most challenging numbers near the first of the program or soon after the intermission. This avoids having an entire section of the program being stressful and fatiguing or placing the numbers in the program at a place when the performer might already be fatigued. Some performers will have two plans: the one they would like to do and an alternative less-demanding program to implement if vocal problems are encountered. A factor, other than the demands of the music, might be the energy expended on stage for choreographic effects. On a long tour, artists might need to pace themselves differently than for a one-night performance.

Coping with the Environment

Loud ambient noise level is one of the more significant environmental factors contributing to vocal abuse. Individuals are known to increase vocal intensity in the presence of noise owing to the Lombard effect that influences all individuals, even laryngectomees (Zeine & Brandt, 1988). Thus, one might attempt to get away to quieter locations when talking. This might mean:

1. Stepping out of a noisy bar when talking to a patron.
2. Moving to a quieter part of a room when giving verbal directions to an associate.
3. Moving away from the TV.
4. Rolling the car windows up before conversing.
5. Waiting for transient high noise level (e.g., as passing traffic) to abate.
6. Wearing ear protection to minimize the sound level and to emulate a conductive hearing loss under which people generally talk quieter.
7. Working with the sound engineer to assure the most prominent feedback is the performer's own voice. Feedback of audience noise, band, and back-up singers should serve merely as reference background for the performer. The artist should not try to adjust vocal loudness to overcome such reference signals. The sound engineers are the persons who should amplify and present the sound properly to the audiences.

Following an indirect counseling approach, individuals might make their own lists of potential communications in noisy environments and itemize alternatives suitable for them.

Airborne irritants represent another area of concern, particularly to individuals with a lot of allergies. Use of Nasalcrom is effective for some individuals in treating allergies before exposure to known allergens. Ensuring maintenance of air filtration or air conditioning systems on a periodic basis is a high priority for some individuals who use leased motor vehicles. Assurance that a performer is not intolerant of certain products released in the making of stage smoke for lighting effects is also important. Some patients favor bare floors to carpeting in the tour bus because of ease in controlling molds and freedom from offensive chemical substances found in fabric floor coverings. Similar consideration could be given to window treatments, bedding, and furniture.

Size of venue (whether classroom, courtroom, theater, arena, or open space) and the distance between the speaker or singer and the listener influence the need for increasing vocal intensity either by physiologic acts or by amplification. One such an amplification system (AudioPack Sound System, 10011 Walford Ave., Cleveland, OH 44102) features a headset microphone for hands-free use in association with the amplifier and two speakers worn around the waist, which makes it effective for use by coaches, auctioneers, tour guides, rangers, and other active professional voice users. For classroom and similar environments, wireless microphones used in association with FM receivers, amplifiers, and speakers (LightSpeed, 15812 S.W. Upper Boones Ferry Road, Lake Oswego, OR 97035) are becoming standard equipment in newly constructed schools. Whereas low level amplification has proved beneficial for students with even mild hearing losses as well as normally hearing children, teachers who use such amplification seem to experience fewer lost employment days because of voice problems (Anonymous, 1990). Several hand-held microphone-amplifiers are available for portable use (LUMINAUD, 8688 Tyler Boulevard, Mentor, OH 44060–4348).

Phone use provides abundant opportunity for potential abuse of the voice. It has been suggested that positioning the handpiece of the phone between the ear and the shoulder produces unnecessary muscle tension and places asymmetric strain on the vocal folds by the resulting head posture. Additionally, nonbusiness phone calls tend to be prolonged beyond necessity, particularly by individuals with time on their hands. This situation is encountered by those who travel great distances between vocational venues, such as those in sales and entertainment. Frequency of calls appears to be a problem for some individuals in telephone marketing. For example, representatives of at least one airline company are expected to take a new customer call within 20 seconds of concluding service to the previous customer and have only one 20-minute break every 2 hours. Any one call is usually quite short but the frequency of calls inclines these individuals to extensive vocal use day after day. It is difficult to convince management of the need for different guidelines such as, for example, 5 minutes between long conversations or 10-minute silence breaks every hour.

Based on the premise that many individuals increase vocal intensity when using the phone, as if the phone attenuated the voice, some laryngologists forbid patient phone use during a period of recovery from vocal fold injury. As an alternative, the counselor might instruct patients on effective phone use and proper intensity levels.

The increasing popularity of mobile phones offers another focus on voice use. Optimizing use by closing car windows, for instance, might incline the user to employ a quieter voice when speaking. There seems to be an association between the difficulty encountered in hearing the speech of others and the loudness of one's own voice. Discontinuing conversation that involves poor transmission and recalling when a new location has been reached is another strategy for cellular phone users.

Personal Factors

There are no data to support the dogma that there is a correlation between efficiency and efficacy of voice use and physical status. Yet, performers have shared their perceived benefits from:

1. Routine exercise (without vocalized grunts; e.g., in weight lifting or striking a tennis ball).
2. Getting adequate rest.
3. Seeking advise from a nutrition expert.
4. Attending to proper eating habits, particularly during performance season
   - scheduling meals to avoid eating just before performance
   - not lying down within 2 hours after a meal
   - avoiding junk food snacks
   - avoiding dehydrating substances such as caffeine (Fig. 7.3), alcohol, vitamin C in excess of 2000 mg, high temperature air as found in smoking, and routine use of antihistamines
   - assuring proper hydration of the body by drinking at least eight glasses of water (approximately one glass every 2 waking hours)
5. Altering typical risky vocal uses during illness to minimize the potential of trauma to the vocal folds when they might be more susceptible to injury.
6. Using a mucolytic agent[1] during periods of high vocal use.

---

[1]The more popular products are Humabid, Organidin (which recently has been reintroduced), Sinubid, and SSKI (supersaturated potassium iodide).

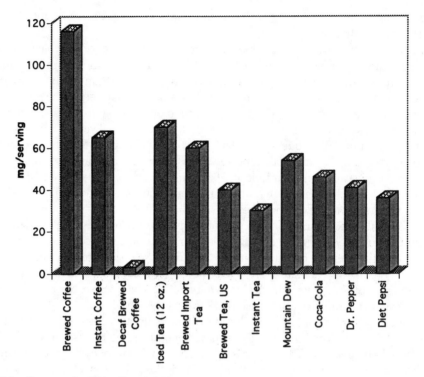

**Figure 7.3.**  Sources of caffeine. (From US News and World Report, 5/22/88.)

Performance Factors (Pampering Procedures)

"The show must go on!" seems to be part of the mores that motivate performers. Wisdom, however, would dictate that when the performer is sick vocal pampering should be accepted. It should be a time when the artist should be permitted not to give the audience 100%. Such pampering might include:

1. Shortening the program.
2. Involving more instrumental pieces between the vocals.
3. Letting others in the group share in carrying the ball.
4. Encouraging co-workers to take care of the task of increasing audience enthusiasm by showing their own enthusiasm and showmanship.
5. Lowering the keys of numbers that involve high notes.
6. Using days off to be off—for rest, recovery, and recreation.

"Walla" Voice Users

The professional who uses voice for special effects may be inclined to use physiologically unhealthy vocal productions that place vocal health at risk. When the counselor assists these individuals to inventory vocal use, special attention might be given to establishing the extent and cost-to-benefit ratio associated with:

1. Character impersonations by an actor or voice-over specialist.
2. Use of a growl as a vocal ornament during singing.
3. Changes in voice characteristics of an auctioneer when crying a sale.

Sometimes the clinician can bring to light in the counseling sessions the fact that vocal tricks or ornaments loose their luster and effectiveness when done too often, which will lead to the client's judicious application of risky productions.

Warm-ups and Cool-downs

Many vocational voice users are beginning to observe vocal warm-ups. Counselors on this topic seem to focus on:

1. Preparing the oral structures for activity with exercises of
   • voiceless and voiced lip trills (that are possible only if the muscles are relaxed and there is an adequate flow of air)
   • alternating between tongue protrusion and retrusion
   • jaw opening and extension
   • head rolls
   • general body stretching
2. Breathing patterns that favor increased
   • dorsal-ventral diameter of the torso at the level of the epigastric area (diaphragmatic breathing)
   • lateral diameter of the lower rib cage (flank or rib-flare breathing)
   • steady flow of air during prolonged exhalations without and with voice
3. Phonatory activities that incorporate
   • humming (to induce attention of voice away from the larynx and foster a sense of vibration in the midface region to signify "placement of the voice . . . in the mask")
   • sustained vowels with lowered larynx during pitch slides (glissando)
   • first line of each song in the concert or some part of each of the actor's lines
   • most vocally demanding activity in the event done at 50% effort with attention to planned techniques of delivery

Recent evidence in exercise physiology (Saxon & Schneider, 1995) suggests that cool-downs are possibly as important as warm-ups. The singer might select some of the warm-up activities and do them in reverse order and with fewer trials. Following the cool-down a performer might use a quiet time for muscular relaxation (Jacobson, 1978) and for signing promotional pictures and other items for distribution back stage. During and after a performance vocal users usually are "pumped." Adrenaline level is high. Jumping immediately into the postperformance "meet and greet" events predisposes the performer to continue vocalizing at performance levels rather than with one-on-one confidential communication characteristics. Thus, in effect, performance is unnecessarily prolonged. Assuring the time for cool-down and quiet time and limiting the length of each visitor's stay, distributing public relations materials to back stage visitors, and coordinating these activities are duties that usually can be assumed by the road manager or other accompanying personnel. To get cooperation from the performer's entourage, the road managers, agents, publicists, promoters, media personnel, and fellow entertainers in the group may need to be educated in matters of voice and its care.

## CONSULTATION IN VOCAL MISUSE—FOSTERING PATIENT RESPONSIBILITY FOR BEHAVIOR IN VOICE PRODUCTION

Dysphonia resulting from other than the presence of abnormal masses, diseases or neurologic control can be presumed to result from misuse, inadequate use of laryngeal muscles, and subglottal air pressures (misuse). There are two facets to intervention. One deals with instating proper mechanics of phonation. Many ploys have been advocated to elicit desired voice characteristics under the rubric of facilitative techniques (Murphy, 1964; Boone & McFarlane, 1994). The other facet involves teaching the client to assume responsibility for the behavior brought to the task of producing voice. Few authors address the aspect of developing behavioral responsibility that most productively is accomplished by direct and indirect counseling. Teaching maintenance of new (or reacquired former) vocal behaviors is influenced by the stories individuals believe about their use of voice.

## The Importance of Behavioral Thematics

People tend to believe and behave in accordance with what they believe about themselves. The importance of such beliefs or themes about self-behavior is brought to light in the writings of Wendell Johnson (1946) who introduced the world of general semantics to the realm of managing stuttering. Dean Williams (1957) showed the fallacy of the "it" of stuttering in his article, *A Point of View about "Stuttering."* About the same time, Hayakawa (1949) wrote *Language in Thought and Action,* which provides information that can influence the counselor's understanding of the language used in clinical counseling. Casteel and Stone (1983) pointed out various language responses that incline clients and clinicians to believe or disbelieve that speaking is self-directed behavior brought to the task of communicating and not something that merely happens. Helmstetter (1982) points out in his book, *What to Say When You Talk to Yourself,* that human beings are the product of the stories they tell themselves. Attention to the content of self-talk, he points out, should be one of man's pre-eminent concerns when change in behavior is desired. These client-based stories often can be influenced by the themes the clinician exhibits during the clinical process.

Clinicians are in the business of changing the way clients behave—of concern here, how they behave in producing voice. Thinking of voice production as an athletic event, speech-language pathologists (SLPs) are analogous to tennis and golf teaching pros or ski instructors. Therefore, their instruction should be physiologically based and they should be aware of their role of a sports psychologist as well. Developing a "can do" attitude is important to the young amateur as well as the seasoned professional athlete. The field of cybernetics is founded on the benefit that imagery and positive thoughts contribute to improved execution of motor acts (behavior). Recent evidence suggests that such imagery influences activity in the supplemental motor cortex and in executing actual behavior that parallels the imagined behavior (Logan, 1996). Neurologic impact of the stories one tells oneself about behavior will continue to explicate and further support the clinically evident validity of self-talk.

## Role of Client Responsibility in Medical and Behavioral Models of Intervention

Two types of themes are prevalent in most clinical environments—those that fit a medical model of intervention and those appropriate to a behavioral model of intervention. In the medical model, the role of the caregiver is active and that of the client is relatively passive. Accordingly, there is the underlying implication that all the patient must do to improve is to take the medicine or receive the surgery. Little is asked of the patient. The caregiver or the medications are the active factor in the therapeutic process. Whatever is causing the condition usually is placed within factors that are external to the patient—a virus or bacteria, a disease process that is not influenced much by what the patient does, or a condition or accident that happens to the patient.

SLPs, however, are not in the business of medicating their clients nor are they into implementing surgical treatment. Instead, they are in the business of ERGs: evaluating, recommending, and guiding practice in adopting new motor skills. The client's role in such ERGs stands in contrast to the role of a patient in the medical model. Success in the behavior modification milieu depends wholly on the client's cognitive activity in recognizing that whatever is wrong lies within the client and the client's ability to do otherwise. In behavioral intervention, the perpetuating cause of the client's problem is internal; not an external factor such as viruses, conditions, or unalterable stimulus-response patterns.

Possibly the most challenging task for the behavioral clinician is guiding a client to implement those skills that are mastered within the clinical environment outside the clinical environment. Typically, maintenance training is initiated after the client has accomplished advanced skills in the clinic. A few clinicians, however, believe that maintenance activities can begin during the early skill-building sessions. In these sessions, maintenance is positively influenced when the client learns that executing skills, be they simple or complex motor patterns, is under his or her control.

The clinician's teaching methods adhere to the principles of learning theory when the clinician influences suitable self-talk in the client through words of instruction and counseling as well as through clinician modeling of appropriate clinical themes.

When implementing a behavioral model, a clinician appropriately should avoid medical model vocabulary and employ behavioral terminology. For example, the term *client* is preferred over *patient*. Dysphonia (of nonorganic basis) and vocal abuse would be discussed in terms of what the client does rather than as a disorder or condition like the flu, a cold, or a disease.

Terms such as *exacerbation* and *remission* are common in the medical model, but would be inappropriate in a behavioral model. Therapy, procedure, and treatment most commonly refer to activities pertaining to the medical model. Thus, the behaviorist might adopt the use of other terms such as *training, intervention, guidance, counseling, management* and *coaching.*

The goal of intervention is another area worthy of consideration in differentiating between medical and behavioral terminology. Behaviorally, the endpoint of intervention is not a cure but rather developing in the client the ability to use improved voice whenever he or she chooses—giving the client behavioral options.

## Thematics and Maintenance of Clinical Performance Outside the Clinic

Unfortunately, empiric evidence is notably lacking that illustrates a correlation between (*a*) language responses as indices of clients belief systems about solutions to their dysphonia and (*b*) maintenance of desired behavior. This may be because of the difficulty one encounters in designing experimental efforts in this area. Nonetheless, Prichard (1971) studied the relationship between changes in the rate of stuttering in one subject and the changes in language themes the person used before, during intervention, and 4 weeks later. Baseline measures showed only 30% of the client's themes were conducive to establishing self-directed speech behavior and a stuttering rate of 21.8 dysfluencies per minute. During the intervention, the dysfluency rate was six per minute and desirable language responses were evidenced at a rate of 95%. Four weeks later stuttering rate had increased to only eight per minute with a decline in number of desirable language responses to 87%. Mathew (1981) found that eleven clients who maintained higher fluency rates after intervention in stuttering demonstrated a greater number and greater variety of what she called "positive language responses" than those five clients who failed to maintain fluency.

Helmstetter (1982) poignantly supports the notion that what we say about ourselves influences our actions:

> Our conditioning . . . has created, reinforced, and nearly permanently cemented most of what we believe about ourselves and what we believe about most of what goes on around us. . . . What we have accepted from the outside world, or fed to ourselves, has initiated a natural cause and effect chain reaction sequence which cannot fail to lead us to successful self-management, or to the unsuccessful mismanagement of ourselves. What we believe determines our attitudes, affects our feelings, directs our behavior, and determines our success or failure:

- Beliefs create attitudes.
- Attitudes create feelings.
- Feelings determine actions.
- Actions create results. (p. 70–71)

  . . . It doesn't make any difference to our internal computer what the problem is or how big it is. But what we tell ourselves about our problems will affect every action we take from that moment forward. (p. 177)

Our self-image, interestingly enough, is largely influenced by other people's stories we hear about ourselves and tell ourselves. These stories or themes incline one either to carry the clinical lessons into the outside world or to abandon the lessons on exiting the clinic. It is the clinician's counseling role to demonstrate language and shape the client's language so that the client uses themes about voicing that fosters client responsibility for behaviors he or she brings to the communicative process.

## Parameters of Behavioral Intervention Thematics

Interviewing clients about successful and unsuccessful accomplishments in generalizing skills to outside the clinic reveals at least four, but not mutually exclusive, thematic areas:

1. Knowledge of right from wrong behaviors.
2. Descriptions of behavior.
3. Responsibility for behavior.
4. Attitudes about complete and partial successes.

Each thematic area has two options for categorizing a client's comments. One can be called *positive language responses* (PLRs) (Prichard, 1971), *desirable language responses* (DLRs) (Mathew, 1981; Casteel and Stone, 1983), or *facilitative language responses* (FLRs). They represent comments that promote client demonstration of being responsible for appropriate behaviors and for the client's choosing to execute them. The other can be called *negative language responses, undesirable language responses,* or *inhibitory language responses* (ILRs). These repress or obstruct the client's using appropriate self-directed behaviors.

KNOWLEDGE OF RIGHT FROM WRONG BEHAVIORS

Most clients enter the clinical process because of ignorance of:

1. The components necessary for normal voice production.
2. What they are doing incorrectly that results in dysphonia.
3. What behaviors to change.

The untrained voice user usually has no more understanding of the phonatory process than of the motoric intricacies required in walking. Both seem to be innate skills that most often are brought to the level of intrigue only when things go wrong. So second nature are these skills that the need for behavioral analysis of both the undesired and desired behaviors go unrecognized. Once the physiology of right and wrong behaviors is understood, however, the processes for learning appropriate behaviors and skill development can be designed.

The clinician's first role is to evaluate the physiologic behaviors of the client that are directly responsible for the undesired dysphonia. Then the clinician can draw on the knowledge in the field of voice production and teach the client more appropriate behaviors. Verdolini and Titze (1995) provide a stimulating approach to the process of recognizing missing ingredients in various types of vocal misuse and choosing those that must be instated. Their approach would seem to hold at least partial answers to the questions clinicians often ask concerning what to work on in voice modification.

In cases of vocal misuse, one generally finds evidence of heightened muscle activity and decreased air flow. Counsel may involve instrumentation to monitor the aerodynamic factors during voice and respiratory movement patterns at various levels of the torso. Electromyography (EMG) of the laryngeal and paralaryngeal muscles with visual and auditory monitoring might assist the client in learning to identify and modify sensations associated with unnecessary muscle activity. Teaching right from wrong behaviors generally is not accomplished in one discrete step of a curriculum nor in one session. Instead, most often, clients become aware of what they are doing and what needs to be done in a gradual process of deepening understanding. In counseling individuals who behave in ways that result in dysphonia, the counselor seeks to replace comments a client has that reflect *lack* of awareness of what to or not to do (inhibiting language responses [ILRs]) with language that reflects awareness of physiologic actions on what to avoid and what to implement (facilitative language responses [FLRs]). This can be taught by attending to descriptions of behaviors.

## DESCRIPTIONS OF BEHAVIORS

One of the principles of general semantics is recognition that a *word* is not a *thing*. Words are merely representations of reality; they are the road maps presenting hints about the territory. When seeking one's way in previously untraveled areas, the traveler appreciates maps that most accurately represent the area. Photographs of the terrain give less chance for misrepresentations than drawings; drawings are generally preferred over verbal descriptions. Sometimes, however, verbal descriptions are the only available medium of presenting information. The words that best convey reality are those more literal and less figurative.

FLRs in counseling behavioral change of voice generally are anatomically and physiologically based rather than obscure abstractions. For example, "Sense the vibrations around the lips and nose when you hum" are better than "place the tone up in the mask." The mask is not an anatomic structure and is not a part of reality. "Avoid speaking down on the cords" seems to have little validity when taken at face value; whereas, "use a higher pitch with less effort and more air flow" seems to more closely address the physiologic response desired in the client. The admonition to "produce voice without tightening the neck muscles" seems more plausible than "let the voice come right out the top of your head." "Bring the vowel sound up behind the soft palate" is sometimes heard from singing instructors but this requests a physiologically impossible accomplishment unless hypernasality results (if, in fact, a vowel can be brought anywhere).

Descriptions of behavior embodying FLRs usually are expressed using active rather than passive voice. Consequently, "our voice just gets stuck once in awhile" should be replace by something like "you squeeze your vocal folds together too tightly." The former statement implies a passive happening and the latter an action.

One of the more common ILRs that often can be heard when monitoring clinical intervention focuses on what to avoid rather than what to do. Admonishments of "Don't" seem less instructive and less appropriate than "Do more of," particularly when eliciting and guiding behaviors for which reinforcers can be dispensed.

## ATTITUDES AND BEHAVIORS

Helmstetter (1982), comments well about the role of attitude and behavioral change. He indicates:

> Attitudes are the perspective from which you view life. Some people seem to have a good attitude about most things. Some people seem to have a bad attitude about everything. . . . Most of us have a combination of attitudes, some good, some not so good. . . . A good attitude is essential to achieve-

ment of any kind! . . . Without a good attitude, a perspective which allows one to see the opportunities ahead and set his sights to reach them, he never will. But even more important is the fact that in order to possess the kinds of feelings which work for us, we've got to have the right attitudes to start with . . . our attitudes are created, controlled, or influenced entirely by . . . beliefs. (p. 67)

In adopting a "can do" attitude one focuses more on success than failures. Accordingly, one might look for partial successes rather than focus on failures to complete a task. Rarely is a failure to execute a behavior devoid of partial successes. For example, with a client who incompletely fulfills an assignment in carryover, the clinician can reinforce the 30% that was accomplished and not focus on the 70% that was disappointing. Focusing on successes rather than failures is facilitated by looking for millimeters of progress toward a goal rather than the 100% accomplishment when the client crosses the finish line. Successful experiences create optimistic attitudes; optimistic attitudes create clients who learn and accomplish goals. Clinicians might well look at a client's dialogue for FLRs associated with optimism built through successes and reject comments that are ILRs based on pessimism fostered by failures. Focusing on successes also forces the clinician to design intervention curricula with small increments of complexity that assure success. The clinician who wants optimistic clients should not ask a client to do something in which there is an element of doubt about successful performance of the requested task.

Self-prophesies regarding the outcome of one's performance may be one of the most critical determinants of that outcome. In reality, most people faced with a challenge seem to respond with something akin to "Oh, I could never do that," when in fact, they really mean "Oh, I never have done that." The implication of "I can't" is equal to a statement of an impossibility. There is little sense in attempting the impossible. When "I can't" is said or heard often enough it fosters pessimism. Few accomplishments stem from pessimism. "I'll never be able to speak this way" is likely to be a defeating self-fulfilling prophesy. Repeated often enough, one gets caught in the trap of "I can't" and then does not. On the other hand, "I think I can at least use this kind of voicing for the first three words" and bespeaks an attitude of impending success. When the success is met, the self-prophesy of a "can do" attitude is perpetuated and the client is inclined to move to the next level of accomplishment. Optimistic attitudes stem from success. A clinician's efforts at carryover, therefore, should be designed for success in sequentially more challenging tasks with each step being at low or no risk for failure.

Another trap foiling carryover is baited by the term *try*. When a client says, "I'll try to," the client is open to an element of possible failure by use of the term *try*. This term stems from the term *trial*, which carries a connotation of unpredictable outcome. Alternatively, "I'll do another sample of" embodies expectation of success and optimism. In reality, the clinician who says "I don't think this will work, but we'll (clinician and client) give it a try" implies a lack of confidence in the technique or in the client's performance. Success is more likely achieved when confidence and optimism rather than insecurity and pessimism are present.

Nothing breeds optimism and success like success itself. Maybe people learn from their failures, but learning from successes is more enjoyable and keeps the person at high levels of performance quantitatively and qualitatively. When people are happy workers, they keep working on what works. When people stop doing what works, they stop working and become unhappy and discouraged with themselves. Accordingly, when clinicians and clients focus on the little successful steps that have brought clients from where they were to where they are now, rather than on crossing the finish line, the clients continue the race. FLRs focus on success, on possibilities rather than impossibilities, and on optimistic rather than pessimistic statements. Furthermore, when a client adopts positive attitudes that person comes closer to believing in success and takes measures to assure success by choosing to be responsible for behaviors.

RESPONSIBILITY FOR BEHAVIORS

Turning again to excerpts from Helmstetter (1982), who on the topic of responsibility states:

> Personal responsibility is at the root of everything we think, do, conceive, fail at, or achieve in our lives. Personal responsibility is the bedrock of all individual action. Responsibility does not mean duty or burden. It is not the measure of our liability or our accountability: it is the basis of our individual determination to accept life and to fulfill ourselves within it (p. 102). . . . We take our first breath by ourselves. And we take our last breath alone.
>
> How then is it that somewhere in between, in that time we call life, we expect someone else to do our breathing for us?
>
> No one will ever breathe one breath for us. No one will ever think one thought that is ours. No one will ever stand in our bodies, experience what happens to us, feel our fears, dream our dreams, or cry our tears. We are born, live and leave this life entirely on our own. That self and the divine spirit which drives it, are what we have. No one else can ever live a single moment of our lives for us. That we must do for ourselves. That is responsibility. (p. 103)

Clients are at the command module of their own being and, like it or not, they are in charge of their own actions. No one person or one thing determines the behavior. The individual is in a position not to accept ILRs (e.g., the ringing phone causes loss of focus on how to speak and makes the person answer it in dysphonic ways). Language reflecting FLRs might resemble "My boss does not make me loose control of intended phonation skills" during such or such encounter. Often, however, individuals under the influence of such stressors, fail to exercise their choice to do what is necessary to produce good voice. FLRs are comments that facilitate a client's awareness of and assuming the responsibility for executing physiologic acts that result in desired vocal production. ILRs, on the other hand, reflect placement of blame for dysphonic voice production on factors outside the individual—external environmental factors.

## Adopting Favorable Thematic Responses (FLRs) and Eliminating Unfavorable Thematics Responses (ILRs)

One may ask at this point, where the client learns FLRs. The answer lies in the clinical process and most often with the clinician. It is the clinician who must counsel the client to exhibit FLRs. This can be done through (a) positive reinforcement of the client's FLR responses, (b) instruction to the desirability of FLRs, and (c) clinician modeling of FLRs.

THE CLINICIAN'S THEMATICS AS A MODEL

One of the first steps in altering a client's language themes from ILRs to FLRs pivots on clinicians' recognizing the ideas and comments in their own dialogue that are desirable and undesirable for teaching client carryover. Such a listing in the area of voice is not typically taught in clinical methods classes. Boone and Prescott (1972) seem to stand alone in the area of content analyses of a therapy session. They, however, dealt with evaluating portions of a session spent in 10 types of activities involving explanations, modeling, evaluation, social interaction, and behavior correction. They did not consider the nature of clinical dialogue that might develop or detract from a client's assuming responsibility for behavior. This apparently was left to other authors such as Sanders (1970) and Williams (1957) who didactically focused on how clinicians should talk about disordered communication. Their guidelines on counseling people who stutter seem commendable to voice counselors and set the stage for self-analysis that also might be used with or by a client. Figure 7.4 presents a schematic of thematic parameters to summarize the foregoing material and to help identify aspects of an analysis protocol. It may be copied and posted on the wall of the clinic room for ready reference.

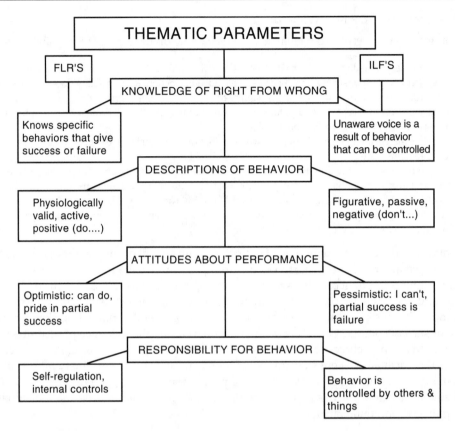

**Figure 7.4.**  Thematic parameters identify aspects of an analysis protocol.

THEMATIC ANALYSES

Formal evaluation of comments used by the client and the clinician increases one's awareness of behavioral thematics. To assist this evaluation, one might audio record a segment
of dialogue in an intervention session. Then, transcribe the sequential utterances of the
clinician or of the client onto a copy of the thematic analysis form (Fig. 7.5).

Next, determine those comments that do not relate to behavioral change and place a
mark in column B and indicate the total number of marks at the bottom of that column. Analyze the remaining comments, first, according to the main thought and to the parameters:
awareness, descriptions, attitudes, and responsibility. Then, for each parameter determine
whether the thought represents an FLR or an ILR. Next, total the number of FLRs and ILRs
in each column. To evaluate the proportion of responses that are ILRs, refer to the formula
at the bottom of the form. The proportion of FLRs will be 100% minus the percent of ILRs
determined and entered in the space provided. Even for good behaviorally based consultants it is unusual to have more than 90% comments that reflect FLRs. For clinicians unfamiliar with behavioral thematics FLRs may be exhibited in less than 20% of the instructional
comments. Setting appropriate counseling models for clients is a challenging task.

When applied to the client's comments, this analysis may give insight to the readiness
of the person to move to another level of the curriculum in learning the mechanics of improved voice. For example, the clinician may choose some level of success (e.g., 80%) with
which the client must maintain targeted physiologic characteristics in vowel production
before moving to syllable or word levels *and* insist that the client's comments reflect 60%

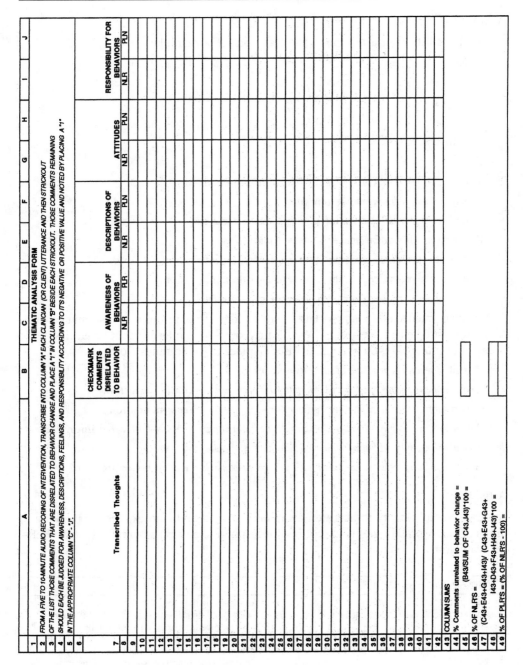

**Figure 7.5.** Thematic analysis form.

FLRs (or whatever present criteria is chosen) of the comments the client gives in describing his or her performance.

## EXERCISES IN NEGATIVE PRACTICE AND CANCELLATION

A clinician may choose to focus attention on developing the use of FLRs and decreasing the prevalence of ILRs by engaging in awareness training. One such possibility lies in the principles of negative practice.

Activity 1

1. Develop a list of terms apropos a medical model. For example:

   Patient:

   Cure:

   Prescription:

   Remission:

   Exacerbation:

   Habit:

2. Next to your list, indicate how each term might be an ILR.

   Patient: *promotes dependence on care giver*

   Cure: *implies removal of causative behaviors; they are overcome*

   Prescription: *initiated by another; recipient's role is passive*

   Remission: *magical improvement, independent of patient involvement*

   Exacerbation: *magical worsening, independent of patient involvement*

   Habit: *automatic response for which patient is not responsible*

3. Negative practice often is associated with a following opposite response that replaces the undesired event. Opposite the indication of how each term might be an ILR, write an *FLR word or phrase* that could be used in place of the stimulus word.

   Patient: *promotes dependence of care giver*—**client**

   Cure: *implies removal of causative behaviors are overcome, not cured*—**correction**

   Prescription: *initiated by another, recipient's role is passive*—**recommendation**

   Remission: *magical improvement, independent of patient involvement*—**cultivated improvement**

   Exacerbation: *magical failing, independent of patient involvement*—**worsen**

   Habit: *automatic response for which patient is not responsible*—**way of behaving**

Activity 2

Another helpful activity to heighten awareness of ILRs and gain experience thinking in terms of behavioral themes is to rephrase or respond to a client's typical ILRs with FLRs, for example:

| Client's ILR Statements | Clinician's FLR Responses |
|---|---|
| My voice just gets stuck! | You're saying that you stop the flow of air? |
| That kind of talking you're teaching isn't going to cut it in real life! | You're building skills now, we'll come to making it sound better using these good skills. |
| I can't do it at the word level! | You've used good flow and relaxed throat both in various vowel and consonant combinations, words are just vowels and consonants used according to more conventional combinations. |
| The phone makes me tense up! | You tighten your stomach or throat muscles when you hear the phone ring? |

**CONCLUSION**

Consultation in the remediation of voice disorders varies with the nature of the problem. In cases of organically based dysphonia, as in vocal abuse, the consultation may assume a role of information sharing. The counselor needs knowledge of how the organicity developed, its general course of events and associated vocal liabilities. Teaching means of suitable compensation for the organic limitations and giving suggestions for achieving vocal well-being through proper hygienic measures and avoidance of vocal abuse often are the counseling tools.

In behavioral manifestations of inappropriate physiology brought to the task of voice production, the counselor must be well grounded in the knowledge of desired vocal physiology and skilled in eliciting such actions from the client. The clinician's counseling skills are put to the test in helping clients recognize that they bring certain behaviors to the task of speaking and they must assume responsibility for choosing what normally must be done to produce normal voice. Success is associated with attending to the client's awareness of which behaviors to avoid and which to use, helping them develop valid descriptions of vocal behaviors, nurturing their optimistic attitudes about change through successes, and helping them recognize their responsibility to effect change. It has been said that the best teaching occurs without words. The challenge to the clinician is to set an appropriate linguistic model through the use of behaviorally compatible themes in clinical dialogue.

## REFERENCES

Anonymous. (1990). The use of soundfield amplification of the teacher's voice in the regular education classroom. Unpublished report. Norris City, IL: Wabash and Ohio Valley Special Education District.

Block, C., Gould, W., & Hirano, M. (1981). Effect of voice therapy on contact granuloma of the vocal fold. *Annals of Otology, Rhinology, and Laryngology, 90,* 48–52.

Boone, D., & McFarlane, S. (1994). *The voice and voice therapy* (5th ed.). Englewood Cliffs, NJ: Prentice Hall.

Boone, D., & Prescott, T. (1972). Content and sequence analysis of speech and hearing therapy. *ASHA, 14,* 58–62.

Buekers, R., Bierens, E., Kingma, H., & Marres, E. H. M. A. (1995). Vocal load as measured by the voice accumulator. *Folia Phoniatrica, 47,* 252–261.

Casteel, R., & Stone Jr., R. (1983). In Filter, M. (Ed.), *Phonatory voice disorders in children.* Springfield, IL: Charles C Thomas.

Chen, X. (1989). Comparative research on vocal polyps and nodules. *Chinese Journal of Otorhinolaryngology, 24,* 53–55, 63.

Clark, J. (1990). Counseling in communicative disorders: A responsibility to be met. *Hearsay,* Spring/Summer, *14,* 4–7.

Colton, R. H., & Casper, J. K. (1990). *Understanding voice problems: A physiological perspective for diagnosis and treatment.* Baltimore: Williams & Wilkins.

Ford, C. N. (1994). Phonosurgery. In Benninger, M., Jacobson, B. & Johnson, A. (Eds.), *Vocal arts medicine: The care and prevention of professional voice disorders.* New York: Thieme Medical Publishers.

Gray, S., & Titze, I. (1988). Histologic investigation of hyperphonated canine vocal cords. *Annals of Otology Rhinology and Laryngology, 97,* 381–388.

Greene, M. C. L. (1980). *The voice and its disorders* (4th ed.). Philadelphia: JB Lippincott.

Harma, R., Sonninen, A., Vartiainen, E., Haveri, P., & Vaisanen, A. (1975). Vocal polyps and nodules. *Folia Phoniatrica, 27,* 19–25.

Helmstetter, S. (1982). *What to say when you talk to yourself.* New York: Simon & Shuster.

Hayakawa, S. (1949). *Language in thought and action.* New York: Harcourt, Brace.

Jacobson, E. (1978). *You must relax.* New York: McGraw-Hill.

Johnson, T. (1985). *Vocal abuse reduction program.* Austin, TX: Pro-Ed.

Johnson, W. (1946). *People in quandaries.* New York: Harper & Brothers.

Lavorato, A., & Mc Farlane, S. (1988). Counseling clients with voice disorders. *Seminars in Speech and Language, 9,* 237–255.

Logan, R. (1996). *Neurophysiologic rationales for goals and procedures in stuttering treatment.* Paper presented at the Twenty-sixth Annual Mid-South Conference on Communicative Disorders, Memphis State University.

Masuda T., Ikeda Y., Manako H., & Komiyama S. (1993). Analysis of vocal abuse: Fluctuations in phonation time and intensity in 4 groups of speakers. *Acta Otolaryngologica, 113,* 547–552.

Mathew, K. (1981). *An analysis of the relationship between the degree of maintained fluency improvement of former Portland State University stuttering clients and the overall language themes they used.* Unpublished masters thesis, Portland State University, Portland, OR.

Murphy, A. (1964). *Functional voice disorders.* Englewood Cliffs, NJ: Prentice-Hall.

Perkins, W., & Curlee, R. (1969). Causality in speech pathology. *Journal of Speech and Hearing Disorders, 34,* 231–238.

Prichard, S. J. (1971). *The structuring of procedures utilized in an adult treatment program.* Unpublished masters thesis, Portland State University, Portland, OR.

Remacle, M., Lagneau, G., Marbaix, E., Doyen, A., & Van den Eeckhaut, J. (1992). Laryngopathies exudatives de l'espace de Reinke. *Annales de Oto-Laryngologie et de Chirurgie Cervico-Faciale, 109*(1),33–38.

Sanders, E. (1970). Talking plainly about stuttering: Guidelines for the beginning clinician. *Central States Speech Journal, 21,* 248–254.

Saxon, K. & Schneider, C.(1995). *Vocal exercise physiology.* San Diego, CA: Singular.

Sieron, J., & Johannsen, H. (1992). Contact granuloma: symptoms, etiology, diagnosis, therapy. *Laryngo-Rhino-Otologie* (Stuttgart), *71*(4),193–197.

Sonninen, A., Damste, P. H., Jol, J., & Fokkens, J. (1972). On vocal strain. *Folia Phoniatrica, 24*(5), 321–336.

Stemple, J. (1993). *Voice therapy: Clinical studies.* St. Louis, MO: CV Mosby.

Stemple, J. C., Glaze, L. E., & Gerdeman, B. K. (1995). *Clinical voice pathology: Theory and management.* San Diego, CA: Singular.

Stone, J., & Olswang, L. (1989). The hidden challenge in counseling. *ASHA, 27*–31.

Stone, Jr., R. (1981). Management of childhood dysphonias of organic bases. In Filter, M. (Ed.), *Phonatory voice disorders in children.* Springfield, IL: Charles C Thomas.

Stone, Jr., R., & Sharf, D. (1973). Vocal change associated with the use of atypical pitch and intensity levels. *Folia Phoniatrica, 25*(1), 91–03.

Stone, Jr., R., & Nuttall, A. (1974). Relative movements of the thyroid and cricoid cartilages assessed by neural stimulation in dogs. *Acta Oto-Laryngologica, 78,* 135–140.

Toohill, R. J. (1975). The psychosomatic aspects of children with vocal nodules. *Archives of Otolaryngology—Head and Neck Surgery, 101*(10), 591—595.

Verdolini, K., & Titze, I. (1995). The application of laboratory formulas to clinical voice management. *American Journal of Speech-Language Pathology, 4*(2),62—69.

Williams, D. (1957). A point of view about stuttering. *Journal of Speech and Hearing Disorders, 22*(3), 390–397.

Wilson, D. K. (1987). *Voice problems of children* (3rd ed.). Baltimore: Williams & Wilkins.

Zeine, L., & Brandt, J. (1988). The Lombard effect on alaryngeal speech. *Journal of Communication Disorders, 21*(5), 373–383.

# 8. Laryngectomy

Stuart I. Gilmore

---

| | |
|---|---|
| **Pathology and Audiology** | **Counseling Laryngectomized Individuals and Their Families** |
| **In the Beginning . . . Changes and Problems** |     Learning to Speak Again—A Major Promoter of Adjustment |
|     The Initial Visit with the Speech-Language Pathologist |     Requirements for Counseling Laryngectomized Individuals and Their Families |
| **Changes Following Laryngectomy** |     • *Clinician Attributes* |
|     Physical Changes |     • *Counseling Skills* |
|     • *Respiration* |     • *A Checklist for Laryngectomee Consultations* |
|     • *Speech* | |
|     • *Nonspeech Communication* | **Postscript** |
|     • *Swallowing and Digestion* |     References and Suggested Readings |
|     • *Sensory Impairment* | |
|     • *Problems Associated with Aging and Previous Lifestyle* | |
|     Social Changes | |
|     Occupational Changes | |
|     Psychological Changes | |

---

The diagnosis of laryngeal cancer precipitates a number of changes that challenge the life-long assumptions, activities, public image, and self-concept of the laryngectomized individual. Functions previously taken for granted, ranging from coughing and blowing one's nose to crying, laughing, speaking, and earning a living, are jeopardized or lost. Crises resulting from being *compelled* to experience, acknowledge, and adapt to multiple, threatening changes generate stresses that compromise the individual's ability to negotiate an ultimate adjustment to those changes. The speech-language clinician's skills, both as an instructor of alaryngeal speech and as a counselor, are critical determinants of the extent to which the laryngectomized individual will resolve the crises and of the amount of stress that will be generated in accomplishing their resolution.

Competence as a facilitator of speech, which is the primary function of the speech-language pathologist, assures selection of appropriate speech mode(s), training goals, and training procedures, as well as early identification and rectification of barriers that can impede speech acquisition. Skillful speech training maximizes the intelligibility and acceptability of alaryngeal speech, minimizes the time required to achieve functional speech, and minimizes speaker anxiety regarding using the new speech mode(s). Competence as a counselor facilitates the laryngectomized individual, and the family, as they learn to cope with the losses, changes, and the rehabilitation process.

The criterion for successful postlaryngectomy rehabilitation is the degree to which the ability to resume life has been restored. Success demands that the speech pathologist be competent in both speech training and counseling. Skilled speech training and counseling are so intertwined in postlaryngectomy rehabilitation that separating them is analogous to trying to understand a tapestry by separating its threads. In keeping with the same analogy, the fabric of rehabilitation requires a strong supporting warp of information, held together by cross threads of the clinician's concern, sensitivity, and skill in interacting with others.

Underlying the present chapter is the premise that the clinician already has an understanding of the speech modes available to the client following his or her laryngectomy, how to train their use, and what factors, anatomic and physiologic in particular, may impede the client's progress. Clinician incompetence in these areas can be a major cause of client frustration, depression, withdrawal, and failure. Moreover, this type of scenario tends to terminate by blaming the negative outcome of therapy on "the client's lack of motivation," leaving neither the client nor the clinician feeling successful or rewarded.

The present chapter is not directed toward developing speech, per se, but toward the accompanying issues subsumed under counseling. The initial objective of the chapter is to clarify the changes and consequent problems associated with laryngeal cancer. These changes, and their associated problems, are the major source of the feelings and behaviors toward which counseling should be directed.

The second objective of the chapter is to describe resources for problem resolution. These resources take three primary, interacting forms. The first to be discussed is the *speech-language clinician,* whose attributes and counseling skills provide clients and their families with opportunities to acknowledge and define feelings and problems and to strategize and refine solutions. The second resource is the *additional information sources* available to the client and family as they seek knowledge, insight, and suggestions for coping with the changes and resolving their problems. The third resource is the *additional support sources* available to the client and family as they cope with the changes, problems, and associated stresses of the laryngectomy. Accessing these resources involves the activities generally acknowledged as counseling.

The third intent of the chapter is to reinforce clinician concern and sensitivity for laryngectomized patients, while supplementing the information and insights needed to apply them effectively to problem resolution.

## IN THE BEGINNING . . . CHANGES AND PROBLEMS

Cancer of the larynx is a disease that generally occurs in late middle age, on the average during the individual's mid-fifties, a time that might well be anticipated as the high point of one's mature life. Children generally have been raised, personal achievements have been recognized, and income is likely to be at its maximum. Individuals may well be anticipating several vocationally productive years prior to retiring to the freedom of relative financial comfort and time to enjoy one's family, friends, hobbies, and leisure. A laryngectomy can be a rude awakening from this dream of the golden years, an awakening to be followed by an array of unknowns and threats, not the least of which is questionable survival.

For the younger laryngectomized individual, the surgery may be the beginning of a nightmare of anxiety regarding life, vocational, and financial assurance, and medical and life insurance: "Will I survive? Who will take care of my family if I don't survive? If I do survive, will I be able, or permitted, to continue the life I have previously known and anticipated?"

These concerns are likely to be the immediate and major ones of the individual who has just been told that he or she has cancer of the larynx, that surgical excision of the larynx is the preferred treatment mode, and that it will result both in breathing through a hole in the neck (the stoma) and the loss of speech as previously known. These are the concerns the individual, the spouse, and the family typically have when they embark on the hopefully life-saving, but immensely life-disrupting, surgery. Along with these concerns, there are innumerable questions and doubts, and great need for information regarding what will happen, clarification, and support.

As a result of the ignorance and misconceptions regarding speaking after laryngectomy, uncovered by a study involving presurgical interviews, Dugay (1966) advocates that the rehabilitation of individuals diagnosed as having laryngeal cancer should begin as soon as the patient is informed of the possibility of undergoing a laryngectomy. Acknowledging that the individual cannot be expected to understand all of the details, Dugay states that the client should be made generally aware of what is about to happen and how the consequent limitations can be minimized.

### The Initial Visit with the Speech Pathologist

The client's initial visit with the speech pathologist, preferably also attended by the spouse or partner and other concerned family members, customarily occurs by referral from the surgeon. Described generally as the preoperative counseling session, its objectives are to provide information, clarification, reassurance, and support.

The session is often initiated with the clinician's request for information regarding what the client and significant others have been told about the surgery, its effects, and the course of rehabilitation. Discussion may then be directed toward clarifying matters that appear to require further explanation, and to answering client and family questions. Depending on patient and family informational status and needs, the dialogue may involve explaining the surgery and its consequences, immediate postoperative care, and the subsequent protocol for accomplishing the return to presurgical functions. Information regarding the various speech modes available following surgery will probably be provided, especially if primary tracheoesophageal puncture has not been elected.

Care is generally taken to refer the client and the family to the appropriate professional resource for explanations that are not within the professional scope of the speech-language pathologist. Reassurance may be provided regarding the availability of needed professional and other resources, equipment and devices, and support. Support includes visitations by a laryngectomee and spouse from the community, and services available from local and national organizations and agencies. Pamphlets and other literature explaining the surgery, its consequences, and resources for managing them may be recommended or supplied (see the bibliography included at the end of the chapter).

The previous brief review of presurgical counseling confirms the need for the speech-language pathologist to be informed regarding the multiple issues facing the laryngectomized individual. Postsurgical counseling is likely to require even broader and more specific and detailed expertise as the client deals with postsurgical challenges. It is imperative that the speech-language pathologist understands the changes and problems associated with laryngectomy to address client and family concerns, anticipate and explain what may follow, help to answer questions, and provide or access the needed support.

### CHANGES FOLLOWING LARYNGECTOMY

The array of changes associated with laryngeal excision can be viewed as falling within four important functional domains: physical, social, occupational, and psychological (See Gilmore, 1994, for elaboration of the topic and review of the literature).

### Physical Changes

Physical changes following a total laryngectomy primarily involve physiologic alterations associated with loss of the larynx and their associated effects on the following functions.

*Respiration.* Laryngeal excision sacrifices airway protection afforded by glottal closure during swallowing, and by coughing. Without surgical construction of a respiratory opening in the neck (the stoma), and surgical direction of the trachea to the stoma instead of the hypopharynx, food and liquids ingested orally would be aspirated, resulting in death. Respiration, coughing, and the clearing of mucus, henceforth, is carried on through the stoma and not the nose and pharynx. Moreover, the filtering, warming, and humidifying functions of the nose and upper airway are also sacrificed.

A number of consequent respiratory complaints can occur, including crusting around the stoma, excessive tracheal mucus, and excessive coughing. These complaints may vary considerably with changes in the (*a*) season, (*b*) temperature, and (*c*) the moisture and foreign matter content of the air, and (*d*) the time elapsed since surgery. Additionally, wheezing, shortness of breath, and fatigue may be symptoms of a stoma that is too small to support adequate respiration.

*Speech.* Loss of the larynx results in the loss of both voice and of pulmonary airflow through the vocal tract to generate pressure sounds, consonant sounds that carry a major portion of the meaning of an utterance. In addition, speaking patterns habituated over years of producing and monitoring one's pulmonary-generated speech may not be readily transferable to alaryngeal speech modes or may even impede learning to use them effectively.

*Nonspeech communication.* Loss of the vocal folds precipitates the loss of audible laughing, crying, moaning, and wailing, all crucial to expressing emotion. Additionally, the ability to whistle is lost following surgical routing of pulmonary exhalation through the stoma.

*Swallowing and digestion.* Swallowing problems may result from constriction of the hypopharynx and upper esophageal sphincter, reduced tongue pressure on the bolus associated with a partial glossectomy, or the presence of a hypopharyngeal pouch. Heartburn and reflux are often reported, especially with a coexisting hiatal hernia, which is not rare in a population of this age.

*Sensory impairment.* Impairment of smell, and consequently of taste, often accompanies the rerouting of the respiratory air stream through the stoma rather than across the olfactory sensors of the nose. Gustatory sensation is impaired as well as awareness of food spoilage, gas leaks, and one's own aroma, with implications for consequent reductions in pleasure, health, and social acceptability.

A high incidence of hearing loss has been found in the laryngectomized population (Robinette, 1994), presumably associated with a combination of age and years of noise exposure. Moreover, as indicated by Robinette, temporary but frustrating conductive hearing losses can occur in individuals confined to bed because of surgery. Not only can a hearing loss impair speech understanding and consequently communicative interaction, it can also impede learning alaryngeal speech.

Because esophageal speech is only about half as loud as laryngeal speech, impaired hearing in an aging spouse or partner also has considerable rehabilitative significance. Hearing impairment on the part of the partner can exacerbate problems occurring between the two individuals, as well as deprive the laryngectomized individual of a needed drill cohort, coach, and source of success and reinforcement while learning a new mode of speech.

*Problems associated with aging and previous lifestyle.* Because laryngeal cancer is typically a disease of older adults, it can be expected that laryngectomized individuals may also have other age-associated physical problems, such as cardiovascular and cerebrovascular disorders, arthritis, dental problems, and so forth. Additionally, the frequent history in laryngectomized individuals of smoking and often of drinking can portend serious respiratory disorders or alcohol dependency that jeopardizes the individual's ability to follow a speech rehabilitation regimen.

## Social Changes

Both the literature and clinical experience indicate that a laryngectomy can severely disrupt one's relationships with spouse, family, friends, and community. Laryngectomized women often report being misidentified as men because of the low pitch of their voices (the mean laryngectomized female fundamental frequency is 85 Hz.). They frequently indicate feeling less feminine and less attractive. Men and women both indicate concern about the presence and appearance of the stoma. Stoma blast is often mentioned as a disconcerting component of passionate lovemaking. Changes in sexual relationships are often a concern for both spouses.

Previously strained marriages may give way completely under the stresses of financial changes and medical costs, impaired communication, and changes in familial roles and lifestyle that attend the loss of the larynx. On the other hand, the gratitude of the laryngectomized individual for the patience and support of the spouse and family is often acknowledged and the spouse's support described as an indispensable facilitator of rehabilitation.

Anticipated, perceived, or real changes in relationships with friends can also occur. Often, social changes reflect difficulties in understanding the laryngectomized individual's early attempts at speech or the friend's discomfort in dealing with the physical changes, the grief being expressed, or even with a fear of cancer. Changes in appearance, notably those associated with the stoma—the presence of a hole in the neck and its being the locus for coughing and clearing mucus—can be dramatic, both in terms of the onlooker's response and the possessor's embarrassment. Research exists that documents the social and vocational stigma associated with being laryngectomized (Gardner, 1966; Gilmore, 1974; Natvig, 1984).

Reports by laryngectomized individuals and their spouses often describe reduced social contacts with friends and decreased participation in church and other organizational activities. These activities may be replaced by participation in a laryngectomee support group, such as a New Voice or Lost Cord Club associated with the International Association of Laryngectomees. Prelaryngectomy activities may be resumed once alaryngeal speech ability is sufficient to support them.

## Occupational Changes

Quite frequently a laryngectomy has dramatic effects on the individual's vocational and avocational activities. Although people often return to their previous positions, some must move to more favorable work environments; for instance, away from the dust or fumes associated with a previous job or to a position where safety does not depend on being heard above noise. Often, those who are approaching retirement decide to do so. In spite of federal legislation prohibiting disability-related employment bias, instances occur when unfair employment practices may be difficult to prove or counteract. Individuals needing to return quickly to activities requiring speech often elect either tracheoesophageal speech or to use an electrolarynx.

Hobbies exposing the individual to noxious airborne materials or those involving water sports, strenuous activity, or wind instruments, may be abandoned. Bidding cards or simultaneously eating and speaking at dinner parties, can prompt retreat from social activities, at least during the early days of rehabilitation. It must be acknowledged, however, that many innovative laryngectomized individuals have found ways to resume their presurgical hobbies, including swimming, running, and playing the saxophone.

## Psychological Changes

As suggested by Gilmore (1994), the sudden and extensive physical, social, and occupational changes associated with surgical removal of the larynx can result in a series of identity crises and accompanying stress as the individual attempts to cope and adjust. Responses often involve a loss of self-esteem; feeling different, disfigured, inferior, rejected, and isolated; and consequent withdrawal. Typical emotional responses have been described in the literature as involving shock, fear, anxiety, worry, and depression. These responses lend themselves to a process of grieving formulation. Shock, denial, bargaining, anger, withdrawal, acceptance, and adjustment are all stages in grieving for a significant loss. In the case of the laryngectomized individual, the loss is one of image of self as known and taken for granted prior to the diagnosis of cancer and consequent removal of the larynx.

A major shortcoming of applying grief theory to loss of the larynx resides in the implicit suggestion that adaptation follows in sequential stages, with little overlapping, reversal, or regression; and that a time exists when the sequence of responses is or should be completed and adaptation accomplished. It is more realistic, perhaps, to view the individual's reactions as components of a normal and variable process of coping, which includes a variety of emotional reactions, any or all of which can be expected in response to the multitude of changed attributes and relationships associated with the laryngectomy.

These emotional reactions occur repeatedly. They are commonly generated by ambivalent return to previous responsibilities and functions associated with increasing demands and desires for independence or by poignant occasions. Emotional reactions evoked by increasing independence occur, for instance, when leaving the routine and familiar environment of the hospital after surgery; when members of the family resume their presurgical attitudes, expectations, and activities; and when the laryngectomized individual returns to work or resumes social activities. Poignant occasions involve briefly enhanced feelings of loss; for example, when the laryngectomized individual would previously have assisted, responded, performed, or directed, but now cannot or feels less than competent. These emotional responses are best understood by the individual and the family not as signs of psychological abnormality, but as phases of an eventual reconciliation following a disability.

## COUNSELING LARYNGECTOMIZED INDIVIDUALS AND THEIR FAMILIES

### Learning to Speak Again—A Major Promoter of Adjustment

Learning to speak again is a major, if not the major, promoter of reconciliation and adjustment following laryngectomy. Recovering speech facilitates expression, recognition, and communication of concerns and feelings, all important to eventual coping. Speaking also enhances obtaining information, and encourages exploring, formulating, and rehearsing coping strategies. In short, regaining speech expedites problem resolution. Moreover, being able to speak enhances opportunities for social exchange and for repairing self-esteem. Intelligible alaryngeal speech serves all of these adjustment functions of laryngeal speech and does so at a time of intense need for those functions.

Besides depriving a laryngectomized individual of the adjustment benefits associated with functional speech, prolonged and unsuccessful attempts to develop alaryngeal speech can erode the individual's confidence, hope, and motivation to continue the pursuit. Failure can result in feelings of frustration and incompetence and, eventually, in withdrawal. Such a scenario in no way enhances psychological status, reconciliation, or adjustment.

It should be evident, for the reasons indicated, that the critical skill required from the speech-language pathologist seeking to enhance the laryngectomized client's psychological well-being is that of being able to develop functional alaryngeal speech in a minimal amount of time.

## Requirements for Counseling Laryngectomees and Their Families

Beyond understanding the changes and problems attending loss of the larynx and having the knowledge and skill required to re-establish speech, certain clinician attributes and counseling skills enhance the speech-language pathologist's contributions to the psychological well-being of laryngectomized individuals and their families.

### CLINICIAN ATTRIBUTES

With respect for the difficulty of stipulating the personal traits necessary to counsel laryngectomized individuals and their families successfully and with equal or greater respect for the impossibility of delineating those traits in the few lines that can be allotted in this chapter to such a complex task, the following five clinician attributes are proposed as salient.

1. Respect and consideration for each client. For instance, it is common for laryngectomized individuals to have histories of smoking and alcoholism and for others to respond with blame and contempt. Although substance abuse has a real and considerable significance for both the physical and the speech prognosis, it should not compromise the client's implicit humanity or needs or the empathy felt by the clinician. Perhaps the primary counseling correlate of respect and consideration for a client is the clinician's ability to ascertain what a client's statements mean *to the client,* a crucial counseling skill.
2. Appreciation for and acceptance of the responsibilities involved in assisting clients to integrate their restrictions, expectations, and function, including investing the required time and physical and psychological energy. Acquisition of the prerequisite information and skills for treating laryngectomized clients is a primary indicator of this attribute.
3. Commitment to understanding and integrating each client's specific restrictions, capacities, functional needs, and expectations when developing his or her treatment objectives and procedures. Whereas the attribute described in number two above relates to general practice, the present attribute relates to treatment individualization.
4. Appreciation of the importance of client concurrence with treatment objectives and procedures. Clinician commitment to equipping clients for active roles in treatment determination stems from this trait. Its counseling relevance lies in the implicit concern for understanding client motivation and assuring the consequent sustained and directed effort required for treatment success.
5. Acceptance of one's own feelings and needs. Inclusion of this attribute reflects the need to assure that the clinician's resources are sufficient to sustain involvement in a client's needs. Knowledge and appreciation of self are, arguably, prerequisites to the previously described attributes supporting counseling effectiveness.

In particular, working with laryngectomized individuals entails confronting associated issues that try the clinician's emotional resources. These challenges include attitudes and fears regarding cancer generally, potential and actual recurrence of the cancer, and mortality, including that of self and loved ones. Dealing with client, family, and one's own grief when cancer recurs or a client dies, is emotionally demanding.

Involvement in very personal concerns faced by laryngectomized clients and their families, such as problems with finances, return to work, marital stress (including sexual problems), and making medical decisions, can stress the clinician, especially if it implies responsibility for determining what to provide, who should provide it, how, and when it is provided. The counseling skills discussed next are as applicable to the needs of clinicians as they are to the laryngectomized client, especially those concerning accessing information and support.

The attributes enumerated above are envisioned as nourishing the counseling skills employed by the clinician to promote the laryngectomized client's reconciliation and eventual adjustment to the changes and problems accompanying loss of the larynx. These counseling skills are presented next.

## COUNSELING SKILLS

Five overlapping and interacting counseling skills are proposed as being crucial for advancing the psychological well-being of laryngectomized persons and their families.

1. *Enabling the client to express, acknowledge, and clarify feelings and concerns.* Underlying this skill is the corollary capacity for the clinician to engender feelings of acceptance, security, and partnership, often referred to as "rapport." Rapport frees clients to disclose information they might otherwise have felt too constrained to divulge and to entertain strategies they might otherwise have been too inhibited to consider or attempt. Client failure to disclose information impedes problem recognition and assessment for both the client and the clinician. Client failure to entertain or to attempt potential strategies jeopardizes problem resolution.

    Expressing feelings has several potential counseling benefits. Emotional catharsis can reduce the stress associated with reconciling changes and coping with problems. It can also facilitate acknowledgement, definition, and appreciation of problems and of underlying attitudes, values, and predispositions to act. These, in turn, can enhance problem resolution.

2. *Ascertaining the client's knowledge, feelings, and attitudes regarding the changes and problems associated with being laryngectomized.* Clinician understanding of a client's condition is the basis for planning and evaluating intervention, including counseling. Familiarity with a client's knowledge base and emotional status is to counseling laryngectomized clients what familiarity with his or her ability to trap esophageal air, prolong phonation, and differentiate speech sounds is to speech treatment. Both have relevance for rehabilitating laryngectomized individuals.

    When discussing the clinician's ability to develop the insights associated with the present skill, it is also important to acknowledge the contributions of a previously described counseling skill, that of enabling expression.

3. *Promoting the client's ability to explore, formulate, evaluate, and execute strategies for problem resolution.* A corollary of this skill is the ability to facilitate problem resolution without engendering client feelings of being compelled to accept specific strategies, the biases of others, or arbitrary deadlines. This skill is analogous to the skills required to assist clients through the acquisition of speech behaviors, from producing simple speech targets through generalization to realistic environments. They also rely extensively on the client's ability to self-monitor and to self-correct.

4. *Accessing, providing, and evaluating needed information.* The skills discussed above facilitate determining the what and when of accessing information needed for problem definition and resolution. On the other hand, the skill presently being described enhances the client's obtaining, evaluating, and using that information. Corollary clinician traits include familiarity with the array of potential resources, networking skills, and acceptance by the professional and laryngectomized communities.

    Information resources include the clinician's knowledge base, publications, video tapes, agencies and organizations, professionals representing associated disciplines, and concerned individuals having potentially valuable knowledge and experience to share. Many of these resources are also cited under the next skill, accessing support for clients and their families.

Among the organizations providing information are the American Cancer Society (ACS) and its affiliated International Association of Laryngectomees (IAL), 1599 Clifton Road, N. E., Atlanta, GA 30329. The national, state, and local cancer societies, as well as state and local affiliates of the IAL, the latter often known as Lost Cord or New Voice Clubs, provide printed matter, trained and knowledgeable hospital visitors (both laryngectomees and spouses), and educational activities. These educational activities include annual national and state meetings and more frequent local meetings, featuring physicians, dentists, psychologists, speech-language pathologists, governmental agency representatives, and others having messages of value for laryngectomized individuals and their significant others. Additionally, the IAL and its state affiliates sponsor national and state seminars designed to enhance the knowledge, skills, and insights of professionals, especially speech-language pathologists. These seminars may also be attended by selected laryngectomees, who, on passing the compulsory examination and a year's supervised "internship," may serve under the direction of a speech-language pathologist as volunteer information and counseling adjuncts and speech assistants.

A representative list of literature designed for laryngectomized individuals, their families, and the community as a whole, is provided at the end of this chapter.

5. *Accessing and providing support for the client and spouse.* Support subsumes a number of components that contribute to comforting and sustaining clients and their families as they deal with the changes accompanying loss of the larynx. Providing support confirms that a client continues to be a person and to be valued while acknowledging and dealing with the changes, concerns, fears, and needs associated with having been laryngectomized.

Both the literature and client reports affirm that the spouse and family are major, if not the principal, sources of support. Salmon's *Guidelines For Those Who Care*, presented in Figure 8.1, represents a practical approach toward nurturing the support provided by family and friends. It offers concrete suggestions, in handout form, that engender an enabling orientation toward the client and promote successful interactions. Although designed for intimates, much of the content is equally appropriate for the professional community.

Other sources of nurturing include hospital visitation by trained laryngectomees and their spouses, support provided by others attending meetings of New Voice clubs, and contributions by physicians, nurses, social workers, and possibly by psychologists. Although often overlooked when listing sources of support, group speech therapy provides opportunities for clients to observe similar problems in others, profit from their models, appreciate that functional speech is achievable, and receive praise for attempts and success.

Additional and separate opportunities for spouse discussion and support are important aspects of postlaryngectomy rehabilitation. Spouses as well as laryngectomees need to express their concerns and frustrations, recognize that others face, feel, and manage similar problems, and learn about how that has been accomplished. They, too, need acknowledgement and praise.

Meeting the support needs of the laryngectomized client and the family requires the same corollary traits as meeting their information needs: familiarity with resources, networking, and clinician acceptance by the communities to be solicited, along with the presumed clinician concern and sensitivity.

## A CHECKLIST FOR LARYNGECTOMEE CONSULTATIONS

Salmon (1994) describes the results of her questionnaire survey of 66 laryngectomees and their 53 spouses, undertaken to ascertain personal experiences and feelings regarding pre- and postoperative counseling sessions. The responses obtained, which Salmon indicates are similar to those reported from more recent surveys, are discussed according to such headings

Guidelines For Those Who Care
Shirley J. Salmon, Ph.D.

1. The laryngectomee's condition is in no way contagious and does not endanger you. Therefore, don't be AFRAID. We are not fearful of contact with people who have had their tonsils, gallbladders, or appendixes removed. The same should be true of those who have had their voice boxes removed.

2. EDUCATE yourself and others to accept the different sound of a laryngectomee's cough and voice. The larynx refines the sound of the cough and voice. After laryngectomy, both are different.

3. Remember having had a laryngectomy does not make a person blind, deaf, or stupid. In all other ways except for speaking laryngectomees are the SAME people after the operation as they were before. When people talk <u>about</u> them instead of <u>to</u> them, laryngectomees see it, hear it, and know it. It is very frustrating!

4. ENCOURAGE self-care of the stoma with clean, healthy, habits that keep it free from mucous and covered at all times. Such habits will prevent the laryngectomee and others from feeling embarrassed or offended.

5. ASSIST the laryngectomee with communication when asked. However, avoid doing all the talking so you do not take away the need to learn to speak well.

6. COURAGE is needed for the first attempts at communication following a laryngectomy. Be sensitive to this fact and be sure you acknowledge good communication style with clear speech, appropriate facial expressions, and meaningful gestures.

7. Allow the laryngectomee TIME to talk. Speech may be slower than it was before. Your manner and attitude will directly affect the laryngectomee. Please help the laryngectomee to relax and not feel rushed.

8. LOOK at the speaker. We all know it is much easier to talk to people who look at us. Besides, lipreading will help fill the gaps when some words are not heard clearly.

9. Tell the TRUTH; never pretend you understand when you don't. The whole purpose of speech is to communicate and it is very frustrating when this is not achieved.

10. Realize the mind and body require a recovery period following major surgery. Adjusting to the loss of voice is harder than you think and the whole family/friend network is affected. Use PATIENCE with the laryngectomee and with yourself. You'll begin to see a light at the end of the tunnel, usually within three to six months.

*Some of this information was taken from the <u>Queensland Newsletter</u>, Australia, April, 1993.

Reprinted with permission of author.

**Figure 8.1.**   Guidelines For Those Who Care*

as (a) information provided and desired, (b) preparation for surgery, (c) whom respondents would like to see, and (d) areas perceived as problematic by the respondents. The speech-language pathologist who participates in laryngectomee rehabilitation should be familiar with Salmon's findings, as well as how they are reflected in the protocol she describes for providing information in incremental steps during the pre- and immediate postoperative period.

The checklist by Salmon, presented in Figure 8.2, delineates her protocol in terms of a proactive sequence of clinician tasks and goals. The descriptor, proactive, is applied in recognition of the author's implicit knowledge and sensitivity regarding the issues underlying successful rehabilitation of laryngectomees. The knowledge and sensitivity reflected in the Checklist For Pre- and Postoperative Laryngectomee Consultations is a concrete example of the requisites promulgated in this chapter for successful counseling of laryngectomees and their significant others.

## POSTSCRIPT

With concern for the gravity of the material dealt with in this chapter, perhaps inherent to the topic of cancer, it must be said that involvement with laryngectomized individuals and

CHECK LIST FOR PRE AND POST-OP LARYNGECTOMEE CONSULTATIONS

Shirley J. Salmon, Ph.D.
Veterans Administration Hospital
Kansas City, Missouri

Patient's Name: _____

                                                        Date Completed  By Whom

1.     Pre-op Consultation with Patient

       A.  Review Medical Chart. Is primary TEP planned?        _____  _____

       B.  Confer with both the patient and spouse.
           Begin by asking facts they can relate about
           the upcoming surgery.                                _____  _____

       C.  Underscore that patient will breathe differently and
           the voice box will be removed.                       _____  _____

       D.  Discuss alternatives for post-op communication and
           test legibility of patient's writing.                _____  _____

       E.  Estimate length of surgery and prepare spouse for
           intensive care unit and patient's appearance.        _____  _____

       F.  Outline post-op services provided by speech-language
           pathologist and set date for first post-op appointment.   _____  _____

       G.  Inform about the availability of a counselor, social
           worker, chaplain, VA pension rep., etc.              _____  _____

       H.  Write consultation report and place in Medical Chart.    _____  _____

       I.  If necessary, investigate referral sources for
           alaryngeal speech therapy.                           _____  _____

II.    Post-op Consultation with Patient

       A.  First Visit

           1.  Give patient packet of selected literature from
               the American Cancer Society.                     _____  _____

           2.  Show to patient and spouse various types of stoma
               covers.                                          _____  _____

           3.  Furnish addresses, prices and patterns for various
               types of stoma covers.                           _____  _____

           4.  Discuss Medic Alert information - "Neck-breather"
               to be engraved on back of bracelet and printed
               on billfold card.                                _____  _____

           5.  Refer to appropriate counselor.                  _____  _____

           6.  Request permission to write I.A.L. and Nu-Voice
               Club to place patient's name on Newsletter mailing
               lists                                            _____  _____

           7.  Record visit in Medical Chart                    _____  _____

**Figure 8.2.**  Checklist for Pre and Post-op Laryngectomee Consultations

Date Completed    By Whom

B.  Second Visit

1.  Discuss literature provided at first visit                          _____    _____

2.  Show film or video-tape that demonstrates
    esophageal speech                                                   _____    _____

3.  Request permission to arrange a visit from a
    laryngectomee (and spouse when appropriate)
    trained by ACS to do hospital visitations.                         _____    _____

4.  Notify head nurse of scheduled time for the visit                  _____    _____

5.  Record in Medical Chart                                            _____    _____

C.  Third Visit

1.  Show film or video tape that demonstrates artifical
    larynx devices                                                     _____    _____

2.  Have various devices displayed during film or video
    tape showing                                                       _____    _____

3.  Record in Medical Chart                                            _____    _____

D.  Other Visits

1.  Discuss visits from alaryngeal speakers and spouses
    who are trained hospital visitors                                  _____    _____

2.  Help select an appropriate artifical larynx device
    and begin instructions about use when NG tube is
    removed                                                            _____    _____

3.  When possible, issue an artifical larynx device after
    instruction but before hospital discharge                          _____    _____

4.  Loan patient, "Self Help for laryngectomees,"
    "Looking Forward," and/or "Hello, Tallulah"                        _____    _____

5.  Schedule patient's outpatient appointment                         _____    _____

6.  Record each visit in Medical Chart and the type
    of artifical larynx device recommended and/or
    issued                                                            _____    _____

Reprinted with permission of author.

**Figure 8.2.**—*continued*

groups is not the morose undertaking that might be anticipated. Arguably, every human experience, even those that threaten life or its most prized elements, has potential for promoting appreciation and growth.

Participation in numerous IAL Voice Institutes and Annual Meetings reconfirms a laryngectomized friend's comment that at no place else in the world are there so many people hugging each other. Another laryngectomized friend confided, after several years of struggle and frequent depression, that she had come to realize that she "had never really lived" until she had cancer.

Another laryngectomized friend once suggested playfully that the world consists of two types of people: those who bemoan the fact that rose bushes have thorns and those who celebrate the fact that thorn bushes have roses. His intent, and mine, are not to rationalize or trivialize the very serious nature of laryngeal cancer, but to affirm that unexpected positives can be found or created if one can look for them.

I have often said, while lecturing about laryngectomee rehabilitation, that if a laryngectomee told me he could fly, my response would be to ask him to show me how he did it. I have come to appreciate that people in general, and laryngectomees in particular, have a wonderful capacity to regenerate. Perhaps what we call counseling is a characteristic of that capacity.

## REFERENCES AND SUGGESTED READINGS

Two types of literature are included in the list of references: chapter and article citations, designed primarily for speech pathologists and other professionals; and pamphlets, booklets, guidebooks, and the like, designed primarily for laryngectomized individuals and significant others. In keeping with the clinician attributes presented, notably the second, *responsibilities,* it is recommended that the clinician become familiar with the items listed, including the "lay" literature, especially if clients are to be referred to those publications. Clinicians should be familiar with the content and aware of the possible ramifications for specific clients as well as the professionals involved. In keeping with the third attribute, *treatment individualization,* it should be recognized that client needs and capacities often support his or her access to the "professional" literature, and the right to question and to dispute.

Some of the information contained in the pamphlets is out-of-date; and there is a notable lack of lay literature dealing with tracheoesophageal speech. A bias toward esophageal speech, reflecting that lack, and a now archaic and untenable prejudice against the artificial larynx, may be sensed in the older literature, both lay and professional. Nonetheless, there is much valuable information to be obtained, especially when the clinician heeds the advice to be familiar with the content and its ramifications.

## REFERENCES

Dugay, M. (1966). Preoperative ideas of speech after laryngectomy. *Archives of Otolaryngology, 83,* 237–240.
Gardner, W. (1966). Adjustment problems of laryngectomized women. *Archives of Otolaryngology, 83,* 31–42.
Gilmore, S. (1974). Social and vocational acceptability of esophageal speakers compared to normal speakers. *Journal of Speech and Hearing Research, 17,* 599–607.
Gilmore, S. (1994). The physical, social, occupational, and psychological concomitants of laryngectomy. In R. Keith, & F. Darley (Eds.), *Laryngectomee rehabilitation* (3rd ed.). Austin, TX: Pro-ed.
Natvig, K. (1984). Laryngectomees in Norway. Study No. 5: Problems of everyday life. *Journal of Otolaryngology, 13,* 16–22.
Robinette, M. (1994). Hearing problems associated with laryngectomy. In R. Keith & F. Darley (Eds.), (1994). *Laryngectomee rehabilitation* (3rd ed.). Austin, TX: Pro-ed.
Salmon, S. (1994). Pre- and postoperative conferences with laryngectomees and their spouses. In R. Keith & F. Darley (Eds.), *Laryngectomee rehabilitation* (3rd ed.). Austin, TX: Pro-ed.

## SUGGESTED READINGS

Blood, G., Luther, A., & Stemple, J. (1992). Coping and adjusting in alaryngeal speakers. *American Journal of Speech-Language Pathology, 1,* 63–69.
Dhooper, S. (1985). Social work with laryngectomees. *Health Social Work, 10,* 217–227.
Gates, C. (1988). The "most-significant-other" in the care of the breast cancer patient. In American Cancer Society, *Psychosocial Issues and Cancer* (pp. 18–25). New York: American Cancer Society.
Lieberman, M. (1988). The role of self-help groups in helping patients and families cope with cancer. In American Cancer Society, *Psychosocial Issues and Cancer* (pp. 34–40). New York: American Cancer Society.
Renner, M. J. (1995). Counseling laryngectomees and families. *Seminars in Speech and Language, 16,* 215–219.
Rice, D., and Spiro, R. (1989). *Current concepts in head and neck cancer.* Atlanta, GA: American Cancer Society. (Note Chapter 1, General Management Guidelines, and Chapter 8, Carcinoma of the Larynx).
Salmon, S. (1986). Adjusting to laryngectomy. *Seminars in Speech and Language, 7,* 67–94.
Shanks, J. (1991). Consequences of total laryngectomy in daily living activities. In J. Salmon, & K. Mount (Eds.), *Alaryngeal speech rehabilitation: For clinicians by clinicians.* Austin, TX: Pro-ed.
Shanks, J. (1995). Coping with laryngeal cancer. *Seminars in Speech and Language, 16,* 180–190.

Snidecor, J. (1971). The family of the laryngectomee, In S. Gerber (Ed.), *The family as support personnel in speech and hearing remediation: Proceedings of the post-graduate course.* Santa Barbara, CA: Training Division, Rehabilitation Services, U. S. Department of Health, Education, and Welfare.

Strasser, M. (1991). Living with a laryngectomee. In J. Salmon, & K. Mount (Eds.), *Alaryngeal speech rehabilitation: For clinicians by clinicians.* Austin, TX: Pro-ed.

## PAMPHLETS

American Cancer Society Publications: these are free of charge, often available through state and local ACS offices and support groups. Among the ones the author has found helpful are the following: *Cancer, your job, insurance, and the law* (ACS, Texas Division, Inc.); *Facts on cancer of the larynx; First steps: Helping words for the laryngectomee; IAL news* (periodic publication of the IAL); *Larngectomee care at home; Talking with the cancer patient; Rehabilitating laryngectomees; Rescue breathing for laryngectomees and other neck breathers; Talking with your doctor; Hello, Tallulah.*

Anti-Cancer Foundation of the Universities of South Australia (24 Brougham Place, P.O. Box 160, North Adelaide, South Australia 5006, Australia): *Cancer and you; Questions you might like to ask your doctor.*

National Institutes of Health, Public Health Service: *Facing forward, A guide for cancer survivors; Talking time: Support for people with cancer and the people who care about them.*

National Institutes of Health, National Cancer Institute: *What you need to know about cancer of the larynx.*

Dabul, B. (1995). *The laryngectomee: A booklet for family and friends* (3rd ed.). Austin, TX: PRO-ED.

Dean, C., & Moidel, B. (1979). *Same face . . . New sound.* Chicago, IL: National Easter Seal Society for Crippled Children and Adults.

Dear, A. (1989). *You can say that again.* Sydney, NSW: Australian Cancer Society.

Kelly, D., & Welborn, P. (1980). *The cover up: Neckware for the laryngectomee and other neck breathers.* Houston, TX: College-Hill Press.

Keith, R. (1983). *A handbook for the laryngectomee* (2nd ed.). Danville, IL: Interstate Printers and Publishers.

Keith, R. (1991). *Looking forward . . . A guidebook for the laryngectomee* (2nd ed.). New York: Thieme Medical.

Lauder, J. (Ed.) (1993). *Self help for the laryngectomee.* San Antonio, TX: Lauder.

Mills, D., & Mills, E. (1995). *Papaw's new voice.* San Antonio, TX: Lauder Enterprises. (A story book for children describing a grandfather's laryngectomy.)

Reynolds, P. (1984). *Living with cancer* (3rd. ed.) West Perth, Western Australia: The Cancer Foundation of Western Australia.

Waldrop, W., & Gould, M. (1969). *Your new voice* (revised ed.). American Cancer Society.

Winstone, H., (1984). *The role of the partner.* Adelaide, South Australia: New Voice Association of South Australia.

## VIDEO TAPES

American Cancer Society. (1988). Code: 4536.05. *Speech after laryngectomy,.*

# 9. Counseling with Parents of Children with Phonological Disorders

Julie J. Masterson and Kenn Apel

The framework and strategies presented in this chapter for counseling with parents of children with phonological disorders are based on the work of Elizabeth Webster in the area of parent and family counseling. Webster's approach to counseling is summarized in her book, *Counseling with Parents of Handicapped Children* (Webster, 1981). Webster's choice of the preposition *with* was not accidental, as it illustrates her view that the professional is not the ultimate authority who hands out prescriptions of what the parent should do to make things right for the child. Rather, the professional works with parents, viewing them as equal team members, and together they determine strategies for effecting change. Webster describes some general principles for facilitating the counseling process and then discusses the primary functions served by the counselor. In this chapter, an overview of Webster's approach to counseling is first provided and then the application of this approach for working with parents of children with phonological disorders is illustrated. Research regarding areas of specific concern to parents of children with phonological disorders is discussed. Finally, an outline is presented of a six-week program based on these principles that might be used with parents and family members of children with phonological disorders.

## GENERAL PRINCIPLES FOR COUNSELING

### Promoting Effective Communication

Webster (1981) highlights the similarities between counselors and the families with whom they work. Although the counselor may not have an individual with a disability in his or her own family, the counselor feels many of the emotions that are associated with this situation. All individuals experience concern, aspiration, guilt, joy, and success, and it is the common ground of experiencing these feeling that can serve as a basis for communication between the counselor and the family members. Counselors should draw on their own backgrounds and personal histories to relate to the needs and wishes expressed by family members of individuals with disabilities.

Counselors should view parents as specialists in relation to their child. Webster suggests the adoption of an "I-Thou" attitude, characterized by the view that the counselee is a whole person who cannot be analyzed or dissected. This does not mean that the counselor does not analyze aspects of the family situation; that is often appropriate and desirable. However, the counselor should not view parents as things to be dealt with or objects to be manipulated (Webster, 1981; p. 25).

Strategies that facilitate open dialogue between counselors and parents are beneficial in the counseling process. For example, counselors need not fear periods of silence. Silence is important in a communicative situation and provides participants the opportunity to think about information and formulate questions or statements. Another beneficial strategy is active listening. After forming hunches, or hypotheses, about the parent's messages the counselor states in his or her own words what he or she thinks the parent is trying to say. These hunches are expressed in a tentative manner, so that the parent is able to agree with or modify the counselor's hypotheses. The use of active listening can be a powerful tool in establishing and maintaining effective communication with parents and other family members.

Finally, Webster suggests that counselors establish a *contract* at the beginning of each counseling session. The contract consists of statements made by the counselor that cover specifics about the current session, including the time allocated, participants involved, and purposes or goals established. This procedure provides security to the parents in that they know what to expect during the session. It also may increase their confidence in the counselor by providing evidence that the session does have a clear purpose and will not proceed haphazardly.

## Receiving Information

It is important to use tactics that facilitate the optimal receipt of information. Written communications are a typical source for clinicians to gather information. Questionnaires are commonly used to gather background or case history data. Written communication offers the advantage of allowing parents and family members time to consider questions and other requests for information. They can consult sources such as diaries or baby books to provide information that may be difficult to recall during a face-to-face verbal interview.

Although written communication is quite valuable, a substantial portion of the information obtained from family members is provided during conversations. This is where the strategies already discussed for optimizing verbal communication become useful. Additionally, different types of questions can be used by counselors to gain knowledge about the client. Questions can be classified as *requests for facts* (RF), *requests for opinions* (RO), *requests for clarification* (RC), and *requests for discussion* (RD). Each type of question can prove to be quite valuable in eliciting the information needed about the client and the family.

## Giving Information

Information can be provided in two general ways: through planned instructional activities and in response to parents' specific questions. Informative sessions should be carefully planned so that counselors do not fall into the trap of giving too much information at once. The appropriate amount of information to be provided depends on individual parents and the experiences they are undergoing at that specific time. When counselors need to respond to parents' questions, they should identify the types of information being requested. This often requires the counselor to form hypotheses about the parents' underlying meaning. For example, a question such as "How will this phonological problem affect Susie's performance in school?" may be not only a request for information, but also a request for some discussion regarding ways in which the parents and teachers can facilitate the child's academic success.

Clinicians would be wise to avoid the use of jargon and to assess continually the parents' understanding of the information being provided. This can be accomplished by asking questions that probe for specific information rather than general questions such as, "Did you understand what I said?" The latter type of question is likely to elicit an answer in the affirmative, even if the parents were unclear about some or all of the information provided. Instead, the clinician might try the following strategy. "I know I've given you a great deal of information. Why don't you summarize it as you will when you get home to your spouse? That way I can check to see whether I've done my job in providing the right information."

## Clarifying Attitudes, Beliefs, and Ideas and Changing Behaviors

Webster (1981) reminds counselors that "clarification precedes action" (p. 120). Before an individual can change a behavior or implement a new strategy, the individual must understand the reason for the change and believe the change is necessary. Assisting parents with clarification is quite effective in helping family members see the need for behavioral change. Webster's suggestions regarding optimal communication and giving information certainly are applicable to parent training. However, counselors are encouraged to proceed with caution when implementing any training program with parents and family members. Again, the target behaviors must be important to the parents themselves. If this is not the case, training may not be very effective. A personal experience illustrates the truth of this principle. One of the authors once left her dogs in the care of some teenage cousins. Not wanting the task to be a burden on the parents, she worked out an elaborate payment system in which each cousin had an assigned duty to be performed by a specific time each day. If the task was not completed, the other cousin had the option to do it and, thus, earn the payment. If neither teen did it, the parent could do it and get the money, thereby causing the teens to lose that day's payment. The charts were detailed and, to be frank, quite impressive (at least to any clinician who had undergone training in behavior modification). The system was explained to the family and questions were entertained at the end of the presentation (there were none). At the end of the vacation, it was time to determine the appropriate recipients of payment. The parents and teens gave a blank look and said, "What chart?" The parents requested payment to be divided equally between the teens. Although it was never really known who took care of the dogs, it was suspected that the parents did. The example is a great illustration of an issue and an associated system that were important to the "clinician" but not to the family.

## IMPLEMENTING COUNSELOR FUNCTIONS: SPECIAL CONSIDERATIONS FOR PARENTS OF CHILDREN WITH PHONOLOGICAL DISORDERS

In this section, Webster's principles for counseling will be applied to working with parents of children with phonological disorders. Additionally, research regarding issues of particular concern for parents of children with phonological disorders will be discussed.

## Receiving Information

CASE HISTORY

One of the first ways in which clinicians gather information from parents and family members is by completing the case history, or background information. The case history should address four main components: (*a*) birth and medical history, (*b*) developmental history, (*c*) speech and language development and present functioning, and (*d*) social and academic functioning. This information is usually first elicited through a written questionnaire and then supplemented with a face-to-face interview. In addition to the typical questions regarding birth and developmental milestones, it is particularly useful to ask parents of children with phonological disorders whether their child babbled. Some parents can offer reasonable descriptions of their child's babbling, which can be useful information in completing a phonological assessment (Bernthal & Bankson, 1993).

Oller, Eilers, and colleagues (Eilers et al., 1993; Oller, Eilers, Basinger, Steffens, & Urbano, 1995; Oller, Eilers, Steffens, Lynch, & Urbano, 1994) reported that parents were quite successful in identifying the onset of canonical babbling in their children. Some parents received fairly extensive training on canonical babbling, but others simply responded to questions about the onset during telephone interviews. The influence of factors such as amount of training, socioeconomic status, type of interview question, and developmental stage of the child were evaluated, and the parent judgments proved to be quite reliable across conditions. The work of Oller and Eilers provides a nice example of how parents can be instructed to watch for specific aspects of development and, as a result, assist in monitoring phonological progress in their children.

It also is helpful to ask parents about their child's present intelligibility and the manner in which others respond to his or her speech. The clinician is interested in determining whether the child is still willing to attempt communication even though intelligibility may be compromised or whether the child has begun to withdraw and avoid talking owing to frustrations over not being understood. Such information is useful in determining whether or not to enroll for treatment.

FAMILY HISTORY

A number of investigators have examined the familial basis of speech and language disorders (Crago & Gopnik, 1994; Shiberg, 1993; Tomblin, 1989). Lewis, Ekelman, and Aram (1989) examined the familial basis of phonological disorders by testing children with phonological disorders, their siblings, and a group of matched children without phonological disorders and their siblings. In addition to differences on measures of speech, language, and reading between the children with phonological disorders and the matched control group, Lewis et al. (1989) found differences between the two sibling groups. The siblings of the disordered children performed more poorly than did the control siblings on phonology and reading measures. Lewis et al. suggested that their results indicate a familial basis for at least some forms of phonological disorders. The results of this investigation suggest that information regarding the speech and language abilities of family members might be useful both in diagnosing children with phonological disorders and in identifying siblings who might also be at risk for them.

REACTIONS TO UNINTELLIGIBILITY

The reactions of the child and others to his or her unintelligibility are important in determining whether to recommend treatment. Sometimes a child might be able to communicate quite adequately, and others in his or her environment are not troubled by the child's speech. If the phonological errors are considered likely to be developmental in nature, the clinician may opt to re-evaluate at a later time rather than immediately enroll the child in treatment. In other cases, a child and/or family members might be quite concerned about the speech errors, and, consequently, a decision to begin treatment may be appropriate.

**Case Example.**   Leigh was a graduate student studying speech-language pathology. Her daughter, Kathy, was three years old. Leigh was taking a course in phonology and asked that her daughter be seen for a phonological evaluation. Kathy's speech errors included velar fronting and liquid simplification. Kathy was stimulable for velars, so the clinician wondered whether to enroll her for treatment or to have Leigh keep track of her velar usage to determine whether it increased without intervention. Such an approach would likely have been appropriate if another factor had not been operating. Leigh reported that Kathy appeared to be so concerned about her speech differences that she had stopped talking in preschool. Even at home, Kathy had begun to avoid words that contained velars. This was somewhat puzzling to Leigh, because neither she nor Kathy's father had been worried about the problem until Kathy showed her concern. Of interest was the fact that Kathy's language skills were quite advanced. After hearing about Kathy's reaction to her phonological problems, the clinician decided to enroll her in treatment immediately. She responded well and her level of communication use returned to normal.

## VIEWS REGARDING INTERVENTION

Parents might also be asked about their views regarding intervention. As stated above, family members must consider treatment to be necessary and important. In the early stages of intervention, the clinician may want to spend some time with family members discussing their attitudes about treatment and, if necessary, helping to clarify the notion that treatment is an important priority for the child. Once the need for treatment is established, clinicians may want to discuss parents' expectations for treatment. Parents sometimes do not have an understanding of the potential timeline for intervention. Some parents expect their child to be "fixed" in two or three months. Occasionally, the clinician encounters a parent who wonders if phonological intervention will be a part of the child's academic activities forever. The clinician needs to discuss these issues with the parents to provide appropriate information regarding the need for intervention and prognosis.

**Case Example.**   Mrs. Jones was a retired elementary school teacher. Her grandson, Greg, was four years old and had delayed phonological development. Both Greg's mother and his grandmother were concerned about his speech and enrolled him in treatment. Mrs. Jones brought Greg to treatment each day and watched the sessions from the observation room. After seeing several sessions, Mrs. Jones expressed concern that Greg was being allowed to take breaks and not using every minute to work on his speech. After some discussion regarding reasonable expectations for young children's performance in treatment, Mrs. Jones said, "I know it may be hard, but I think it's necessary for him to do the work now. He needs to clear up this problem this year or he won't be able to start kindergarten." This statement gave the clinician an opportunity to talk about factors that affect children's rate of progress in treatment. Interestingly, Greg's early academic (literacy) skills were quite strong, likely due to being read to by Mrs. Jones and by playing rhyming and letter games at home. The clinician pointed out this fact to Mrs. Jones and also highlighted Greg's willingness to communicate with others. Mrs. Jones seemed to relax after that conversation, although the clinician continued to ensure that Mrs. Jones was aware of the progress that Greg was making toward his phonological goals.

## Giving Information

### MOTORIC VERSUS CONCEPTUAL PHONOLOGICAL DISORDERS

One of the first tasks facing the clinician is to explain what a phonological disorder is to parents. The nature of children's speech-sound disorders continues to be a topic of lively debate among speech-language pathologists. Although there may not be total consensus on the subject, most professionals believe that errors can be generally classified into two types, motoric and conceptual. Motoric, or phonetic, errors are those that are due to be the child's inability to readily articulate a target sound or sound class. Conceptual, or phonemic, errors are those that are due to a child's inappropriate sorting, organization, or representation of the phonological system. Most clinicians have seen a child who substitutes a [θ] for an /s/, yet also substitutes [f] for /θ/. The [f] for /θ/ error is not due to the child's inability to produce an /θ/, but rather is due to faulty organization or use of the phonological system. A basic description of these two types of errors is useful for parents. It helps them to understand the intervention process and it also can be useful when they implement activities the clinician sends home.

This dichotomy also can be helpful in describing intervention techniques. Some techniques, such as minimal pairs, are primarily conceptual in nature; and they are used to facilitate appropriate organization and use of the phonological system. Others, such as phonetic placement instructions and drill, are primarily motoric; and they are used to facilitate and stabilize correct articulation of the target sound(s).

**Case Example.**    Caleb, a five-year-old boy, was seen for a phonological evaluation. He fronted velars consistently; however, he was readily stimulable for velar production. The clinician decided to use a conceptual approach to treatment and labeled the target class (velars) as throat sounds and the intruder class (alveolars) as tippy sounds. He explained to Caleb's parents that Caleb could produce the /k/ and /g/ sounds, but just needed help in determining when to use them. Word sorting and minimal pair activities were used in treatment. At first, Caleb's dad, Eric, wondered why Caleb was not being asked to practice /k/ and /g/ words repeatedly. Eric mentioned that he had considered having Caleb say the /k/ and /g/ sounds several times each night before going to bed. The clinician realized that his original explanation of the nature of Caleb's error was likely not sufficient. He asked Caleb to repeat some of his productions of words that contained velars, which Caleb was able to do readily. He then illustrated how minimal pair activities allowed Caleb to see the consequences of using the tippy sounds. Eric seemed to understand the rationale for the treatment approach and reported that he had begun pointing out words with throaty sounds in them at home.

RELATIONSHIP BETWEEN OTITIS MEDIA AND PHONOLOGICAL DISORDERS

Another common question heard from parents is whether frequent middle-ear problems might have caused their child's phonological disorder. There have been several investigations regarding the relationship between otitis media (OME) and phonological disorders (Paden, Novak, & Beiter, 1987; Roberts, Burchinal, Kock, Footo, & Henderson, 1988; Shriberg & Smith, 1983). The issue is cloudy owing to the fact that there are children who have suffered almost continuous bouts of otitis media yet do not have phonological disorders, and there are children with phonological disorders who have no documented history of otitis media. Paden, Matthies, and Novak (1989) followed children who were seen for insertion of pressure-equalization (PE) tubes to determine which children would ultimately need phonological intervention. They found that three factors held primary predictive value: (*a*) the severity, or number of phonological errors at the time of PE tube placement, (*b*) the severity, or number of phonological errors four months after surgery, and (*c*) the amount of time between the surgery and the first six-month period during which the child was free of otitis media. In addition, they found that velar deviations and cluster reductions tended to occur in children who ultimately required treatment. Although these results do not clarify the specific relationship between otitis media and phonological disorders, they do have implications for parents and clinicians who are making decisions regarding treatment for children who suffer from OME. It seems that children whose phonological systems are already significantly compromised at the time of surgery should be considered at risk. Further, children should be monitored after surgery and those who do not show sufficient phonological improvement after four months should be considered candidates for intervention. Finally, children who do not experience remission from otitis media following surgery should also be considered at risk for phonological problems and perhaps enrolled in treatment.

RELATIONSHIP BETWEEN PHONOLOGICAL DISORDERS AND ACADEMIC PROBLEMS

One of the most frequent concerns voiced by parents of children with phonological disorders is the impact that the problem may have on the child's performance in school. A variety of studies have suggested a link between early speech and language disorders and later reading and spelling problems (Catts, 1989; Clark-Klein, 1994; Lewis & Freebairn; 1992; Robinson, Beresford, & Dodd, 1982; Stackhouse, 1982; Webster & Plante, 1992). Clark-Klein (1994) analyzed the spelling errors of children with and without histories of severe speech-sound disorders. The children with histories of phonological disorders demonstrated more spelling errors than did the other group. Lewis and Freebairn (1992) reported similar findings regarding reading and spelling during the elementary, adolescent, and adult years. The nature of the link between phonological disorders and academic problems is not without controversy (Bishop, 1985). The types of phonological errors present may possibly play a role in determining whether or not there is a link. Perhaps children with phonological disorders characterized by a greater number of conceptual errors are more likely to show problems in reading and spelling than those whose disorders are characterized by articulation errors (e.g., phonetic distortions).

Given the potential link between phonological disorders and reading and spelling skills, it is likely a good idea to discuss with parents ways in which they may facilitate the development of literacy skills in their children. The time-honored practice of reading to children is especially important for parents of children with phonological problems. Games that foster the development of metalinguistic skills, such as rhyming and initial and final sound identification, also can be provided to parents. For parents of older children, activities such as interactive journal writing and taking turns reading book chapters can be fun.

**Case Example.** Caitlin was a four-year-old child enrolled for phonological intervention. Her parents, Patty and Lee, expressed concern about Caitlin's future performance in school. Originally, they were mainly worried that she would not be understood by the teacher and the other children. After observing treatment, they commented on the use of written words and letters as part of the intervention materials and asked the clinician why they were working on reading. The clinician explained the potential link between early phonological problems and later reading and spelling performance. She also indicated that Caitlin's treatment was not really targeting reading skills, but instead literacy materials were being included so that Caitlin might get a head start in discovering sound-symbol relationships. Patty and Lee responded, "We didn't realize that Caitlin's speech would affect her reading." The clinician clarified that the relationship between speech and reading was probably not unidirectional. However, reading and speech do seem to share a common foundation. Patty, Lee, and the clinician then discussed some activities that could be used at home to facilitate Caitlin's phonological awareness. Patty remembered playing a game in which the first player names a word and then the second player has to identify the last sound and provide a word beginning with that sound. The clinician remarked that final sound identification might be somewhat difficult for Caitlin initially, but she might be able to provide another word that had the same initial sound. Lee remarked that rhyming games might also be helpful. The clinician responded that those activities would be beneficial. She reminded them that Caitlin would likely give them feedback about whether the activity was at the right level or too difficult and also whether the activity was fun, and encouraged Patty and Lee to take their cues from Caitlin. Lee and Patty left the session excited about the opportunity to do some activities at home that might be both enjoyable and helpful for Caitlin.

PARENTS AS THERAPISTS

Another common request heard from parents is in reference to what they can do to facilitate their child's acquisition of necessary phonological skills. Most of the published literature regarding services with families of children with phonological disorders concerns the efficacy of programs designed to train parents to work on their children's phonological skills (Broen & Westman, 1990; Carrier, 1970; Dodd, McCormack, & Woodyatt, 1994; Dudzinski & Peters, 1977; Eiserman, Weber, & McCoun, 1992; Eiserman, McCoun, & Escobar, 1990; Sommers et al., 1959). These programs have been used for the past several decades. For example, Sommers et al. (1959) compared the progress of children whose parents were involved in a training program with those whose parents were not. The two groups of children were described as having functional articulation deficits, and all children were seen for speech therapy. The parents of the experimental group of children were told that they should come to the clinic with their children each day. During their visits, they attended lectures and discussions regarding speech problems in children. Afterwards, they observed their children in therapy. They were also given home assignments and feedback regarding implementing these activities. The parents of the children in the control group were not asked to attend therapy with their children and were not given information specific to their children's speech goals. At the end of the clinical period, both groups of children were re-evaluated. In spite of the increased parental involvement, the children in the experimental group made no more progress in reducing speech errors than did the children in the control group. Parents in both groups completed a questionnaire regarding their attitudes toward the therapy program. Both groups responded favorably; however, the parents in the experimental group tended to respond somewhat more positively. Sommers et al. suggested that group differences may have emerged if the treatment had been longer.

Sommers (1962) did a follow-up study and compared the progress of children whose mothers were trained with those whose mothers were not. He considered additional factors such as intelligence and type of therapy (group vs. individual). In this study, the children whose mothers were trained generally made greater improvement than did the children of mothers who were not trained. Sommers et al. (1964) later conducted a related investigation to determine whether the effects of training would vary based on maternal attitudes regarding child rearing. The results indicated that children whose mothers underwent training reduced the number of articulation errors present in their speech to a greater degree than did the children of untrained mothers. This pattern was present regardless of maternal attitude.

Eiserman and colleagues (1992; 1990) conducted a series of studies to evaluate the efficacy of parent training with children who have moderate speech and language disorders. The studies were conducted during a two-year period with comparisons made at the end of each intervention year. Half of the children were assigned to a clinic-based program and attended weekly sessions with a speech-language pathologist. Parents of this group attended a parent support group that focused on general knowledge about child development. These parents were offered homework activities; however, only two parents made such requests and each did so only once. The other half of the children were assigned to a home-training program. The mothers of these children received in-home bimonthly sessions designed to train them in therapeutic techniques. Instruction included information regarding both phonetic (motoric, targeting individual sounds) and phonemic (contrastive, targeting error patterns) approaches to phonological intervention. After each training, the mothers were given worksheets, activities, and written instructions to follow during the next two-week period. The mothers were urged to work with their children in 20–30 minute sessions, at least four times per week. Pre- and post-treatment measures of family functioning and the children's speech and language skills and general development were recorded. The children were comparable at the pre-test; however, the parents in the home-training group demonstrated higher levels of stress than did the parents in the clinic-based program. The intervention programs lasted seven (first year) or eight (second year) months. At the post-test, family stress levels were comparable between the groups.

Additionally, the children undergoing each approach made comparable gains in speech and language development. In a few areas of general development (e.g., the expression of feelings or affect), the children undergoing the home-based program actually made greater improvement than did the children in the clinic-based group. Eiserman and his colleagues concluded that home-based programs do offer a viable alternative to traditional clinic-based intervention. The authors cautioned that such an approach is not necessarily less expensive. The fees associated with the two interventions in these studies were comparable. Further, if monetary charges were associated with parental time invested, the home program was actually more expensive. Eiserman and colleagues further highlighted the fact that their subjects had mild to moderate disorders and the families were generally middle-class, with sufficient financial resources and well-educated mothers who did not work outside the home. They cautioned about generalization to other groups. The authors encouraged future research regarding the usefulness of home-based programs for children with more severe disabilities or other types of family constellations.

Broen and Westman (1990) recently described "Project Parent," which was designed to increase the effectiveness of parents as teachers of speech production skills. This program provided parents with information regarding their children's specific phonological error patterns and assisted them in setting appropriate goals for target behaviors. Additionally, parents received instruction that covered optimal teaching techniques. Consequently, the program provided training in both *what* and *how* to target skills that would result in improvement in their children's phonological systems. Broen and Westman highlighted the importance of considering parents as equal team members and allowing them to take the lead and responsibility for direct work with their child. Broen and Westman studied two groups of children with delayed phonological development. Children who scored two or more standard deviations below the mean were enrolled in the Project Parent program, and children who scored between one and two standard deviations below the mean were not seen for any intervention. This Project Parent program included weekly parent-child sessions attended by a small group of children and their parents. These sessions included time for parent discussion and individual time for each parent-child pair to work with the clinician. Additionally, parents were given home activity kits, which were designed to target each child's particular phonological patterns. At the end of six months, both groups of children were re-evaluated. Children seen in the Project Parent program made significant phonological progress during the intervention period. This degree of change was greater than the maturational change made by the group who did not receive intervention. Although the two groups did differ somewhat in the extent of the children's phonological delay, Broen and Westman's results support the efficacy of parent training. Further, their study compared the outcomes of parent treatment with no treatment. They did not compare treatment that included parent involvement with treatment that did not. Consequently, it is difficult to determine the role that parent involvement per se played in the progress made by the children.

Dodd, McCormack, and Woodyatt (1994) described a program for parents of preschoolers with Down syndrome. The parents attended twelve three-hour sessions led by speech-language pathologists. Half of each session consisted of training on a specific topic: (*a*) listening skills, identification of errors in child speech; (*b*) how to elicit acceptable productions of target functional words; (*c*) how to provide specific feedback about production; and (*d*) how to selectively reinforce acceptable productions. The other half of each session included small-group discussions or sessions with a psychologist about relevant issues such as educational services, behavior management, and family dynamics. Dodd et al. reported that the parents' skill in using the facilitative techniques was correlated with the degree of improvement in their children's phonological abilities.

These studies indicate that there are some benefits associated with training for parents whose children have phonological disorders. Given the vast amount of literature that supports the involvement of families in any intervention program, clinicians should strongly consider involving parents in the treatment program. The final section of this chapter includes some specific ways in which parents might be trained to facilitate the acquisition of phonological skills by their children.

## Clarifying Attitudes, Beliefs, and Ideas and Changing Behaviors

As the clinician works with family members to clarify attitudes and change behaviors, it is important to keep in mind that change rarely happens if an individual does not recognize the need for it. Consequently, successfully providing information for parents of children with phonological disorders serves as a necessary foundation for effecting change.

INFLUENCE OF PARENTAL MODELS

There is little published research regarding the effects of parental input on phonological development. Perhaps this is due in part to the emphasis on the child's innate abilities to acquire a linguistic system, even when confronted with input that is far from consistent and precise. That is, children appear to be able to develop a reasonable phonological system despite the limitations of the input provided, so study of the input may not be particularly significant. Bernstein-Ratner (1987; 1993; in press) has challenged this idea, arguing that it is the nature of the input that determines whether specific innate skills will be useful in language acquisition. For example, infants show adultlike categorical perception and discrimination of voice onset time (VOT) differences. Although the display of such skills at such an early point in life may be somewhat amazing, the importance of this ability for categorization of stops (plosives) in conversation depends on how consistent the VOT differences are between stop categories. Malsheen's (1980) data indicate that over half of the initial stops produced in conversation are ambiguous in their VOT characteristics. Apparently, adults rely on other cues (i.e., lexical, syntactic, grammatical) to identify stops in conversation. One may conclude that VOT discrimination is not so important in sorting and establishing stop phonemic categories. Bernstein-Ratner (1984a) reports, however, that the degree of overlap drops to approximately 10% when adults address young children who are at the one- or two-word utterance stage. Consequently, the infant's perceptual skill with VOT has an opportunity to be of some value to the language learner. The treatment of VOT in child-directed speech is an example of how modifications in parental input can facilitate the development of an appropriate phonological system. Bernstein-Ratner reported that child-directed speech (CDS) is often more precise than adult-directed speech. For example, mothers were reported to use optional rules, such as dental deletion, deletion of voiced dental fricative, and conversion of /ts/ to [s], less frequently in the speech directed to children than in speech directed to adults (Bernstein-Ratner, 1984a). Vowel production was also more consistent in mothers' CDS, with less overlap among vowel categories (Bernstein-Ratner, 1984b). These increases in precision and decreases in variability are thought to occur during the stages in which such modifications would be most useful, such as the one- and two-word utterance stage.

Bernstein-Ratner (in press) cautions that even though it may be reasonable to associate more precisely articulated parental speech with a more rapid pace of child language acquisition, there are no conclusive date to support such a relationship. There is some support for the notion that overarticulation by the parent does have an effect on the developing child's phonological system. Bernstein-Ratner describes her daughter's use of an epenthetic vowel with final nasals. The child had previously deleted most final consonants. When the tapes were re-analyzed, it was apparent that the mother had begun to exaggerate final consonant articulation. This pattern included full release of the nasals, which was acoustically similar to vowel epenthesis. Bernstein-Ratner offered similar instances of parental influence, such as the use of vowel length changes to mark the presence of final consonants, final consonant replication, and epenthesis within consonant clusters. All of these patterns, which characterized young children's utterances, were also seen in the speech of their mothers. Bernstein-Ratner emphasized the paucity of information on parental articulatory style and the effects it may have on a child's phonological development.

Plunkett (1993) describes two Danish children's language development between ages one and two. Plunkett focuses on the segmentation problem experienced by language learners; that is, the child must learn how to segment the running stream of speech input into individual lexical items. The two children used different segmentation strategies. Although the developmental rate for both children was within normal limits, one child was somewhat more precocious. That child's mother was found to use exaggerated prosodic contours and repeat her child's linguistic units more often than did the mother of the other child, who tended to use a higher proportion of articulatorily imprecise expressions. Although there are certainly other factors that may influence the strategies children adopt in acquiring their language systems, Plunkett's findings suggest that environmental factors do play a role in rate and quality of development.

There is a need for additional studies regarding the effects of parental input on phonological development. The evidence so far seems to indicate two principles that might be communicated to parents of children with phonological disorders. First, parents should avoid underarticulation or the use of simplification processes in speech to their children. The old adage, "Don't talk 'baby talk' to your children" seems to indeed have some truth value. Second, parents should avoid overarticulation because the resulting prosodic and articulatory patterns may not be optimal models. Characteristics associated with child-directed speech, such as use of short utterances that are articulated with clarity and frequent repetitions and expansions of the child's utterances, may have positive effects on phonology just as they do on other aspects of language acquisition.

**Case Example.** Melissa was an 11-year-old student diagnosed as having a mild language disorder. She was enrolled in treatment at her local school to target grammatical errors and figurative language. The clinician had just been assigned to this school, so when she met Melissa for the first time, she noticed that Melissa used an inappropriate prosodic pattern. Her pitch was too high and she used exaggerated inflectional patterns, resulting in a sing-song quality. The clinician thought that if a listener heard Melissa speak but did not see her, the listener would likely think that she was a preschool child. As the clinician visited with Melissa, she revealed that she often felt "ignored" and "left out" by the other students. Classroom and playground observation confirmed that Melissa was often not included in group activities. The clinician noticed that Melissa did make some attempts to interact with her classmates; however, they typically responded minimally and then did not continue the conversation. Melissa appeared frustrated and concerned about her lack of friends. The clinician suggested to Melissa that they work on having her sound more like her friends. Treatment subsequently included role-played activities in which Melissa's prosodic patterns were contrasted with patterns that were more age-appropriate. Melissa's current prosodic patterns were eventually labeled, "high voice" and the target patterns were labeled, "low voice."

After a month of intervention, the clinician scheduled a conference to talk with Melissa and her mother, Cindy. Melissa had begun to show some progress during intervention sessions, but the clinician had not observed any significant gains outside of the treatment room. Cindy arrived early and the clinician indicated that they would be discussing the areas that Melissa had been working on as well as some new goals being addressed in treatment. Cindy indicated that she was very interested in doing anything that would help Melissa. Melissa was Cindy's only child and they lived alone. When Melissa arrived for the conference, the clinician was surprised to hear the way that Cindy communicated with Melissa. When speaking to Melissa,

Cindy's pitch and degree of inflection increased and her communication patterns were consistent with the characteristics of child-directed speech often used by mothers of toddlers. Cindy referred to Melissa with terms such as "Baby" and "Sweetie." The clinician used open-ended questions to gather information about Cindy's perceptions of her daughter. The clinician's hypotheses were confirmed as Cindy described her treatment of Melissa at home. It was fairly clear that Melissa was given limited responsibilities and Cindy's expectations of Melissa were more consistent with those appropriate for a younger child. For example, Cindy indicated that she selected Melissa's clothes each day. After some discussion, the clinician described the kinds of activities that she and Melissa had been using in treatment to target Melissa's prosodic patterns. Cindy was a little surprised and indicated that she had not really been aware of the manner in which she was speaking to Melissa. The clinician then asked Melissa to share her thoughts regarding her use of the new "low voice." Melissa remarked, "It makes me sound bigger, more like the other girls. Maybe they'll start noticing the difference, too." Cindy seemed to see the importance of changing the manner in which she interacted with her daughter and indicated that she and Melissa could use some of the same activities at home. In subsequent sessions, the clinician and Cindy were able to brainstorm about other ways to encourage Melissa to function at a more age-appropriate level.

VALUE OF INTERVENTION

The value of early language intervention has been established by several researchers (Feldman, Sparks, & Case, 1993; Fey & Cleave, 1990; Nye, Foster, & Seaman, 1987). We sometimes encounter parents who may not be convinced that intervention is necessary for their children with phonological disorders. This attitude may be due to family members or even professionals who have advised the parents to not worry because the child will grow out of it. Once the speech-language pathologist has determined that intervention is necessary because the problem is not developmental or because the child is showing significant concern about his or her speech patterns, some time should be spent discussing with parents how this conclusion was made. It seems logical that parents who are convinced that intervention is necessary are more supportive of the clinical process. This can mean increased attendance, as well as increased utilization of home-based activities.

**Case Example.**   Joy was two years old when seen for her original evaluation. During the parent interview, Joy's mother, Chris, indicated that she was not really concerned about Joy's speech. However, her sister thought she should bring Joy in for an evaluation, so she had done so just in case her sister was right. Chris indicated that the family physician had determined that her hearing was okay and said that children that young were not seen for speech therapy. The clinician found that Joy produced only four vowel sounds and the consonant /n/. Joy was, however, using some of the vowel sounds in a consistent manner to refer to a few specific referents. The clinician explained to Chris that although many children were only beginning to use words at age two years, they usually produced a variety of consonant and vowel sounds by that time. Chris remarked, "Joy is so young, though. Won't time just take care of this?" The clinician responded that there were no reliable predictors for determining which children would mature sufficiently without intervention and recommended that Joy be enrolled in treatment. Chris agreed and commented, "I guess I just didn't realize that children Joy's age could be helped by treatment."

**CONCLUSION**

This chapter has illustrated the use of Webster's (1981) principles for effective counseling in working with parents of children with phonological disorders. Several specific topics about which clinicians may want to gather information from parents or provide information for parents have been presented. Finally, topics such as the need for early intervention and the effects of parental input on phonology were discussed as potential areas that may require clarification or change in parental behavior. Additional information is provided in Appendix 9.1. Outline for Six-Session Counseling Program. This is a program that could be used with parents of children with phonological disorders. These six outlines are meant to serve as guides for the way in which a clinician might organize a similar program. Clinicians can modify any of the information that does not fall within their theoretic framework of phonological disorders and their approaches to assessment and intervention. A series of pre- and postcounseling questions are also provided so that the clinician can tailor some of the topics to individual parent needs and evaluate the effectiveness of the program.

## REFERENCES

Bernstein-Ratner, N. (1987). The phonology of parent-child speech. In K. Nelson & A. van Kleeck (Eds.), *Children's language* (Vol. 6). Hillsdale, NJ: Lawrence Erlbaum Associates, 159–174.

Bernstein-Ratner, N. (in press). From signal to syntax: But what is the nature of the signal? In J. Morgan & K. Demuth (Eds), *From signal to syntax*. Hillsdale, NJ: Lawrence Erlbaum Associates.

Bernstein-Ratner, N. (1993). Interactive influences in phonological behaviour: A case study. *Journal of Child Language, 20,* 191–197.

Bernstein-Ratner, N. (1984a). Patterns of vowel modification in mother-child speech. *Journal of Child Language, 11,* 557–578.

Bernstein-Ratner, N. (1984b). Phonological rule usage in mother-child speech. *Journal of Phonetics, 12,* 245–254.

Bernthal, J., & Bankston, N. (1993). *Articulation and phonological disorders* (3rd ed.). Englewood Cliffs, NJ: Prentice-Hall.

Bishop, D. (1985). Spelling ability in congenital dysarthria: Evidence against articulatory coding in translating between phonemes and graphemes. *Cognitive Neuropsychology, 2,* 229–251.

Broen, M. A., & Westman, M. J. (1990). Project Parent: A preschool speech program implemented through parents. *Journal of Speech and Hearing Disorders, 55,* 495–502.

Carrier, J. K. (1970). A program of articulation therapy administered by mothers. *Journal of Speech and Hearing Disorders, 35,* 344–353.

Catts, H. (1989). Speech production deficits in developmental dyslexia. *Journal of Speech and Hearing Disorders, 54,* 422–428.

Clarke-Klein, S. M. (1994). Expressive phonological deficiencies: Impact on spelling development. *Topics in Language Disorders, 14,* 40–55.

Crago, M. & Gopnik, M. (1994). From families to phenotypes: Theoretical and clinical implications of research into the genetic basis of specific language impairment. In R. Watkins & M. Rice (Eds.), *Specific language impairments in children*. Baltimore: Paul H. Brookes, 35–52.

Dodd, B., McCormack, P., & Woodyatt, G. (1994). Evaluation of an intervention program: Relation between children's phonology and parents' communicative behavior. *American Journal of Mental Retardation, 98,* 632–645.

Dudzinski, D. & Peters, D. L. (1977). Home-based programs: A growing alternative. *Child Care Quarterly, 6,* 61–71.

Eilers, R. E., Oller, D. K., Levine, S., Basinger, D., Lynch, M. P., & Urbano, R. (1993). The role of prematurity and socioeconomic status in the onset of canonical babbling in infants. *Infant Behavior and Development, 16,* 297–315.

Eiserman, W. D., McCoun, M., & Escobar, C. M. (1990). A cost-effectiveness analysis of two alternative program models for serving speech-disordered preschoolers. *Journal of Early Intervention, 14,* 297–317.

Eiserman, W. D., Weber, C., & McCoun, M. (1992). Two alternative approaches for serving speech disordered preschoolers: A second year follow-up. *Journal of Communication Disorders, 25,* 77–106.

Feldman, M., Sparks, B., & Case, L. (1993). Effectiveness of home-based early intervention on the language of mothers with mental retardation. *Research in Developmental Disabilities,* 387–408.

Fey, M. & Cleave, P. (1990). Early language intervention. *Seminars in Speech and Language, 11,* 165–181.

Lewis, B. & Freebairn, L. (1992). Residual effects of preschool phonology disorder in grade school, adolescence, and adulthood. *Journal of Speech and Hearing Disorders, 35,* 819–831.

Lewis, B. A., Ekelman, B. L., & Aram D. M. (1989). A familial study of severe phonological disorders. *Journal of Speech and Hearing Research, 32,* 713–724.

Malsheen, B. (1980). Two hypotheses for phonetic clarification in the speech of mothers to children. In G. Yeni-Komshian, J. Kavanagh, & C. Ferguson (Eds.). *Child phonology* (Vol. 2). New York: Academic Press.

Nye, C., Foster, S., & Seaman, D. (1987). Effectiveness of language intervention with the language/learning disabled. *Journal of Speech and Hearing Research, 52,* 348–357.

Oller, D. K., Eilers, R. E., Basinger, D., Steffens, M. L., & Urbano, R. (1995). Extreme poverty and the development of precursors to the speech capacity. *First Language, 15,* 167–188.

Oller, D. K., Eilers, R. E., Steffens, M. L., Lynch, M. P., & Urbano, R. (1994). Speech-like vocalizations in infancy: An evaluation of potential risk factors. *Journal of Child Language, 21,* 33–58.

Paden, E. P., Matthies, M. L., & Novak, M. A. (1989). Recovery from OME related phonologic delay following tube placement. *Journal of Speech and Hearing Disorders, 54,* 94–100.

Paden, E. P., Novak, M. A., & Beiter, A. L. (1987). Predictors of phonologic inadequacy in young children prone to otitis media. *Journal of Speech and Hearing Disorders, 52,* 232–242.

Plunkett, K. (1993). Lexical segmentation and vocabulary growth in early language acquisition. *Journal of Child Language, 20,* 43–60.

Robinson, P., Beresford, R., & Dodd, B. (1982). Spelling errors made by phonologically disordered children. *Spelling Progress Bulletin, 22,* 19–20.

Roberts, J. A., Burchinal, M. R., Kock, M. A., Footo, M. M., & Henderson, F. W. (1989). Otitis media in early development and its relationship to later phonological development. *Journal of Speech and Hearing Disorders, 53,* 416–424.

Shriberg, L. (1993). Four new speech and prosody-voice measures for genetics research and other studies in developmental phonological disorders. *Journal of Speech and Hearing Research, 36,* 105–140.

Shriberg, L. & Smith, A. (1983). Phonological correlates of middle-ear involvement in speech-delayed children: A methodological note. *Journal of Speech and Hearing Research, 26,* 293–297.

Sommers, R. K. (1962). Factors in the effectiveness of mothers trained to aid in speech correction. *Journal of Speech and Hearing Disorders, 27,* 178–186.

Sommers, R. K., Furlong, A. K., Rhodes F. E., Fichter, G. R., Copetas, F. G., & Saunders, Z. G. (1964). Effects of maternal attitude upon improvement in articulation when mothers are trained to assist in speech correction. *Journal of Speech and Hearing Disorders, 29,* 126–132.

Sommers, R. K., Shilling, C. D., Paul, C. D., Copetas, F. G., Bowser, D. C., & McClintock, C. J. (1959). Training parents of children with functional misarticulation. *Journal of Speech and Hearing Research, 2,* 258–265.

Stackhouse, J. (1982). An investigation of reading and spelling performance in speech disordered childrenn. *British Journal of Disorders of Communication, 17,* 53–60.

Stewart, J. (1978). *Counseling parents of exceptional children.* Columbus, OH: Charles E. Merrill.

Tomblin, B. (1989). Familial aggregation in specific language impairment. *Journal of Speech and Hearing Disorders, 54,* 167–173.

Webster, E. (1981). *Counseling with parents of handicapped children.* San Diego: College-Hill Press.

Webster, P. & Plante, A. (1992). Effects of phonological impairment on word, syllable, and phoneme segmentation and reading. *Language, Speech, and Hearing Services in Schools, 23,* 176–182.

# Appendix 9.1.   Outline of Six-Session Counseling Program

### Session I: Introduction

1. The counselor opens the session with an overview of parents' views on intervention obtained from the parent questionnaire.
2. The importance of intervention is discussed and clarifications made in regard to the parental views.
3. Discussion of PL 94-142 and PL 99-457
   - Handouts are given of PL 94-142 and PL 99-457
   - The rights of the child and parent are discussed
4. Discussion of Public School Criteria in regard to School Speech services
   - Criteria handout is given
5. The role of the SLP under ASHA guidelines is discussed
   - Guidelines handout is given
   - Intervention time frame is discussed
6. Question and Answer period
7. Lead into next week's session
   - Types of Phonological Errors and Intervention

## Session II: Overview of Phonological Disorders and Approaches to Intervention

1. The counselor defines the term "phonological disorder" as a broad-based term that applies to a system in which any non-developmental errors in speech sound production occur.
   - These errors can be caused by two basic types of problems: motoric and conceptual
2. Motoric errors are characterized by a child being unable to readily articulate, or produce, a target sound or sound class.
   - Examples are given of motoric errors
   - Questions are answered and discussed
3. Conceptual errors are characterized by inappropriate sorting, organization, or categorization in the phonological system. These errors occur even though the child is able to articulate the target sound class.
   - Examples of conceptual errors are given
   - Questions are answered and discussed
4. The assessment process will be described.
   - Discussion of the procedures, including single word inventories, conversational sample, stimulability tasks, receptive measures, hearing screening, and speech mechanism evaluation
   - Description of deriving phonetic inventories and determining operation of simplification processes and other substitutions
   - Use of the results to form hypothesis about nature of each error pattern
5. Review information and group discussion.
6. Lead into next session: The Cause: Separating Fact vs. Fiction

## Session III: Causes of Phonological Disorders: Separating Facts from Fiction

1. The counselor opens the session with a discussion of the parental views regarding the cause of their child's phonological problems stated in the questionnaire. What did they blame?
2. Clarification: Separating fact from fiction.
   - The relationship between otitis media and phonological problems
   - The sex of the child does not cause the phonological problems
   - Socioeconomic status has not been proven to be the cause
   - A certain personality or emotional behavior has not been shown to cause phonological problems
   - Familial link to phonological problems
3. Question and answer period
4. Lead into next session: Phonological Disorders and Academic Performance

## Session IV: Phonological Disorders and Academic Performance

1. The counselor discusses possible links between phonological disorders and later academic problems.
   - Discussion of the children's academic problems noted on the parent questionnaire
   - Discussion of studies addressing relationships between phonological disorders and academic skills

2. Discussion of ways to facilitate literacy skills
   - Reading to your child (provide a list of recommended children's books)
   - Examples of games to elicit literacy skills focusing on metalinguistics and phoneme recognition
   - Interactive journal writing
   - Taking turns reading chapters in books
3. Question and answer period
4. Lead into next session: Responding to Your Child

## Section V: Responding to your Child

1. The counselor discusses the parents' views and attitudes regarding responding to the child. This discussion begins with information that was provided on the pre-test.
2. Clarification of how you should respond to your child
   - Responding to specific portion of an utterance that was understood
   - Teaching parents how to request clarification from their child
   - How parents can teach others (siblings, teachers, and so forth) to respond to their child
   - How to reinforce your child
3. Discussion of fine-tuning phonological input
   - Highlighting targeted sounds as they appear in conversation
4. Discussion of how to encourage the child to recognize and respond to signs that suggest his/her message was not understood (e.g., blank looks in listener, replies that do not make sense)
5. Question and answer period
6. Lead into next session: Parental Role in Treatment

## Session VI. Parental Role in Treatment

1. Overview of information regarding the studies showing parental role in treatment to be beneficial.
2. Tips on how to be involved in treatment
   - Ask the clinician questions
   - Observe treatment sessions
   - Request activities to do at home to reinforce the concepts the clinician is targeting in treatment
   - Make sure information given to the clinician is up to date
   - Be an active participant with the teacher and clinician to ensure the academic success of your child
3. The counselor provides an overview of treatment tasks parents can do at home
   - Those dealing with motor errors (placement cues)
   - Those dealing with conceptual errors
   - Give illustrations of tasks
4. The counselor discusses when parents should get involved in treatment activities at home.
5. Discuss some practical activities parents can do to help (based on Stewart, 1978)
   - Admit there is a problem
   - Accept your child as he or she is
   - Praise your child
   - Be there when he or she needs you
   - Learn to have patience

- Don't deprive your child of appropriate discipline
- Be honest with your child
- Take a positive approach
- Support those who are trying to help your child
- Don't give up

6. Final remarks

## Pre-Counseling Questions

1. How do you view the clinician's role in intervention?
2. How do you view your role in intervention?
3. What is a phonological disorder?
4. How did you feel when you discovered your child had a speech problem? What did you think was the cause of the problem?
5. What do you think could cause a phonological disorder?
6. Do phonological disorders relate to academic performance? If so, explain.
7. How would you react if you weren't able to understand your child?
8. Does your child appear to be aware when he or she is not being understood? If so, how do you think your child feels about that?
9. How do others (siblings, teachers, children) react to your child's speech problem?
10. Are there ways you can be involved in your child's treatment?
11. What would you like to learn the most about from these sessions?

## Post-Counseling Questions

1. How do you view the clinician's role in intervention?
2. How do you view your role in intervention?
3. What is a phonological disorder?
4. What do you believe to be the cause of your child's speech problem?
5. What do you think could cause a phonological disorder?
6. Do phonological disorders relate to academic performance? If so, explain.
7. How would you react if you weren't able to understand your child?
8. Are there ways you can be involved in your child's treatment?
9. Do you feel the sessions caused changes in your beliefs and responses? If so, please discuss.
10. Was there a subject or information you would have liked to know more about?
11. Do you feel that the information was presented in an organized manner?
12. Did you feel that the counselor was knowledgeable and related to you as a parent?

# 10. Child Language-Learning Disorders

Kenn Apel and Julie J. Masterson

---

**Implementation of the Four Functions of Counseling: Special Considerations for Parents of Children with Language-Learning Disorders**
- *Receiving Information*
- *Giving Information*
- *Clarifying Attitudes, Beliefs, and Ideas and Helping to Change Behaviors*

**Implementation of the Four Functions of Counseling: Special Considerations for School-age Children with Language-Learning Disorders**
- *Receiving Information*
- *Giving Information*
- *Clarifying Attitudes, Beliefs, and Ideas and Helping to Change Behaviors*
Conclusion
Epilogue

---

Barbara is the mother of Adam, a five-year-old boy with a language-learning disorder. She also is a member of a counseling group for parents of children with language disorders. In past sessions, she has been a great support to many of the other parents, relating her experiences dealing with her child's disorder and the professionals with whom she has come in contact. She has even related how she has worked through her feelings of anger, helplessness, and guilt to get to a point where she can be an active participant in the treatment process. On this particular day, however, she comes to the meeting, and announces that she has been told Adam needs glasses. She bursts into tears, stating that she does not know how she can possibly get him to the ophthalmologist in addition to all the other errands and appointments she has to keep.

This scenario, although unique to Barbara, is not unique in the types of feelings and thoughts that are expressed by parents of children with language disorders. Clinicians often find themselves faced with similar situations in their daily interactions with parents of children with language disorders and, when working with older children, the child as well. It is for this reason that clinicians also must function as counselors. Whether in an initial interview, during a speech and language evaluation, within a treatment session, or in a special counseling group, clinicians find the need to use their counseling skills on almost a daily basis.

Counseling, in its broadest sense, is an endeavor between two or more people (Webster, 1981). As counselors, clinicians must be prepared to give and receive information, and help others clarify thoughts and feelings and change their behaviors (Webster, 1981). These functions were described in Chapter 9. Although these functions are used in all clinical situations with all clinical populations, there are some situations and issues that are unique to children with language disorders and their parents. In this chapter, each of these counseling functions is discussed in relation to the concerns specific to language-learning disorders, both in the preschool and school-age populations. Note that we have combined the discussion of two of the functions under the heading, *Clarifying Attitudes, Beliefs and Ideas and Helping to Change Behaviors*.

## IMPLEMENTATION OF THE FOUR FUNCTIONS OF COUNSELING: SPECIAL CONSIDERATIONS FOR PARENTS OF CHILDREN WITH LANGUAGE-LEARNING DISORDERS

### Receiving Information

DEVELOPMENTAL INFORMATION

As most clinicians know, it is important to obtain accurate information concerning the developmental history of a child being seen for a speech and language evaluation. With a thorough knowledge of developmental history, hypotheses for possible causes can be formed (Owens, 1995). There is an art to requesting information regarding development. Clinicians should be aware that some questions may cause parents to feel they do not know enough about their child's history. Most parents diligently record information about their child's development during the first several months, but day-to-day duties often prevent the continued attention to developmental details. Consequently, parents often must rely on memory when questioned about development. Unfortunately, those memories are not always readily retrievable. It is possible, then, that some parents may feel guilty or embarrassed when unable to remember certain milestones. Clinicians need to balance their desire for details with a sensitivity of parents' feelings of being unaware.

As clinicians gather developmental information, they may think it necessary to confirm or question information provided by a parent on the case history form or during a personal interview. However, confirmation for confirmation's sake may cause parents to feel the clinician does not trust the information given or, even worse, that the clinician has not listened carefully to the parents' responses. Therefore, information about mundane or unremarkable events should not be questioned. At the same time, the clinician needs to be certain that understanding of the information given matches the intent of the reporting parent. The use of *clarifying questions* or statements is crucial to ensuring this match. The manner in which questions are asked can determine the success or failure of an interview. Clinicians should use general or leading statements (Webster, 1981) followed by specific questions. As they receive information, clinicians should ask themselves," Do I have the same understanding of the information as the parent?" This question often leads to the use of clarifying statements or questions such as, "I want to make sure I understand this. Did you mean by 'late' that Johnny was learning to say words later than you thought he should?" or, "I think I know what you mean, but could you give me an example?"

As they clarify, clinicians need to be cautious about asking multiple-part questions (e.g., "Do you think Johnny was late in development or okay? You know, do you think he talked like other children, or do you think that he was just a little behind, or maybe where he should have been, in your opinion?"). Run-on questions only confuse parents and reduce the possibility of getting the information desired (Webster, 1981). Extended questions usually arise when clinicians feel they have not asked a question clearly or assume that parents did not comprehend the first question. Because this lack of parent comprehension is just an assumption and may not be true, it is important for the clinician to wait and determine whether the first question was clear before proceeding. If a question was clear, the parent will provide an answer. If a question was not clear, as evidenced by a parent's off-topic response or request for clarification, the clinician then can rephrase the information.

Providing opportunities for silence when receiving information from parents can be helpful to all of the people involved (Webster, 1981). Parents are able to collect their thoughts and perhaps think of other examples of their child's behaviors to report. Likewise, clinicians can think about how to phrase a question or determine which information needs to be requested next. For example, we often use statements such as, "Let me think about how I want to ask this next question," or, "I want to follow up on what you just said, but I need to take a few seconds to decide how to ask it." There is no shame in pausing to decide how to phrase a question. Many parents appreciate both the honesty of the statement and the model of taking some personal thinking time as well.

In addition to providing silence, clinicians should give evidence of active listening. *Active listening* involves developing hunches, or hypotheses, about what parents are feeling or thinking about a current topic and then stating those hunches (Webster, 1981). For example, as a mother reports on the success of integrating her child into a regular education kindergarten class, the clinician might acknowledge this information as well as the probable joy the mother is feeling. Such an acknowledgment might sound like the following: "Okay, Johnny is now in the kindergarten at his home school. Wow! That must be so great for you! It sounds like you are very proud of him." When parents feel that a clinician is interested in their thoughts and feelings, rather than only the factual information, tense situations seem to become much less so and cooperative bonds begin to form.

Parents often do not know what to expect during a meeting with a clinician. This may cause apprehension. Most parents have no idea what will be asked nor what is involved when they initially interact with a speech-language pathologist. A formal meeting with a professional can sometimes cause anxiety even for parents whose children have received services in the past. The clinician's role is to ease that anxiousness by telling the parent what to expect during the interview. Webster (1981) talks about providing parents with a contract that describes the format for the meeting. A *contract* typically states the information to be covered in the interview, the participants who will be involved, the parents' role (e.g., only providing information or both providing and requesting information), and the expected length of time for the interview. Also, the clinician should state the topics to be covered in the interview and then announce those as subheadings as the interview proceeds. This technique orients parents to the clinician's plan. For example, a typical contract might sound like the following:

> Ms. Zeine, we have the next 20 minutes to cover some additional information about Joey's developmental history. I have some questions or clarifications about the history form you completed. I'd like to ask a few questions, but feel free to jump in with your own questions as we proceed. I plan to ask about his developmental, medical, and educational history. I'd like to start with some questions about his speech and language development.

Once certain information is obtained, the clinician can state that a new topic will be addressed and proceed with questions dealing with that topic (e.g., "Now, I'd like to shift to his medical history. Did Joey ever have any ear infections?"). With this kind of procedure, the parent is aware of the clinician's plan and where within that plan they are currently operating.

Finally, clinicians should not overlook the fact that children are often in the care of other adults for considerable amounts of time during the day. Children may spend large portions of the day with day-care workers or grandparents. If the child is in another adult's care, it is helpful to observe and or get information from these individuals as well (Owens, 1995).

FAMILY HISTORY

Whether in the case history form or during the interview, it is important to gather information about immediate family members. Specifically, clinicians should be interested in determining whether siblings, parents, and extended family members (e.g., uncles, aunts, cousins, grandparents) had some identified learning disorder. However, obtaining this information and understanding its significance, can be challenging. The terminology currently used in the field today differs from that used 10 to 20 years ago. For example, what might have been called a speech problem 20 years ago could be either a phonological disorder or dysfluency in today's terminology. Similarly, dyslexia, which often is reported when parents are asked whether any remarkable learning problems have occurred in the family, is a term with multiple connotations (Kamhi & Catts, 1989). Usually, no matter what the exact behaviors were that led to a family member's diagnosis, the common underlying symptom was a lack of success in learning to communicate or in academic performance (most often reading and spelling). Although such reports alone do not give a clinician the answer to the etiology puzzle, they provide some evidence that the child's disorder may be linked to others within the family (Tomblin, 1989; 1991).

## CURRENT COMMUNICATION SKILLS OF THE CHILD

Although parents can be quite reliable in providing information about their child's language skills, the terms used to label the behaviors can be interpreted in different ways. For example, some children produce what appear to be two- or three-word utterances that, for the child, function as single units (e.g., whadat? ) (Peters, 1977). If parents consider such productions to be more than a single unit, the result might be a misunderstanding of linguistic capabilities. Similarly, parents may be attributing meaning to nonlinguistic productions. For example, babbles consisting of reduplicated syllables of *ma* or *da* may be interpreted as true productions of *mama* or *daddy*. Consequently, the information provided by parents needs to be balanced with the observations made by the clinician. Unfortunately, children will not always produce language, given a strange setting (clinical room) and an unknown adult (clinician). One strategy that can be used to supplement parental reports of the child's current level of language use is to have parents tape record their child at home. The expectation is that the child will produce language as he or she customarily does. The outcome of these tapings can be informative in two different ways: (*a*) If the child is producing language at or above the level reported by the parents, then the clinician has confirming evidence on which to base the diagnosis and, if appropriate, treatment goals. (*b*) If the child's language skills are below the level reported by the parents, it may open some dialogue between the parents and clinician regarding the exact level of the child's language abilities. That is, the discussion may lead to clarification of parents' thoughts or understanding of their child's capabilities and, possibly, a change in their style of interaction.

## STRATEGIES ATTEMPTED TO ENCOURAGE COMMUNICATION

As children begin to develop speech and language, parents modify their language input in a way that is thought to facilitate learning (James, 1990). However, when a child does not meet parents' expectations for speech or language development, some parents reduce or alter their input to their children (Girolametto & Tannock, 1994; Millet & Newhoff, 1978; Schodorf & Edwards, 1983 ). At times, in their attempts to help their children, parents' language input may become less conducive to language learning for the child with language disorders. This may be most apparent when they and their children are observed in a diagnostic setting. Often, it seems parents hope to show off their children for the clinician and the conversation between parent and child becomes a question and answer format. The following dialogue is not unusual of parent-child interactions occurring during a language evaluation:

Parent: "What's that?"
Child: "Cow."

Parent: "What does the cow say?"

Child: "Moo."

Parent: "What color is it?"

Child: "Brown"

This exchange, unfortunately, may not show the child's true linguistic capabilities, given the type of questioning used and the directiveness of the parent. In addition, parents may state their child is able to say all the colors, numbers, or alphabet and then commence to have the child demonstrate. Although these may be useful as children approach school-age, they alone hold little communicative strength. Similarly, parents may direct their children to imitate their language models. This type of imitation plays little to no role in the acquisition of language (Lahey, 1988). As a whole, these parental attempts to facilitate language learning need to take a back seat to strategies that facilitate more functional language skills. It is important, therefore, for the clinician to know how and when parents interact with their child. If needed, other ways of interacting that might be more conducive to developing language skills can be identified and shared.

Many parents naturally provide appropriate language models for their children, responding to their child with simple, contingent utterances that are expansions of the child's utterances. Clinicians should be prepared to praise parents whose style of interaction seems facilitative for language development. Parents need to hear that the strategies they are using to encourage language development are useful. By making them aware of these skills and the positive benefits of their use, parents may feel comfort in the fact that they are contributing to their child's learning of language.

**Case Example.**   Virginia was the mother of an 18-month-old girl, Audrey. She brought her daughter to the clinic after reading about common developmental milestones in a popular parent magazine. She was concerned that her daughter only spoke a few words. On the case history form, Virginia reported that Audrey produced some single word utterances but mostly sounds that "aren't like the words." During the interview, the clinician attempted to clarify Virginia's statement by asking the following question: "In order to best understand your concerns, I'd like you to provide some examples of what you mean when you say her sounds 'aren't like the words.'" Virginia obliged, by stating: "Well, when we play peekaboo, she says it wrong when it's her turn. She's not saying a word. It's not all the right sounds." The clinician then used a second clarifying question, asking whether it was the actual sounds that seemed to be in error. Virginia affirmed that, stating that Audrey said, "dee-doo for peekaboo" during the game. The clinician then observed Audrey and her brother playing. Although many of her speech sound productions were incorrect, most of her one-word utterances were intelligible in context. Asked whether this was the behavior Virginia questioned, she responded affirmatively. The clinician then clarified the information that had been presented in the parent magazine, stating that children at one and a half years of age often mispronounce words, yet the productions are still considered to be words. Virginia seemed relieved that she could consider these incorrect productions as words and stated that her fears had been eased.

## Giving Information

### POSSIBLE CAUSES OF LANGUAGE-LEARNING DISORDERS

Interest in the search for an explanation for the cause of language-learning disorders has risen and fallen over the past several years. A few years ago, there was an excellent forum in *Language, Speech and Hearing Services in Schools* (Kamhi, 1991) in which the cause of language-learning disorders was debated. In fact, the debate even addressed whether the question was worthwhile. Aram (1991) argued that clinicians cannot ignore the search for a cause of language-learning disorders, because otherwise they then risk becoming technicians. In addition, Aram pointed out that parents often are consumed with the search for the cause. To ignore the search for a cause then diminishes parents' need for an answer to the question regarding cause.

Why do parents search so avidly for a cause? It seems that for many parents the drive to find a cause develops out of feelings of guilt or anger (Webster, 1981). Many times, parents report directly or indirectly the feeling that they may have caused the disorder (Webster & Ward, 1993). Parents also sometimes feel anger about the disorder, questioning whether someone could have done something sooner to help prevent it. Unfortunately, it is often difficult to state why such a disorder occurred. Symptoms such as family history of learning problems and negative factors in the medical history (e.g., recurrent bouts of otitis media) may provide some idea of a possible cause. There is no guarantee, however, that these or other factors are true causative agents (Owens, 1995). Nevertheless, it is important for their sake to address parents' desire to know the cause. If parents begin to understand what might have caused the disorder or, at the very least, understand that there is no evidence to suggest they caused the disorder, they then may begin to move toward acknowledging the problem and helping the clinician in the remediation process (Webster, 1981).

## SCHOOL READINESS

"Will my child be ready for school?" is one of the most frequently asked questions clinicians face in working with parents of children with language-learning disorders. This is truly a loaded question. This question might be to determine whether the child is academically ready for school or it may be a request regarding the general intellectual capabilities of the child. When a diagnosis of language-learning disorder is given, parents may not distinguish this diagnostic label from other labels (e.g., mental retardation, autism, and developmentally delayed). This might cause quite a bit of confusion and anxiety for the parents. To such a question, the clinician might first respond with a clarifying question, such as, "I want to do my best to answer that question, but I need to clarify what you mean by it. Are you asking whether he has the skills that are required in a kindergarten class?" Or the clinician might say, "Are you asking whether he is smart enough to attend school?" Other professionals, such as psychologists or academic diagnosticians, may need to be consulted to provide the requested information adequately. Once the true meaning of the question is known, however, the clinician can try to answer the question truthfully and in a manner that reflects personal expertise and acknowledges that of other professionals (Webster, 1981).

## APPROACHES TO TREATMENT

As mentioned, parents generally have little to no understanding about the type of treatment provided by speech-language pathologists. Any knowledge of the profession is generally based on their experiences when they were in elementary school. Because the type of treatment of speech-language disorders and the range of targeted speech-language skills have increased dramatically over the last 10–15 years, parents' knowledge may be incorrect. Thus, it is important for parents to hear what the plan of treatment is for their child, especially as they may play an integral role in the treatment process. Providing goals in lay terms, utilizing examples, and providing a theory behind the approach for treatment not only educates parents, but it helps them become knowledgeable allies when they are asked to support the treatment through in- or out-of-session work. An illustrative example of this is a case in which a supervisor began to oversee a graduate student who was treating a preschool-age client. The client, who had been seen previously in a different clinic, had received a traditional behaviorist approach to treatment. Imitation had played a major role in treating the child. However, the supervisor and the graduate student were providing treatment that was communicatively based and emphasized the use of models with little, if any, direct imitation requested. The approach matched the supervisor's theories of language development and learning and, quite frankly, seemed perfectly logical. However, an important piece of the intervention plan—providing information to the parents regarding the approach and its rationale—was inadvertently omitted. Within two weeks, the supervisor found himself backpedaling to provide this information as the parents threatened to remove their child from the clinic. In their words, all they saw was play. Once the rationale about the treatment approach and its theoretical underpinnings were provided, the parents appeared to feel better about the approach and actually became quite involved as partners with the clinician in the remediation process.

## PARENTAL ROLE IN THE TREATMENT PROCESS

The role of the parent in the treatment process cannot be over emphasized (Crais, 1991). Parental involvement is essential, although its form may vary depending on the parent-child dyad and the situation (Conti-Ramsden, 1993). Experience has shown that most parents wish to be involved. Involvement can range from encouraging their child to complete homework assigned by the clinician, to being a partner within the treatment session, to being the major agent of change via a home program. Conti-Ramsden (1993) and Tannock and Girolametto (1992) provide reviews of several possible parent-clinician partnerships. No matter the type of partnership undertaken, the clinician must determine the appropriate level of parent involvement and then encourage the parents to take that role.

There are two points to be considered as the clinician asks for parent involvement. First, the clinician should be aware that parental involvement may not always be appropriate. At times, parents need to be asked to separate from their child for part of the treatment process because their presence encourages the child to remain silent. Second, some parents may not be ready to help with the treatment plan, owing to their feelings regarding the disorder itself (Webster, 1981). Parents sometimes need time to move through feelings of anger, resentment, helplessness, and the need for distancing to a point of acknowledging the disorder and their role in helping to remediate it. It is important that clinicians recognize this and through encouragement, active listening, and acknowledgment of positive steps (e.g., bringing the child to the session), help parents begin to understand what role they might want to undertake in their child's treatment. Through the clinician's recognition and support, parents may feel they can better cope with their child, the disorder, and the strategies and plans to remediate it.

## ROLE OF OTHERS IN THE TREATMENT SESSION

Whereas parents are usually the adults most involved in their child's treatment, other individuals may serve as partners in treatment as well. Siblings, grandparents, and day-care caregivers can be equally important in addressing the needs of the child. The clinician must understand that the child may be part of several social units, only one being the family (Stone, 1992; Webster, 1981). Thus, it may be appropriate to include caregivers or siblings in the counseling process so that a true understanding and appreciation of the methods and goals for change are clearly understood by those who interact with the child. By involving in treatment these other significant individuals in a child's life, the possibility of all the social units helping to remediate the child's disorder increases.

## LENGTH OF THE TREATMENT PROCESS

Along with wondering about the cause of the disorder and school readiness, parents often question the length of treatment time. Clinicians do not have a method of pinpointing the amount of treatment any given child might need and it would be unethical to promise a cure in a specified period of time. In discussing the potential length of treatment time with the parents, clinicians should be open and honest, remaining within the boundaries of their expertise, experience, and comfort. Although they can be given some guidelines regarding approximate length of treatment, parents respect the fact that the clinician avoids empty promises.

## LONG-TERM RAMIFICATIONS OF LANGUAGE-LEARNING DISORDERS

There are enough data at this point to suggest that preschool children with language disorders are, at the very least, at risk for language-learning disorders during the school years (Aram, Ekelman, & Nation, 1984; Bishop & Adams, 1990; Catts, 1993). The most common school-age language-learning disorders are in the areas of literacy: reading, writing, and spelling. Children with language-learning disorders are also at risk for difficulties in social interactions within and outside of the classroom (Nelson, 1993). There are no data at this point to suggest that all children with language disorders during the preschool years will experience literacy or social difficulties in the school years. Neither are there any data linking severity or type of language disorder with school-related difficulties. With this in mind, it is important for the clinician to inform parents about the possibility of later language-based, literacy disorders in the school years. Although it is important to relay this information to parents, the clinician may prefer to wait until the child has been in treatment for some time and the parents appear open to new information. At best, the clinician can only suggest that a child is at risk for literacy problems. It is hoped that increasing parental awareness of the at risk nature of language disorders, implementing preventative activities that focus on emergent literacy skills (e.g., rhyming, print awareness), and consistently monitoring literacy development, academic difficulties can be prevented or addressed earlier than they have been traditionally.

**Case Example.** Nick was a two-year-old boy referred for evaluation and treatment after an evaluation at a large, urban speech language hearing center. At the time, Nick had no expressive language. Results of the first evaluation included a diagnosis of developmental apraxia of speech (DAS), based on the fact that he did not use any identifiable words and produced a limited number of sounds. An alternative communication system (e.g., sign language) was recommended because oral language might prove to be fruitless. There was a history of learning problems for Nick's siblings. One brother was being seen for learning disabilities in the schools and another was receiving speech services for a phonological disorder. The new clinician diagnosed the problem as a language disorder. He explained the implications of the two diagnoses and recommendations for treatment goals and activities. The former diagnosis required implementing an alternative communication system, whereas the present diagnosis focused on developing a verbal first lexicon. In addition, the possible etiology of the disorder was discussed which, in this case, other than family history of speech-language problems, was not very concrete. Nick's mother was extremely concerned that he would stand out if she were to enroll him in a preschool program and wondered whether other children would mock him. She stated, "Well, you know, because he's different. Kids might pick up on that. They are mean to, well, those kind of kids." After acknowledging the mother's frustration of hearing other children mock a loved one, the clinician verbalized a hunch that the mother was really concerned about her son's intelligence. Tearfully, she confirmed that hunch. The clinician then brought out a report from the former evaluation in which a developmental psychologist had stated that cognitive skills appeared age-appropriate. After the clinician explained the psychologist's results again and provided examples, Nick's mother expressed relief. Re-addressing her concern about preschool, the clinician also suggested that she consult the preschool teacher and determine her experience in dealing with nonverbal children and what techniques she had used for effectively integrating these children with their peers.

Nick was subsequently enrolled in treatment with the clinician. Nick's parents were told the purpose of the treatment and the initial goals. In addition, his mother was encouraged to watch and, after several sessions, to interact with him and the clinician as treatment was provided.

After Nick had been enrolled in treatment and had begun to make progress in acquiring language, Nick's mother was informed that there was a connection between early language disorders and later literacy difficulties. Because her eldest son was currently experiencing literacy problems, she was very interested in receiving information that might circumvent or lessen the possibility of reading and writing problems for Nick. Early emergent literacy activities (i.e., rhyming, book reading, and print awareness tasks) were integrated into Nick's treatment as he reached three years of age. His mother was present for these activities and she was encouraged to duplicate them at home. When Nick was dismissed at three and one-half years of age, she was again reminded of the at risk nature of his disorder and given further, more developmentally advanced emergent literacy activities to use at home. Further, she was advised to monitor his reading and writing skills as they began to develop in the early elementary school years.

## Clarifying Attitudes, Beliefs, and Ideas and Helping to Change Behaviors

### DISCUSSING EMOTIONS

Most parents do not expect nor are prepared to parent a child with a disorder, language or otherwise. The emotions that are expressed by parents of children with language-learning disorders, either directly or indirectly, include anger, guilt, despair, feelings of being overwhelmed, and confusion (Webster & Ward, 1993). By actively listening to parents (i.e., attempting to listen for the emotions that underlie their statements or questions), the clinician can help parents identify these feelings as well. Once these emotions are acknowledged, then a number of different avenues are open. Simply identifying and acknowledging frustrations and guilt can help parents feel supported and normal and allow them to focus on other issues and concerns. Likewise, if a clinician senses that parents are feeling anger toward professionals, their spouse, or even God, verbalizing this hunch may help parents clarify the issue or issues that have contributed to these feelings. Subsequently, both the clinician and the parents can start to address the issue(s) in a constructive manner.

It also should be recognized that parents express joy about their children. Joy is an emotion that often is not acknowledged by clinicians because it is not a negative or interfering emotion. Many parents find joy in their children's progress, no matter how slow or how minimal it might seem to professionals, friends, or family. It is important to share in that joy with parents, acknowledging the happiness they receive from their children. Parents need to know there is a professional who is interested and cares about hearing their emotions, whether positive or negative. The wise clinician realizes that it is through this ability to identify and clarify parents' emotions that parent-clinician bonds are strengthened, thus promising a better integrated team to treat the child with the language disorder.

### PARENT-CHILD INTERACTIONS

It has been some time since Nelson (1973) identified different styles of language acquisition used by children. Nelson reported on two different types of language-learning styles, expressive and referential. Among other differences, Nelson noted that expressive children tend to produce greater numbers of personal-social and function words (e.g., "Hi," "more," "all gone") and prefer socially oriented activities (e.g., "This Little Piggy"). Referential children, on the other hand, produce a greater number of nouns and prefer naming games.

Although not every child has a definite, well-defined style, it is helpful to identify whether one exists and how well matched the parents' style of interaction is to the child's. Some children appear to prefer one learning style, whereas the parents seem to be operating under the other style of learning. The mismatch is not the cause of the language-learning disorder; however, it may be a maintaining factor that needs to be changed. Clinicians can help parents recognize the mismatch and understand the benefits of changing their style of interaction in a number of ways. Discussions of the child's interaction style and viewings of videos emphasizing the traits that seem to suggest such a preference can be very helpful in highlighting a particular style. Additionally, by clarifying parents' ideas of what creates an adequate environment for language learning and actively listening to the frustrations they have about past attempts to interact with their child, the clinician may be able to increase their awareness of their child's preference for learning. Through this increased awareness, parents may be open to changing their interaction style to better match their child's apparent preference (Webster, 1981). The skillful clinician helps parents identify behaviors that do not seem to match their child's language acquisition style so that they understand that a change may be beneficial to their child.

## IMPORTANCE OF EARLY INTERVENTION

Clinicians often hear parents question whether treatment should be implemented during the preschool years or whether a wait-and-see attitude is more appropriate. Some parents verbalize this question directly. With other parents, clinicians may pick up on this feeling by actively listening to the parents' statements. For example, some parents may say, "Well, he seems so young. I wonder if it will be too difficult for him." Parents may use this statement to question whether treatment should begin early for their child. The clinician who discerns this message in parents' statements should attempt to help them clarify their thoughts and feelings on this issue. First, clinicians can clarify this statement by asking whether the parent is concerned about starting the child at a preschool age. If this parent concern is confirmed, the clinician might utilize data from recent research (Paul, 1991) that suggests that many slow-to-develop children continue to manifest language-learning problems in later years. In addition, a statement regarding success with other children's early treatment might be appropriate. Most experienced clinicians are aware that many children who do not undergo treatment fall farther and farther behind their peers in their ability to communicate.

**Case Example.**    Jill brought her two and one-half year-old son, Jesse, in for a speech and language evaluation. The clinician provided a number of different familiar toys (e.g., doll house with people, food and kitchen materials) and began interacting with Jesse as he played. Jesse appeared to prefer games that necessarily involved a social interaction between the two participants, suggesting an expressive style of language acquisition. Jesse was observed to produce two- and, infrequently, three-word utterances. The longer utterances were typically produced after the clinician repeated and expanded on his one- and two-word utterances. Jill then was observed interacting with her son in the same setting with the same toys. As Jesse began to play with the toys, Jill began to ask him to name objects, colors, and the number of items she held, suggesting a more referential style of interaction. During this parent-child interaction, most of Jesse's utterances were one-word utterances.

During the postevaluation conference, Jill and the clinician observed a video of the two play situations. Jill was asked whether she noticed any difference between the two settings. Jill reported that her son seemed to talk longer sentences when interacting with the clinician. The clinician noted that Jesse seemed to produce higher level language when his utterances were repeated and expanded. In addition, he stated that Jesse seemed to produce more language when engaged in games that called for social interactions. Jill acknowl-edged these points. However, she felt that her questions to Jesse allowed him to practice his colors and numbers. She expressed concerns that Jesse might not perform well in preschool if he did not know his colors and numbers. The clinician confirmed this feeling, stating, "We all want our children to do well in school. It's a scary thought to think our chil-dren might not know some facts that other children might know." He then stated that lan-guage skills, such as talking in complete utterances, were quite necessary for children in preschool as well because children use language to play and socialize. He asked whether Jill might consider trying the strategies of repeating and expanding on Jesse's utterances and engaging him in more interactive games in order to prepare him for the social aspects of preschool. Jill agreed to try these strategies, stating that she could work on the colors and numbers maybe later.

## IMPLEMENTATION OF THE FOUR FUNCTIONS OF COUNSELING: SPECIAL CONSIDERATIONS FOR SCHOOL-AGE CHILDREN WITH LANGUAGE-LEARNING DISORDERS

As mentioned, the basic principles of counseling apply in any clinical situation with any population. However, when dealing with school-age children, especially with students who are in the upper elementary grades, middle/junior high school, and high school, the situations that lead to the need for counseling can change. In addition, the individuals with whom counseling is conducted include other professionals (teachers, specialists) as well as the student. This, then, raises additional issues and concerns.

### Receiving Information

ACADEMIC HISTORY AND CURRENT ACADEMIC FUNCTIONING

Clinicians need to determine previous events in a student's life that were important for communication and education. In some cases, the student in question will not have been seen by a speech-language pathologist before reaching school. As parents are interviewed to determine whether any difficulties existed earlier in development, clinicians should be aware that the lack of an identified language disorder during the preschool years does not negate the possibility that one might have existed. Conversely, the lack of an identified preschool language disorder does not nullify the possibility that a student's academic dif-ficulties may be language related (Nelson, 1993). Once again, careful questioning and fo-cusing to understand the meaning of the responses given by parents and other profes-sionals will help the clinician best understand the factor or factors that may be causing academic difficulties. Terminology may be a hurdle to overcome when receiving informa-tion regarding students in this age range because some terms, such as *dyslexia*, have dif-ferent meanings to different individuals, and other terms, such as *metalinguistics*, are fa-miliar to only a small group of professionals. Thus, as the clinician receives information, he or she needs to clarify the use of terms that may have one connotation for parents and yet another for professionals.

For the school-age student, special attention should be devoted to performance in written language. If portfolios have been maintained of the student's work, then this set of documents should be surveyed for information. A portfolio, which is a compilation of a student's work gathered by the teacher and the student, can be a rich source when deter-mining possible language-learning disorders. Dialogue journals, which are ongoing writ-ten dialogues between students and teachers, also are wonderful sources of information (Silliman & Wilkinson, 1991). Both sources represent a student's work over time. Using material from either of these two sources may provide the clinician with insights into a student's written language skills. For example, a student's written report that demonstrates poor spelling may suggest poor phonological awareness skills or a lack of morphological knowledge. Written summaries of books or events may provide evidence of poor narrative skills. Most students will not have had their metalinguistic, narrative, and complex syntax skills assessed, and the clinician will want to determine whether deficits in these areas are adversely affecting the student's academic performance. One cautionary note is in order, however, for the use of portfolios. When examining a student's portfolio, the clinician should determine whether the work represents the student's own abilities or whether teacher help was given to the final product. Both types of data can be helpful, as long as the source of authorship is clear.

## INTERVIEWING THE STUDENT

The clinician needs to determine the current academic functioning of the student to best serve the student's needs. Many times, the student him- or herself can serve as an excellent information source. One of the many benefits of working with school-age children is that they are able to provide insights into their learning challenges and successes that may not be obtainable through other means. However, interviewing students, particularly those who are middle- or high-school age, can be a challenge. There are several strategies to keep in mind as one attempts to interview the school-age child.

First and foremost, the clinician needs to recognize the student as a partner in the process of receiving information (Larson & McKinley, 1985). The student should be informed of the purpose of the meeting, his or her role in the meeting, and the amount of time that is expected to be devoted to obtaining the information. The language that is used can be crucial in determining the effectiveness of the interview. For example, it is not uncommon for some adults to feel they need to get at the level of the student. In doing so, professionals try to use common idiomatic expressions that students use. This can be a mistake because these expressions are generation-specific. Typically, the use of these expressions by others outside the restricted age range is considered inappropriate or, at the very least, silly. Instead, an adult can enhance the effectiveness of an interview by showing respect for a student and using language that the adult normally uses, modifying or explaining terms as needed for understanding.

A second consideration for interviewing the school-age child is the time and location of the interview. Unfortunately, time is not always under the control of the clinician. There may be a small window of opportunity during which the clinician can gain access to the student for interviewing. Every effort should be made to interview the student at a time during which a favorite subject or peer program is not in conflict. Location, however, can be manipulated. Some students prefer to be taken out of the class for an interview, whereas others wish to be seen in a separate area of the classroom. Again, only by respecting the student and treating the student as a partner in the clinical process will such factors lead to successful receipt of information.

As with the techniques used with parents already mentioned, listening for meaning and trying to clarify statements that may be interpreted a number of ways will lead to a favorable interview. Even more so, addressing the feelings or attitudes students have as they describe their histories, successes, and failures in academia creates a more productive clinical interaction. This can be difficult because some school-age children distrust professionals. Others may feel less like cooperating owing to past experiences with professionals who have been one-sided and dogmatic. The clinician must balance respect for the student's feelings and style of interaction with the need to obtain information that will aid in determining an accurate plan of treatment.

**Case Example.** Georgetta was a twelfth grade student at a local high school. She was in a remedial reading class, non-discreetly disguised as a literature class. She and all the other students in the class knew why they were there, as did most of the senior class. Activities in the class focused on reading simplified versions of classics and completing formulaic worksheets that required students to interpret meanings of words, the authors use of phrases to relate underlying themes, and so forth. Georgetta was one of seven or eight students who had volunteered to receive additional help from a graduate clinician in speech-language pathology. Although this small group of students had been told they would meet regularly as a small group in the library, each was asked whether he or she would prefer to meet separately with the clinician initially to determine the skills each wanted to improve. Georgetta chose to meet separately.

The initial conference started with the graduate clinician informing what seemed to be a somewhat reluctant, belligerent young woman about the purpose of the meeting (i.e., to determine what tasks were difficult or easy for her to perform in the remedial class), her responsibilities during the meeting (i.e., to answer some questions and then voice some of her questions or concerns), and the amount of time to be spent on this endeavor (i.e., approximately 15 minutes). Georgetta's first few comments were less than helpful. When asked what was difficult for her to do in class, her only response was "everything." Similarly, when she was asked what was easy, she answered, "nothing." The clinician, who sensed that Georgetta was feeling that the new program was just another class for students who were not successful in school and would involve more work on paper, voiced this hunch. Georgetta confirmed that hunch, reporting that she was tired of having to do work that seemed to go nowhere and that was obviously busy work. The clinician then asked Georgetta what she might choose to have, should she be able to design a program to meet her needs. Her response included working on real-life paperwork, like job forms. She stated that she was worried that she was only eight months away from graduating and unable to read and write adequately, which might prevent her from getting a job once she was finished with high school. The clinician affirmed her feelings, stating that it must feel like time is running out quickly. Once Georgetta confirmed this feeling, the clinician began asking for more information that would help define the specifics of a program to meet Georgetta's needs and also aid her in other areas of her life (e.g., reading for pleasure and understanding an essay examination). As Georgetta began to see she could be a partner in the process of constructing the program and that her opinion was being heard and integrated into the developing program, her participation began to improve. Eventually her attitude became quite facilitative.

## Giving Information

RELATIONSHIP BETWEEN LANGUAGE SKILLS AND ACADEMICS

As mentioned, sufficient literature exists that supports the strong relationship between language skills and academics (Aram, Ekelman, & Nation, 1984; Bishop & Adams, 1990; Catts, 1993). All academic subjects rely on adequate receptive and expressive language skills (Wallach & Butler, 1994). Although most elementary, middle, and even high school curriculums involve courses or subjects labeled variously as "language" or "language arts," the use and understanding of language cannot be divorced from other subjects. Instead, language cuts across the entire curriculum (Wallach & Butler, 1994). Thus, any deficiency in language skills, at the very least, creates an at risk situation for academic difficulties or failure.

Unfortunately, this relationship between language and academics and the overwhelming impact of a language-learning disorder on academic performance do not always seem apparent to other professionals. It is not uncommon in the schools for children to be identified and receive individualized learning plans without any consultation with a speech-language pathologist. Thus, any possible underlying language-based cause or maintaining factor for reading and writing difficulties, such as poor metalinguistic skills or inefficient use of more complex syntactic structures, may very well be overlooked. Thus, it becomes the job of speech-language pathologists to inform others about what their role can and should be in identifying and planning services for children experiencing language-learning disorders.

## ROLE OF THE CLINICIAN

It may be necessary for clinicians to provide information to other professionals about the expertise and knowledge base each brings to the task of helping school-age children with language-learning disorders. When educating other professionals, the clinician must be aware of different options that can be used to relay the information, as well as the manner in which it is relayed. These two factors can make for a successful or less successful experience in giving information.

As clinicians know, they are not alone in feeling the pressure of time commitments within the work space. Other professionals are equally short of time, which, unfortunately, sometimes leads to shortness of patience as well. The creative clinician realizes that there are both verbal and written ways of communicating information about services and skills in identifying special needs of the school-age child. For example, clinicians can establish good working relationships with other professionals by attending general staff meetings, serving on site-based school councils, volunteering for school committees, and even chatting over lunch. By participating in this way, a relationship can be established so that there will be later opportunities in which the clinician can provide information about his or her expertise in language and learning. More directly, clinicians can offer thoughts and ideas during multidisciplinary team meetings that might not have been addressed. Workshops or in-services are other avenues for dissemination of information.

Written materials that can be used to inform colleagues of the clinician's skills and knowledge base include a staff newsletter or, as more and more schools and clinics become part of the information highway, through electronic mail. Some clinicians in the past have informed their colleagues, parents, and other members of the school community by providing fliers at Parent Teacher Association and faculty meetings that outline what they do, their expertise, and so forth. In each of these examples, the main purpose is to educate colleagues and others about the skills and knowledge the clinician can bring to the task of identifying and helping a child with language-learning disabilities. Marketing one's expertise remains essential because it still seems that many professionals assume the clinician is able to work only on speech sounds.

**Case Example.**   Genevieve is a speech-language pathologist in a local school district who serves students at the elementary and middle school levels. Frustrated over what seemed to be a lack of awareness of her expertise regarding language and learning, she attempted to inform other staff members by conversing with them at lunch. However, progress seemed slow and somewhat cumbersome because, frankly, most teachers wanted lunch topics to be non-educationally related. Then, after a discussion with the principals at her two schools, Genevieve posted information about her services and skills on the main bulletin boards of the two schools. During each of the four weeks in November, she dressed the boards with information relating her background, the kinds of testing she could conduct, and the types of school problems for which she might be able to offer assistance. The response to these bulletin boards was overwhelming. Teachers, parents, and even students began to talk more with Genevieve about her services and her help.

## Clarifying Attitudes, Beliefs, and Ideas and Helping to Change Behaviors

As mentioned, clarification is a crucial tool to use in the counseling process because it allows all members of a group to understand best what each is saying. This is certainly true when working with the school-age population. The clinician must actively listen to parents and teachers to understand best what is being said and what feelings or attitudes are being related. In addition, when working with school-age children, clinicians will find they may need to use their clarification skills when serving as a team member of a multidisciplinary teams and working with students themselves.

SERVING AS A TEAM MEMBER

Becoming a team member should theoretically be a natural step after the clinician has provided information to colleagues so they understand his or her role in the area of learning and language disorders. However, as in any work area involving adults who have different backgrounds, and sometimes different goals, conflicts may occur. Words used by one individual to make a point may be misunderstood or misinterpreted by another (Webster, 1981). Through *clarification,* these misunderstanding and misinterpretations may be cleared. It is not uncommon for any professional who has a clear idea of a specialized plan for a student, to take any information that suggests a different plan as a challenge of the original idea (Fisher & Ury, 1981). It is important for clinicians to recognize that they come to any task or meeting with specific ideas of what they believe to be important and certain perceptions of other professionals and their capabilities. These perceptions may interfere with what a clinician hears from others. Likewise, the clinician also must accept that others come with their own perceptions. Clarification can be the means through which all parties come to understand the true intent of messages. By asking for clarification (e.g., "I'm hearing you say . . . , Am I right in understanding this about what you said . . . ?"), all team members should have a better grasp on the issues confronting the team.

At times, clarification may involve *confronting* another individual about information that person has given or an action performed. The clinician can clarify in a constructive manner by using "I" statements (e.g., "I'm feeling frustrated because it seems I am not being heard.") as opposed to "You" statements (e.g.," You aren't listening to me."). I statements tell the other members what the clinician is thinking and feeling (Webster, 1981). You statements, on the other hand, may cause a listener to become defensive because the speaker is telling the listener something about the person that might not be correct. Although many individuals are nervous about confronting others or are afraid of stirring up trouble or hurting feelings, constructive confrontations can and often do lead to clarification and better understanding among team members.

FACILITATING STUDENT RESPONSIBILITY

One goal in working with school-age children and adolescents is to help them understand their role in the intervention process and become actively involved in the services they receive. Consequently, the ability to clarify their thoughts, feelings, and attitudes is critical. Clinicians will find that it often is necessary to clarify the thoughts and feelings school-age children have about the services they are receiving. Sometimes, clinicians need to reiterate the purpose of the treatment and the long-term goals set for the student. Perhaps even more importantly, a clinician who actively listens to concerns that may not seem immediately relevant may prove to be the best facilitator for self-change. Students will not change their behaviors, or be willing to work toward changes, until they understand the importance of the change. Discussion with students about their ideas regarding treatment and their concepts of the long-term objective may enable the clinician to clarify false assumptions, misconceptions, and unrealistic goals and to make appropriate and pragmatic changes to the remediation plan.

At times, older school-age students may behave in ways that cause a clinician to feel frustrated and unappreciated. It is not unlikely that some students will cause the clinician to want to give up and just abandon work with them. This is a natural reaction and a perfectly legitimate feeling. On one hand, the clinician needs to remember his or her responsibility is to motivate students to become part of their own intervention services. However, it is also important for the clinician to verbalize, as a means of clarifying difficult situations, what his or her thoughts and feelings are about the manner in which treatment is proceeding and how the partners (the clinician and the client) are interacting and working toward those goals. Again, it may mean the clinician needs to temporarily put intended work aside and listen with an open mind and active ear to the feelings that the student may have that are interfering with progress. Students, especially during the adolescent years, have a great deal on their minds. It is foolish for any adult to assume that these students can easily set aside their day-to-day concerns to work toward a goal that may seem to only impact a distant future. Sometimes, the best treatment is for a clinician to listen to the issues confronting a student, determine how they are affecting the student's progress, verbalize hunches about the student's thoughts and feelings, and demonstrate to the student that there is an individual who is willing to listen and to help better understand the student's thinking and feelings. Through this process, more progress may actually be made toward the student's long term-goals.

**Case Example.** Lynda was diagnosed with a language-learning disorder. Although her oral language abilities were adequate, her literate language skills (reading and writing) were considerably below age expectancies. Lynda, who at the time was in third grade, was receiving services in her school (including Chapter 1 reading services) and resource room for written language deficits. Because of these services, she was pulled out of the classroom twice a day and seen within the classroom once a day. In addition, she was seen by a speech-language clinician in private practice twice a week. One day, in a session with the clinician, Lynda put her head down and refused to participate in an activity. Sensing there was a problem, the clinician stated that she seemed frustrated and asked whether she wanted to discuss it. Lynda then listed all the different services she was receiving and suggested that she was getting too much information and most of it seemed to be unimportant. To put it bluntly, she was tired of going to all of the special classes. The remainder of the session dealt with acknowledging her feelings of being overwhelmed and clarifying the purposes of the services. In addition, a plan was devised to talk with her parents about her feelings and ask whether they had any ideas for how to make meeting her challenges less frustrating.

Once Lynda's parents were apprised of her feelings, much to Lynda's delight, they agreed with her and suggested that all professionals involved in her case meet to discuss ways to streamline her services while still creating a plan of treatment that would best help her academic skills development. Lynda was overjoyed.

A subsequent meeting was held with all the professionals involved (the parents, the speech-language pathologist, the resource room teacher, the Chapter 1 teacher, the regular education teacher, and the principal). Because the speech-language pathologist was the only professional not from the schools, he was asked to explain his program and the purpose of the goals and procedures. After completing that task, the resource room teacher suddenly said, "Well, I do things like that, but just tell me what you want me to do and I'll do it." Taken aback, the speech-language pathologist first attempted to clarify by stating that the teacher seemed upset about something he had said. The resource room teacher stated that she was responsible for many children, not just Lynda, and that she could not just do "everything that I'm asked to do for every single child." The speech-language pathologist then stated that he was reporting on what he had done. He affirmed that it probably would seem overwhelming if it appeared that he was asking the resource room teacher to modify everything she was doing. He also explained that he was not attempting to tell her what to do. He proceeded to question whether all the professionals involved would feel comfortable discussing how their services might be duplicating each other so that services might be cut back or different services offered. Once that suggestion was made, all the professionals agreed, and the resource room teacher's frustration diminished as the situation was clarified. In the end, Lynda's services were cut back to classroom pull-out only twice a week, with some services within the classroom and some continued through the private practice. All involved, including Lynda, were pleased with the outcome.

## CONCLUSION

In this chapter, Webster's (1981) suggestions for effective counseling have been used as a framework for counseling parents of children with language-learning disorders, as well as other professionals and the children themselves. Three crucial points were made throughout the chapter. First, the basic functions of counseling can and should be used by clinicians when working with clients of any age and disorder, with their parents, and with the professionals who serve them. Some clinicians may assume that they only need to pay attention to the needs of their client. However, those adults that teach, serve, or nurture that child also are influential and, therefore, necessarily need to be involved in the counseling process.

Second, certain issues and concerns arise that are particular to children with a language-learning disorder and their parents and teachers. Clinicians should be aware of parents' fears regarding academic success for their children with language-learning disorders. Additionally, they should remember that the professionals who serve these children also may have ideas and concerns that differ from the clinician. Through the use of effective counseling skills, the clinician should find that he or she can work productively with all adults involved.

Finally, and perhaps most importantly, clinicians should be aware that their counseling skills will be used on almost a daily basis. Whether engaged in a clinical task or discussing an issue with a colleague or parent, their ability to actively listen, clarify, and understand others is crucial to the success of any interaction. As clinicians begin to use these skills on a day-to-day basis, they soon discover the benefits of being an effective and caring counselor.

## EPILOGUE

And what about Barbara, the mother of the five-year-old boy with a language-learning disorder who needed glasses? Although the clinician did not expect her to be the focus of counseling for the day, attention was quickly turned to Barbara. The clinician and the other parents actively listened to her tearful explanation of her son's need for glasses and her seeming inability to get to all of her appointments. Then, verbalizing a hunch, the clinician asked whether the glasses made her feel that professionals were telling her "one more bad thing about Adam." With a sigh, she replied "yes." The remaining portion of the meeting was devoted to acknowledging her feelings of anguish and hurt and then discussing with her ways she thought she might be able to attend an appointment with the ophthalmologist. By the end of the session, Barbara had clarified her feelings of disappointment about the recent diagnosis, thought more about the implications of glasses for her son, and decided on a plan that enabled her to make an appointment for him. As she left the meeting, her final comment was, "Thanks for listening. I owe you one."

## REFERENCES

Aram, D. M. (1991). Comments on specific language disorder as a clinical category. *Language, Speech, and Hearing Services in the Schools, 22,* 84–87.
Aram, D. M., Ekelman, B., & Nation, J. (1984). Preschoolers with language disorders: 10 years later. *Journal of Speech and Hearing Research, 27,* 232–244.
Bishop, D., & Adams, C. (1990). A prospective study of the relationship between specific language disorder, phonological disorders, and reading retardation. *Journal of Child Psychology and Psychiatry, 21,* 1027–1050.

Catts, H. W. (1993). The relationship between speech-language disorders and reading disabilities. *Journal of Speech and Hearing Research, 36,* 948–958.

Conti-Ramsden, G. (1993). Using parents to foster communicatively-impaired children's language development. *Seminars in Speech and Language. 14,* 289–295.

Crais, E. (1991). Moving from parent involvement to family-centered services. *American Journal of Speech-Language Pathology, 1,* 5–8.

Fisher, R., & Ury, W. (1981). *Getting to yes: Negotiating agreement without giving in.* New York: Penguin Books.

Girolametto, L., & Tannock, R. (1994). Correlates of directiveness in the interaction of fathers and mothers of children with developmental delays. *Journal of Speech and Hearing Research, 37,* 1178–1191.

James, S. L. (1990). *Normal language acquisition.* Newton, MA: Allyn and Bacon.

Kamhi, A. G. (1991). Specific language disorder as a clinical category: An introduction. *Language, Speech, and Hearing Services in the Schools, 22,* 65.

Kamhi, A. G., & Catts, H. W. (1989). *Reading disabilities: A developmental language perspective.* Austin, TX: Pro-Ed.

Lahey, M. (1988). *Language disorders and language development.* New York: Macmillan.

Larson, V. L., & McKinley, N. L. (1985). General intervention principles with language impaired adolescents. *Topics in Language Disorders, 5,* 70–77.

Millet, A., & Newhoff, M. (1978). *Language disordered children: Language disordered mothers?* Paper presented at the American Speech, Language, and Hearing Association, San Francisco.

Nelson, N. W. (1993). *Childhood language disorders in context: Infancy through adolescence.* New York: Macmillan.

Nelson, K. (1973). Structure and strategies in learning to talk. *Monographs of the Society for Research in Child Language, 38,* 11–56.

Owens, R. E. (1995). *Language disorders* (2nd ed.). Newton, MA: Allyn and Bacon.

Paul, R. (1991). Profiles of toddlers with slow expressive language development. *Topics in Language Disorders, 11,* 1–13.

Peters, A. (1977). Language learning strategies: Does the whole equal the sum of the parts? *Language, 53,* 560–573.

Schodorf, J. K., & Edwards, H. T. (1983). Comparative analysis of parent–child interactions with language-disordered and linguistically normal children. *Journal of Communication Disorders, 16,* 71–83.

Silliman, E. R., & Wilkinson, L. C. (1991). *Communicating for learning: Classroom observation and collaboration.* Rockville, MD: Aspen Systems.

Stone, J. R. (1992). Resolving relationship problems in communication disorders treatment: A systems approach. *Language, Speech, and Hearing Services in the Schools, 23,* 300–307.

Tannock, R., & Girolametto, L. (1992). Reassessing parent-focused language intervention programs. In S. F. Warren & J. Reichle (Eds.), *Causes and effects in communication and language intervention.* Baltimore: Paul H. Brookes.

Tomblin, B. J. (1989). Familial concentration of developmental language disorder. *Journal of Speech and Hearing Disorders, 54,* 287–295.

Tomblin, B. J. (1991). Examining the cause of specific language disorder. *Language, Speech, and Hearing Services in the Schools, 22,* 69–74.

Wallach, G. P., & Butler, K. G. (1994). *Language learning disabilities in school-age children and adolescents.* New York: Macmillan.

Webster, E. J. (1981). *Counseling with parents of handicapped children.* San Diego: College-Hill Press.

Webster, E. J., & Ward, L. M. (1993). *Working with parents of young children with disabilities.* San Diego: Singular Press.

# 11. Adult Neurogenic Communication Disorders

Paul R. Rao

The counseling role requires a healthcare professional to have an inner sense and genuine grasp of what confronts the person and family with a disability. This professional and personal virtue can be termed "compassion" or "empathy," both etymologically meaning "to feel inside." The layperson's operational definition of this sense can be captured with the maxim to "walk a mile in my shoes." In an effort to assist the reader in gaining such a sense, this chapter begins with a consumer perspective that conveys the utter horror of becoming incommunicado, of having been injured in a "brain attack" that unalterably changes one's life. America was dramatically introduced to stroke or a "brain attack" by Koppit's (1978) award-winning play *Wings,* in which Edith Stilson, a former aviatrix, is portrayed as having had a stroke with resultant aphasia. When her doctor asks what happened to her, she turns to the audience and responds, "Near as I can figure it, I was in my brain and crashed." Eleven years later, Joseph Chaikin (1989), an off-Broadway playwright, suffered a brain crash and subsequently wrote the following consumer perspective on receiving an award presented by the National Aphasia Association:

> I am aphasic.
> After the stroke, I could only say one real word—"yes."
> When I wanted to say "no,"
> I could only say "yes."
> When I wanted to say "I love you," or "I hate you,"
> I could only say "yes."
> Now I discover more and more about aphasia every day.

Sometimes each hour. Each hour is precious to me.

There are one million Americans who live with the disability of aphasia.

There are trillions and zillions of stars, magnificent spirals of majestic violence in the Galaxies.

I am working on a new play. A woman, an astronomer, researching the planets, while driving on a road, has an accident.

She is aphasic.

Human communication should be simple—but it is difficult to talk at all.

Some things are not important. And some things are important.

Conversation is important to me—social conversation, talk about art, even gossip.

Talking is also important for my work. I have worked in theater, all my life. To work, I need to talk, to be *understood*.

I have worked with many actors . . . African, Chinese, European, Japanese, Arab, Jewish, and American Indian. Together, we have made theater. To understand.

My future is devoted to my work. I will direct "Waiting for Godot." There are more projects.

Now that I am aphasic, I am "the other." We must understand others and talk to them. I understand more about vulnerability, about being different, about not fitting in. What is normal? Who sets the standard?

I have a new family . . . another sphere. Aphasia brings us all together in a new way.

Communication is important. Each of us has a different voice, a new mother tongue for us. I have energy to work for aphasics. Our communication is PRIMARY.

As the American Speech-Language-Hearing Association's bicentennial motto aptly states: "Human Communication Is Essential To Life." Clearly, people with neurogenic communication disorders must struggle with their loss and not lose the struggle to regain the essence of humanity—communication. The speech-language pathologist (SLP), with expertise in the exchange of information by individuals with communication problems and extensive training and education in the theoretic and practical approaches to being a change agent, is ideally suited to serve in the helping role of counselor for persons with neurologic injury who need support, information, and hope.

## MODELS TO CONSIDER WHEN SERVING PERSONS WITH NEUROGENIC COMMUNICATION DISORDERS

Speech-language pathologists are well-trained in the management of the various communication disorders affecting adults. How well prepared are they to manage the psychosocial sequelae of a "brain-attack?" Clearly their knee-to-knee, eyeball-to-eyeball, and heart-to-heart profession is one that entails assisting the communicatively impaired and their immediate circle of family and significant others to cope and possibly recover from a devastating trauma. By definition, it entangles SLPs in a charged and complex web of human emotion. In his foreword to *Counseling the Communicatively Disordered and Their Families*, Luterman (1991) writes:

Most of us soon discover that, ready or not, the field of communication disorders brings us into frequent contact with a broad range of emotional issues. It is true that although most SLPs and audiologists receive little guidance in how to deal with these issues, they exist nonetheless and often have an enormous impact on the outcome of our clinical efforts. (p. 18)

Stone and Alswang (1989) suggest that, although the literature reveals that counseling has always been seen as a crucial component in speech-language pathology and audiology, professionals in these fields continue to experience confusion and anxiety about such work. They attribute this confusion to the fact that other healthcare professionals have worked without clarity about the range, depth, or style of counseling appropriate for a specialist in communication disorders, a problem of poorly defined boundaries. Clearly, SLPs are not psychologists or trained counselors, and clinicians may indeed feel justifiably confused and anxious if a person with stroke is becoming verbally abusive to the spouse. In this case, the SLP may be unable to serve appropriately and safely the patient and the spouse. The SLP may have infringed on a gray but dangerous boundary. Besides strict boundary issues, Yudkovitz (1992) attributes whatever failure we may experience in the counseling realm to an absence of tools with which to set appropriate boundaries.

> What we want is for them to be better SLPs and audiologists. For that to happen they must begin to understand and take into account in their work the fact that, in addition to a particular dysfunction, there is something basically and deeply human that must be attended to. (p. 6)

The following models are designed to arm the clinician with the prerequisite tools to provide holistic SLP treatment to persons with adult neurogenic communication disorders and their significant others. The models in order of presentation and scope range from a simple hierarchy of need to the World Health Organization's (WHO) model of consequences of pathology and to finally a model of aging with a disability.

## Hierarchy of Need

Clinicians need to be sensitive to the need level of their patients along the recovery continuum. Maslow (1968) provided a popular pyramid (Table 11.1) that explains much of human behavior. SLPs can find clear applicability of Maslow's hierarchy with most of their patients; for example, why a person with traumatic brain injury (TBI) who feels physically threatened might dispense with social niceties and attack the real or imagined aggressor.

Maslow's hierarchy of need starts at a person's most basic need (physical) and assumes that until that need is met, the individual struggles to satisfy the physical need. Only when that need is met does the person strive to meet the next most pressing need (safety). Patients with severe physical impairments may be so overwhelmed by their hemiplegia or hemianopsia that they are quite literally unable to attend to the SLP's exhortation to try to say "cup." Once the patient feels like the physical impairment no longer puts him or her at risk for life and safety, then the SLP may begin to foster social communication and prod for pragmatics. Once the physical anxieties are allayed, the therapist might begin to hear between the lines the patient's wish to "go home for the weekend" (social) or "to dress him or herself" (self-esteem), or to "go back to work" (self-actualization). Although individuals seldom evidence a neat progression up or down the hierarchy of need, a stair step progression up the need-based pyramid has been illustrated here as it makes sense when dealing with loss following a traumatic illness and knowing the stages of recovery that have been well documented in the literature (Hagen, 1981; Ylvisaker & Szekeres, 1994) for persons with TBI. However, it is important to stress that needs vary and therefore the place one finds the patient on the pyramid fluctuates depending on circumstances, physical condition, and other contributing variables. Treatment must be at the level where the SLP finds the patient and not where he or she wants or expects the patient to be. Following an acute illness, such as stroke, patients initially have very little time and energy for what

**Table 11.1**
**Maslow's Hierarchy of Need**

| |
|---|
| Self-Actualization |
| Self-Esteem |
| Social |
| Safety |
| Physical |

might be termed enrichment activities such as hobbies; their needs drive the therapeutic regimen.

## Model of Consequences of Pathology

The World Health Organization (WHO) (1990) outlines a model of consequences of pathology that assists consumers and professionals in appreciating the differences between an *impairment* (dysfunction at the organ level, e.g., brain), *disability* (functional consequences of an impairment that affect performance of daily tasks, e.g., can't use the right hand to eat due to paralysis), and *handicap* (social disadvantages resulting from an impairment or disability, e.g., can't go back to work). Patients and families often arrive at rehabilitation medicine with an acute care medical model in mind, expecting that there is a drug, surgery, or other medical intervention that will "fix" the hemiplegia or the aphasia. Modern medicine has given us many miracles, so it is not surprising that our patients and their families not only hope for a medical miracle, but expect that a transplant, an injection, a surgical intervention will remediate the disabilities that are caused by an impairment. Generally a person with a *hemiplegia* (paralysis of the arm and leg on one side of the body) due to a stroke begins receiving physical therapy (PT) that involves both active and passive range-of-motion and strengthening exercises, and a host of other modalities that are designed to help the patient recover as much movement as possible. PT also assists the patient to compensate for any residual paralysis via the use of orthoses (e.g., leg brace, arm sling). The person with hemiplegia may require a wheelchair to get around and maybe later will use a quad cane. There is no sudden and miraculous ability to walk again. Usually there is lingering paralysis and pain, sometimes for the rest of the patient's life.

Patients must be immediately disabused of the notion of a medical "quick fix" and advised to expect the arduous and long struggle that is "rehab" with the pay-off of increased independence and a lessening of the handicap! Once the patient and family adopt the rehab mind set, real physical and psychological progress can be made. In this context, it is important to point out to the patient that SLPs do not address the organ level of pathology; a stroke or head injury has happened and once the patient is neurologically stable, there is little that can be done at the impairment (organ) level. Tests help measure degree of disability: a person may have a Broca's aphasia that affects talking more than any other modality. Treatment may make some in-roads in reducing the language or cognitive disability following a stroke or head injury, but the most critical role of all the team players—patient, significant others, and rehabilitation team members—is actively to pursue reducing the handicap.

Handicap can be defined as a "limitation of choice." A person with a stroke that results in damage to the brain (impairment) has *aphasia* (disability) that results in a handicap (can't order a cheeseburger). The crucial ingredient of the WHO model is to convey to consumers the element of "choice." How does rehab work? How does one "come back?" Generally, in persons with significant neurologic injury, no great gains can be expected at the impairment or disability level. Rehabilitation helps close the gap between pre- and post-neurotrauma status by helping the person with a disability exercise more options. The greater the degree of choice, the lesser the handicap! The person with aphasia may minimize the handicap by having a communication book, a pad and pencil, and a repertoire of functional gestures; more options and less handicap. Most SLPs have treated persons with a mild disability (e.g., a person with a mild stuttering problem) but a major handicap (e.g., afraid to talk on the phone or go out on a date) and vice versa (e.g., a person with severe aphasia who volunteers at a hospital visiting other persons with stroke), so clinicians can immediately appreciate the difference between disability and handicap. A person with a neurologic impairment must understand the distinction between the disability and its social consequences. Thus, the major thrust of the rehabilitation effort must be directed toward reducing the handicap. A person with stroke may have relatively few choices right after the stroke and therefore be quite "handicapped." However, with the assistance of family, friends, therapists, doctors, and nurses, the patient learns many ways to bathe, walk, talk, and, therefore, become more "abled" and less handicapped. The overview of "closing the gap" is a patient education tool that has been available to clinicians the past decade (Appendix 11.1). Patients cannot begin actively and intelligently to participate in rehabilitation if they have unreasonable medical expectations and unrealistic rehabilitation goals. Counseling begins by educating the consumer regarding the nature and cause of the illness and the treatment expectations. The educated consumer can then become a key player on the treatment team and his or her own best advocate for setting personalized rehabilitation goals. The patient and family might take solace in the fact that: "over 80% of persons receiving rehabilitation services return to their home, work, schools or an active retirement. Rehabilitation can lengthen life, improve the quality of life, and reduce subsequent illness" (Medical Rehabilitation Education Foundation, 1993, p. 3).

## Aging with a Disability

Trieschman (1987) states that "aging is a process of adjusting to a constantly changing internal and external environment and as a result there is no definable point of being aged." A person with a neurologic impairment that results in a disability and a consequent handicap must not only cope with the neurotrauma but also with the added challenge of aging with a disability. Each person aging with a disability must be viewed in the context of change and its consequent challenges.

The essential problem of aging is not only how to treat declining biologic-organic function, but also how to adapt the environment to allow the person to be as functional as possible—to work around or compensate for the altered biologic function. (Trieschman, 1987, p. 3). Trieschman espouses a system approach to intervention as the strategy most suited to meet the challenges of aging, whether disabled or non-disabled. For the SLP the implications for counseling the person with a disability are to reinforce a practical approach to coping with life's changes and stressors. Trieschman (1987) establishes a conceptual framework for counseling the person who is aging with a communication disability:

> The concept of health or adjustment is defined as the balance achieved among three major influences in life: psychosocial (P), biological-organic (O), and environmental (E). Behavior, health or adjustment (B) is the interactive result of these three influences (i.e., $B = F [P,O,E]$). Aging is viewed as a change in the balance, often the result of the alteration of biological-organic (O), which then has an impact on the psychosocial (P) and environmental (E) influences in life. (p. 4)

Thus, as a person experiences a communication disorder resulting from head injury or stroke, he or she will have problems when altered biologic-organic (O) function tips the health and adjustment balance. This communication disability thus places stress on the psychological realm of function (P) and often requires additional environmental support services (E) to keep the person with a disability functioning satisfactorily in his or her own milieu.

Table 11.2 presents a menu of variables that interact and influence all of our lives. The dynamic balance among these variables is a major factor in determining health and communication status at any given moment. American society tends to focus on health and clinicians must be sensitive to the behavioral component of health, especially when counseling persons with health problems. Trieschman (1987) observes that living entails at least three major categories of behavior (see Table 11.3 for an outline of the behavioral components of health):

**Table 11.2**

**Behavior (B) as a Function of the Interaction of Psychosocial (P), Organic (O), and Environmental (E) Variables**

| Psychosocial Variables (P) | Organic Variables (O) | Environmental Variables (E) |
|---|---|---|
| Take responsibility for self | Intelligence and cognitive ability | Income |
| Will to live | Endurance | Transportation |
| Social skills | Strength | Architectural and geographic barriers |
| Style of coping with stress | Perceptual motor coordination | Access to knowledgeable health professionals |
| Locus of control | Aptitudes | Educational and vocational resources |
| Self-confidence | Amount of physical impairment | Financial disincentives |
| Judgment | Sensory abilities | Family and interpersonal support |
| Problem solving ability | Bladder and bowel control | Socioeconomic status |
| Education | Respiratory function | Availability of physical assistance (if needed) |
| Work history | Pain | Behavioral supervision (if needed) |
| Job skills | General health status | Payment for medical care |
| Cultural and ethnic group | | Role models |
| Gender | | |
| Creativity | | |

Table from Trieschman, R. (1987). *Aging with a Disability.* New York: Demos: 47. Reprinted by permission.

1. Survival activities (e.g., promotion of wellness).
2. Harmonious living and working environment (e.g., family relationships).
3. Productivity (e.g., community service) (p. 49).

Rao (1992a) illustrates the application of this model to a person with stroke: Let us assume that Mr. Jones is a 70 year-old person who sustained a left cerebrovascular accident (CVA) with resultant aphasia. He cannot dress himself independently (Category 1) and must rely

**Table 11.3.**

**Behavioral Components of Health (B)**

| Survival Activities |
|---|
| Promotion of wellness |
| Prevention of medical problems |
| Activities of daily living (bathing, grooming, dressing, eating) |
| Housekeeping |
| Mobility |

| Harmonious Living and Working Environment |
|---|
| Family relationships |
| Friendships |
| Relations with service personnel and coworkers |
| Relations to authority figures |
| Financial management |
| Management of personal affairs |

| Productivity |
|---|
| Employment in or out of the home |
| Educational activities |
| Family and social roles |
| Community service |
| Avocations |
| Scholarly pursuits |
| Artistic endeavors |
| Athletic endeavors |

Table from Trieschman, R. (1987). *Aging with a Disability.* New York: Demos: 49.

on his wife to assist him. He resents his wife always telling him to try to say things when he can't. This tends to distort their relationship from a prestroke husband-wife relationship to a poststroke mother-child relationship (Category 2). Finally he no longer wishes to go to the local stroke club to be around all those other individuals who can't help themselves either (Category 3). (p. 22).

As is evident in this patient sketch, there is a definite and powerful interaction between his three major categories of behavior. Severely reduced independence in conducting survival activities has a destabilizing effect on one's life satisfaction and productivity. If one feels unproductive, unneeded, and useless then the drive to survive stalls. As Trieschman (1987) puts it, "if one has no real reason for getting out of bed each morning, there is less reason to take care of one's body." Thus how one performs these behaviors ([B] survival activities, harmonious living, productivity) is influenced by the (P), (O), (E) interaction, which in turn influences the (P), (O), and (E) variables. Hence, according to Rao (1992a), it becomes a person system when applied to an aging person with a communication disorder who must struggle, consciously or unconsciously, to maintain or reassert homeostasis. The juggling ability that the disabled adult must daily demonstrate in keeping life in the balance gives new meaning to the expression "stressed out." The SLP would be wise to consider Trieschman's model when counseling persons with a disability; the more the patient attempts to push for independence without resources, the greater the likelihood that the patient will become "stressed out" and burdened by failure to meet unrealistic expectations.

The person with a disability is in a constant struggle to maintain homeostasis of (P), (O), and (E). It is clear from the literature and from the experience of SLPs working with adults with disabilities that they pay a penalty every day. Paying this penalty means stress; the alarm cycle sets in where there is an alarm (e.g., you forgot to take your blood pressure medicine), you then gradually adapt (you finally calm down when you realize that taking the pill is only delayed an hour), but then fatigue and perhaps exhaustion sets in (e.g., you collapse on the sofa and decide not to go for your walk). This vignette can be multiplied many times on a daily basis with minor and major stressors and barriers facing the person with a disability. Gradually, the energy and enthusiasm erodes and the prospect of a life-long struggle against these barriers saps the soul and exasperates the psyche. Rao (1992a) adds a caveat to all clinicians to rethink the concept and importance of independence for persons with a disability.

> Based on the stress model and the consequent penalties that must be paid, is it all that important for our patients to walk from the waiting room to the treatment area if doing so drains his time and energy? The person with a disability must be empowered to decide what is important and what is not important in his or her life at a given point in time. If it is important that the SLP warrants his complete attention, energy, and effort, then the laborious "independent" walk back to the treatment area should be waived and a quick and easy ride in a wheelchair entertained. (p. 24)

The need to educate patients in stress management and in self-empowerment to make healthy choices that will likely bring the greatest dividends cannot be overstated. Helping the patient to inventory his or her new self with all of the acquired limitations and resources is a *sine qua non* to "smelling the roses" and "seizing the day." The models and discussion above suggest that pre-crisis intervention with patients involves knowing what their needs are; explaining the rehabilitation process with sufficient detail so they can appreciate their individual goals, choices, and roles in recovery; and finally to sensitizing them to the need for balance, energy conservation, and establishment of priorities in their lives.

## COUNSELING AS AN INTEGRAL COMPONENT OF MANAGEMENT

A consumer perspective and several theoretic and practical models have been introduced to provide a framework for SLPs engaged in counseling persons with neurogenic communication disorders. The presumption here is that counseling is indeed an integral part of managing persons with communication disorders. This is not a new concept. As early as 1969, the literature discussed the attitudes of families of persons with aphasia (Malone, 1969). According to Webster and Newhoff (1981), the following four services should be provided by the professionals who intervene:

1. Receiving information the families wish to share;
2. Giving information to family members;
3. Helping individuals clarify their ideas, attitudes, and emotions; and
4. Providing them with options for changing their behavior and also for changing the behavior of the spouse. (p. 234)

This is pretty basic information. Clinicians should give and get information (and SLPs should be the very best at this among all the team members). SLPs counsel clients, their families, and significant others (SO) regarding the nature and impact of communication disorders. Professionals assist in developing appropriate goals for recovery from or adjustment to a communication disorder by establishing an effective interpersonal relationship in which client change and growth are realized. The SLP assists clients in understanding their feelings and the varying options that they might face in coping with a catastrophic illness. In addition to these services, counseling roles may also include developing strategies for manipulating the environment and developing coping mechanisms and systems for emotional support. As recommended in the *Preferred Practice Patterns* (PPPs) (ASHA, 1993), counseling procedures are designed to facilitate the patient's or client's recovery from or adjustment to a communication disorder. Specific purposes of counseling may be to " provide patients/clients and their families with information and support, make appropriate referrals to other professionals, and help patients develop problem-solving strategies to enhance the rehabilitation process" (ASHA, p. 19). The *Preferred Practice Pattern* (ASHA, 1993) that pertains to provision of counseling by speech language pathologists is:

I.  Expected Outcome
    A. Professionals assist patients/clients and their families to develop appropriate goals for recovery from, adjustment to, or prevention of a communication or related disorder by facilitating change and growth in which patients/clients become more autonomous, more self-directing, and more responsible for achieving their potential and realizing their goals to communicate more effectively.
II. Clinical Indications
    A. Counseling services are offered as part of speech, language swallowing, hearing, or balance screening, assessment, or treatment, or upon request or referral.
III. Clinical Process
    A. Counseling services for patients/clients and their families include:
       1. Assessment of counseling needs
       2. Provision of information
       3. Use of strategies to modify behavior and/or the patient's/client's environment
       4. Development of coping mechanisms and systems for emotional support
       5. Development and coordination of patient/client and family self-help and support groups
    B. Professionals are responsible for ensuring that the patient/client and family receive adequate counseling. Referrals to and consultation with mental health professionals may be an integral component of counseling.

IV. Setting/Equipment Specifications
   A. Counseling is conducted in a setting conducive to patient/client and family com-
      fort, confidentiality, and uninterrupted privacy.
V. Documentation
   A. Documentation includes a statement of pertinent background information, results,
      and recommendations, including the need for further counseling or referral. (p. 20)

Simmons (1990), in a chapter on aphasia treatment, is even more explicit than Webster
and Newhoff (1981) when she states that a major issue that must be addressed early on
and continue throughout treatment is counseling and educating the client and the family.
In her view, this should include:

1. A general discussion of characteristics of brain damage, possibly with relevant literature
   and referral to outside sources such as stroke clubs or support groups;
2. Facts on the nature of the disorder with specifics about what is wrong and what is right
   with the patient;
3. Information on goals and expectations, which includes the aphasic person's (sic) input
   in goal setting and treatment planning;
4. Acquiring information on family interaction, and how their strategies promote or hin-
   der communication;
5. Direct family training in ways to facilitate communication, such as recognizing when to
   allow the patient more time to elaborate or when to stop and ask for clarification. (p. 68)

These issues are applicable to the adult population with a communication disorder. Clearly,
the implication of Simmons' sage advice is that counseling must be integrated into treatment so that the family can immediately appreciate the problem and learn how to enhance
both the patient's communication and their own coping skills. Counseling should not be a
separate session but should be part of the holistic treatment session. When family members
are present in therapy, it is a "golden opportunity" to model, train, observe, and challenge
the participants in the act of communication. Counseling is treatment and good treatment
is counseling. For a description of a family-centered approach to SLP treatment that is designed to enhance the family's understanding of both the communicative and emotional
ramifications of the aphasia and, thereby, indirectly foster emotional adjustment and support while enhancing communicative recovery see Andrews and Andrews (1990). A general rule and practice that enhances the possibility of effecting a counseling treatment session is, with the patient's consent, to invite accompanying family member(s) to observe a
treatment session, thus making the family a part of treatment. Certainly there are caveats to
this advice that must be considered. Observations should not be attempted if a family member's presence would be disruptive for a highly distractible patient, or if their presence precipitates an episode of anger or lability in the patient, or if the patient does not wish anyone
to observe his or her attempts in therapy. However, more often than not, an experienced
SLP will accomplish more in therapy with the family present than with the patient alone.

## FUNCTIONAL COMMUNICATION ASSESSMENT AS A PRELUDE AND
## PREREQUISITE TO COUNSELING

With each new referral, the SLP is charged with conducting a complete assessment of the
client's communication ability. Rao (1994) outlined the diagnostic-specific assessment
process that results in a treatment plan and a tact for counseling. A comprehensive diagnostic test protocol should consist of the following areas of assessment:

- Subjective complaint and reason for referral
- Background information, including medical, biographic, and behavioral history

- Sensorimotor screen (e.g., hearing and vision test results)
- Oral motor examination of structures and function of the speech and swallowing mechanisms
- Standard voice and speech evaluation
- Standard language evaluation
- Standard cognitive screen
- Functional status assessment of communication
- Patient and family participation and contribution
- Environmental prosthetic and device inventory
- Pragmatic performance and potential (p. 297)

Having completed the comprehensive assessment, the SLP is expected to arrive at a communication diagnosis and prognosis. The prognostic challenge facing the clinician is to estimate the potency of the various prognostic factors pertinent to a given case and make the best clinical estimate about the patient's overall prognosis. Clearly, the patient and SO are most concerned about the prognosis for return of communication skills. The SLP will be unable to begin providing counseling and support to the family and SO until the assessment, diagnostic, and prognostic processes have been completed. Only then will the SLP be truly conversant with the facts and functional ramifications of the findings. Then and only then is the SLP able to share honestly and professionally with the patient the desired diagnostic and prognostic information that can begin the post-traumatic healing process for the family unit. The key word and concept in all of this discussion is "functional." Increasingly, SLPs are being asked to assess the patient's functional communication abilities, to identify functional treatment goals, and to achieve functional outcomes. In short, various customers—payors, patients, physicians—want a bottom line "functional" and factual report of findings. Thus SLPs will be best positioned to serve in their role as counselors once they have truly conducted a functional assessment wherein the SLP "evaluates one's communication, manifested in the performance of daily life activities despite noted speech, language, cognitive, or hearing impairment." (Frattali, Thompson, Holland, Wohl, & Ferketic, 1995, p. 4). A particularly helpful functional communication tool that also serves as a framework for functional counseling is the *Communicative Effectiveness Index* (*CETI*) (Lomas et al., 1989). The CETI is an index of 16 situations that the significant other is asked to rate the patient's performance in particular situations on a 10-cm visual analog scale with the anchor at one end of the scale being "not at all able" and at the other end being "as able as before the stroke." Figure 11.1 shows a few examples of the CETI.

The CETI, although designed to be rated by significant others, is an excellent tool to administer both to the SO and to the patient who has functional sentence level reading. The completed CETI provides clear instances of lack of correlation and, as a consequence, probable miscommunication on the parts of the SO and the patient. If the patient feels that he or she participates in conversations with strangers just as well as before the stroke and the spouse rates the patient as not at all able to do so, clearly there is an opportunity to discuss with the family unit the concept of pragmatics or initiative or self-awareness or a variety of other communication concepts that once clarified and understood will most likely result in better communication awareness and consequent family adjustment.

**Case Report.** C.R. was a 37-year-old who experienced a stroke with aphasia nearly two years earlier. His stroke recovery was surprising in its breadth and depth. His initial status was severe in all vital spheres. He could not walk, talk, bathe, or toilet. The prognosis was fairly grim for such a bright young man with a wife and two young children. C.R. desperately wanted to get better and at the outset was assertively a

NOT AT                                                         AS ABLE AS
ALL ABLE                                                       BEFORE STROKE

1. Getting somebody's attention.

2. Getting involved in group conversations that are about him/her.

3. Giving yes and no answers appropriately.

4. Communicating his/her emotions.

5. Indicating that he/she understands what is being said to him/her.

6. Having coffee-time visits and conversations with friends and neighbors
   (around the bedside or at home.)

7. Having a one-to-one conversation with you.

**Figure 11.1.**   Examples of items from the Communicative Effectiveness Index. (From Lomas, J., Pickard, L., Bester, S., Elbard, H., Finlayson, A., & Zoghaib, C. (1989). The communicative effectiveness index: Development and psychometric evaluation of a functional communication measure for adult aphasia. *Journal of Speech and Hearing Disorders, 54,* 13–124.)

part of the team's planning and implementation process. C.R., an avid sports fan, moved from "yes" and "no" questions and a single communication book, later to an alphabet board, and finally to self-motivated internal coaching to arrive at his message and intent in a complete, coherent, and cogent manner. His daily outpatient treatment program was totally vocationally focused because the patient demanded that the team assist him in returning as a customer service agent for a major United States airline. " I have two children, I have to get better." His daily regimen of SLP, vocational rehabilitation, and occupational therapy was designed to assist C.R. to return to his work environment with several occupational adaptations (automatic paper cutter, stapler, and a phone head set). The airline was willing to consider C.R. for re-employment, but he had to be able to perform as well as before the stroke. The team was thus challenged by the hard driving, goal-oriented patient. The SO (Caroll) and the CETI became helpful companions to C.R.'s rehabilitation program and eventual return to work. Caroll completed the CETI at monthly intervals during C.R.'s outpatient therapy regimen. However, besides rating how well C.R. was able to function in the 16 CETI situations C.R.'s wife provided additional commentary that became crucial to the succeeding stage of treatment. Caroll's "post-CETI sharing" with the SLP assisted the SLP in fostering positive change in C.R. during his struggle to strike back at stroke.

"I hope this questionnaire is helpful to you. I do want to qualify some of my answers. While Craig's conversational abilities are coming along, I do notice that he is not as active a participant in debates/discussions as he was before the accident. He definitely does not shy away, but is somewhat reserved in the number of responses and their complexity. I also find that Craig has a more difficult time talking to 'strangers' on the phone than he does in person. If it's possible, could you or Janet work with him on telephone communications? If you have any questions or want to discuss this further, please give me a call. Caroll" Feedback 1/18/92.

"Craig's speech and ability to communicate continue to improve every day. He is getting much better at phone communication and no longer checks to see if I'm around before making a call. He is also improved in his ability to interact with strangers (i.e., clerks at the Giant, etc.) and the ability to write checks has done a lot to further his independence (a mixed blessing as now we have to co-ordinate daily to avoid the problems some members of the house have had). While his ability to write has improved, I feel it has not kept pace with the improvements in his speech. He continues to struggle with the spelling of even the most familiar words. Are there any strategies or ways I can help Craig improve in this area? While he was never a prolific writer, I do worry about the level of frustration that this lack of improvement causes him. Thanks for all your help. Caroll" Feedback 3/15/92.

"Sorry this is so late. Craig's communication, both verbal and written, continues to improve. He still struggles with spelling, but he can now write notes/phone messages that can be understood by all. For a while, Craig had difficulty dealing with the kids in stressful/disciplinary situations. He would often yell to get their attention or to correct them. As a defensive measure, they had begun to yell back at him and at each other. Because of the work you're doing with him, and the discussions we've had with the psychologist, Craig has made remarkable progress in this area. He is able to control his response to the kids and in turn they are listening to him and not yelling at us or each other as much as before. It has made life for all of us that much happier. From time to time, I still note that Craig's auditory memory is slow, but he continues to work on it. Please let me know if you need any additional information. Caroll" Feedback 3/30/92.

The above three insightful vignettes provide ample evidence of three key counseling principles: (a) The SO can be the key liaison and player in a patient's recovery from the trauma of being "incommunicado"; (b) the SLP cannot treat what the SLP does not know; and (c) success begets success. What a wonderful commentary of Caroll's clinical insight from C.R.'s use of the phone, speaking with strangers, spelling, parenting, and remembering—all functional skills that were addressed in therapy once Caroll suggested or more tactfully asked if "there was anything she could do to work on" a given skill. The functional assessment and ongoing use of a functional communication rating tool such as the CETI became the foundation for a trusting and therapeutic relationship with Caroll and C.R. This ongoing dialogue permitted all parties in the treatment equation to express goals, anxieties, expectations, and accomplishments. (See Appendix 11.2 for a copy of C.R.'s consumer testimony before the Agency for Health Care Policy and Research.)

## CURE-CARE CONUNDRUM

The above case of C.R. illustrates another challenge for the SLP: When is enough, enough? C.R. was engaged in some form of treatment for nearly two years and the data suggested that when C.R. finally returned to work full time as a customer service agent for a major U.S. airline that he still exhibited some chronic, residual language deficits, particularly in the areas of secondary language skills, fluency, and auditory retention span. Clearly, treatment could have continued. C.R. was industrious, motivated, and dedicated to excel, but he was even more focused on "getting on with his life." Wertz (1983) capsulizes this treat-terminate counseling dilemma in his philosophic discussion on aphasia therapy:

> It is possible for clinicians and patients to be confronted with a cure-care conundrum. If one views aphasia as existing over a period of time, from its onset to the death of the patient, one can divide time into periods. How one divides the time and what one does during each period is influenced by one's values. In the care of the terminally ill, one value, preservation of life, may eventually give way to another value, alleviation of suffering. Similarly, in the management of aphasia, one value, the quality of language, may eventually give way to another value, the quality of life. (p. 7)

Wertz (1983) believes that there are at least two time periods in the management of aphasia, and the duration of these periods varies depending on the needs, desires, and abilities of individual patients. Wertz further believes that SLPs need to be attuned to the existence of these periods and the appropriate duration of each for each person with aphasia. Finally, Wertz believes that the duration of each period is negotiable between the SLP, the patient, and SO.

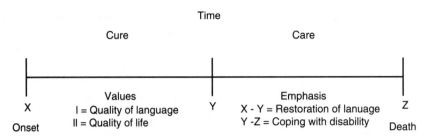

**Figure 11.2.** Temporal model for managing aphasic patients that indicates therapeutic values and emphasis may change over time. (From Wertz, R. T. (1983). A philosophy of aphasia therapy: Some things that patients do not say but that you can see if you listen. In R. T. Wertz (Ed.), *Communicative Disorders*, p. 7. Reprinted by permission.)

Refer to Figure 11.2 for an illustration of Wertz's (1983) temporal continuum of the cure-care conundrum. This framework has been suggested as a useful tool for managing persons with aphasia, but is potentially applicable to all persons with adult neurogenic communication disorders. Early on in a case, the SLP as clinician and counselor needs to determine for an individual patient when the focus should switch from "cure" to "care," from emphasizing restoration of language to stressing coping with a disability. This is a terribly practical and realistic model for a number of reasons. First, few persons who suffer some sort of "brain attack" ever completely recover from the communication problem and there is always some residual disability with which to cope. Second, some patients make significant improvement, whereas others make none. Third, the first phase (the search for the "cure") is multifactorial and cannot be predicted with any degree of precision. Finally, in truly patient-focused care, the consumer determines the amount of care being sought and when to emphasize learning to live with a devastating disability (the search for the "care"). The SLP as counselor can be the crucial change agent in assisting the patient and SO to adapt to and cope with the injury and ultimately to separate from treatment. Refer to Appendix 11.3 for a list of suggestions to the person with aphasia and the family (Wertz, 1983) that were intended to prevent psychosocial problems from developing. C.R. clearly knew that he had residual communication problems but he also knew that "it was time to move on" or as is stated in Appendix 11.3, "Must prepare for independence, for an end to treatment." If the SLP as counselor addresses the suggestions with the patient and SO, the family unit will be able to move more smoothly and confidently from the "cure" to the "care" phase of coping.

## CAVEATS TO COUNSELING IN SPEECH LANGUAGE PATHOLOGY

It must be stressed that the counseling role that SLPs play with communicatively impaired clients is one that entails provision of education and support. It is a role borne of people in crisis who need information and support for where they are and when they need it, not unlike the counseling that is indicated in a rape crisis center hot line. The patient and SO may know next to nothing about the etiology, nature, prognosis, and treatment of the sequelae of the "brain attack." They may be unsure about where to receive services in the community, about the benefits of a stroke or head injury support group, and about when and if they may be able to return to work. The SLP should be able to respond to most of these types of questions in an honest, matter-of-fact, and timely manner. However, the

SLP must also know when to request help and when to refer, when the subject matter and counseling needs begin to encroach on territory in which the SLP has insufficient training, education, and experience. Moreover, to relate back to the Stone and Alswang (1989) idea about anxiety reduction through maintenance of boundaries, it is much easier to recognize red flags or boundary issues, including the need for consultation or referral, if the SLP knows about:

1. How relationships work.
2. How therapeutic relationships work.
3. How people may feel and may enact their feelings.
4. How people may feel about being different, having a disability, having a family member with a disability, and how they may enact their feelings.
5. How we, the clinicians, may feel and how we may enact our feelings (Yudkovitz, 1992, p. 6)

SLPs are *not* trained social workers, psychotherapists, or counselors and the ethics of the profession requires that the SLP stay within his or her scope of practice and abide by all local and state licensing laws. It is illegal and unethical to advertise oneself as a counselor except as that role falls within the practice parameters of speech-language pathology (see ASHA, 1993). It should be apparent that indeed there are boundaries that SLPs must respect as they keep primary the needs of the patient. For this reason, SLPs *do not* provide marriage, bereavement, sex, or other special needs counseling. Patients who present with a communication disorder overlaid on a personality or psychiatric disorder present special challenges to the SLP. Persons with adult neurogenic communication disorders often can be effectively treated with a companion psychotherapist who can use the SLP's communication expertise to interface and collaborate with the patient with serious psychological problems (e.g., spousal abuse, marital discord, child abuse, transvestitism, depression, and suicidal thoughts) and his or her family. Although not psychologically based, issues dealing with divorce, child rearing, abortion, and other such social issues have come up in clinical practice and the SLP's charge is always to know and recommend the resources in the community that might best serve the pressing needs of the patient and the family. All of these problems and issues are very real and all may hamper the SLP therapeutic process. Finally, all of these problems and social issues may require the expertise of a professional other than an SLP for a satisfactory long-term solution. Social workers, psychologists, and chaplains are often better suited to assist the patient and SO to deal with deep underlying psychological problems and family-related issues. The SLP is often the key person who detects the psychosocial issue or problem and successfully encourages the patient to seek outside consultation and support.

## COUNSELING CONSIDERATIONS FOR ADULTS WITH A SPECIFIC NEURO-COMMUNICATION DISORDER

### Aphasia

Persons with aphasia typically present with a language disorder that crosses all language modalities but with intellectual abilities generally intact. A person with aphasia generally has trouble with both reception and expression during communication and, therefore, is a challenging subject to counsel. Frequently the clinician must resort to yes or no questions to discover the true nature of what could be bothering the person with aphasia. When addressing comprehension and expression activities in therapy, the SLP might uncover episodes of sadness, anger, or displays of other human emotions. The SLP might then find it opportune to combine counseling with treatment. If the clinician deals with the patient's emotion that is on line, he or she is frequently able to defuse the situation and also able to appreciate exactly what the patient was emoting because of the context in which the emotional disruption was found. It might be that the patient wants to go home, or is worried about bills, or is concerned that his son quit his job and moved back home. Each day, life brings change and challenges with which mere mortals often cope by simply ventilating. The person with aphasia cannot simply ventilate. This is where the adept SLP can begin to talk in behalf of the patient (ventilate) and obtain patient reaction to the various scenarios described by the descriptive SLP.

In short, the person with aphasia generally has normal memory and emotions, but because of the language disability, cannot problem solve or vent as can most stressed normals. This is where clinically sensitive and empathic SLPs can be of utmost value to the team, by applying their communication expertise to help their patients sort out their feelings. Tanner (1987) stresses the importance of engaging the support of the family when counseling the person with aphasia, because sorting out their feelings and dispelling their myths can have a salutary impact on the patient's overall post-stroke adjustment. Stroke is a family illness and, therefore, it behooves professionals to treat it as such. Some families of stroke patients have reported that they were still struggling to cope with the changes in their lives three to five years after the onset of the illness (Christensen & Anderson, 1989). Burns, Dong, and Oehring (1995) conjecture that this is the reason that speech-language treatment following stroke continues in some form for more than four years post stroke in 32 to 63% of aphasic persons (Doyle & Holland, 1984). Measurable benefits can be obtained when families are provided information and counseling on the following issues (Tanner, 1987):

Definition of aphasia and related disorders

Types of aphasia

Framework of communication

Paraphasia

Word finding behaviors

Jargon

Random naming errors and neologisms

Emotional lability

Awareness of errors and self-correction

Catastrophic reaction

Tip of the tongue phenomena

Perseveration

Recall versus recognition of correct words

Echolalia

Slow rise time and auditory fade

Disorders of perception

The value of therapy

Choosing a therapist

Rao (1982) reported on the results of a family discussion program that found additional issues that were of frequent concern to families of persons with stroke:

Physical function

Personality changes

Increased use of profanity

Increased fatigue

Euphoria

Role changes

Withdrawal and depression

Changes in lifestyles

Prognosis

Role of the family

Resources in the community

Seizures

Visiting with the patient

Community re-entry

This menu of post-stroke concerns will aid the SLP in assisting the family in adjusting to the trauma that may have befallen a family member. Even in this era of the educated consumer, the SLP should assume consumer ignorance about how best to respond to the multiplicity of issues that daily confront the patient with aphasia and the family. Despite the catastrophic effects of aphasia on the individual and family, some persons with aphasia and their family members do seem to cope with the inevitable changes (Sarno, 1993). This ability to adapt is obviously very important in its own right because it permits the individual to redefine "the quality of life in an altered state" and attain a sense of "self-actualization" (Sarno, 1993, p. 326).

## Motor Speech Disorders Dysarthria and Apraxia

Persons with motor speech disorders generally present with speech intelligibility problems, but with language and intellectual skills intact. In addition to the aforementioned issues that might be raised with stroke families, Tanner (1987) lists additional issues that are particularly germane to patients with motor speech problems and their families:

Sensation deficits to the mouth and face as well as accompanying drooling

Cosmetic and intelligibility aspects of dysarthria

Evaluating sucking, chewing, swallowing, and motor speech disorders

Families often are most struck and stuck by their inability to understand what the patient is saying. Frequently, the most effective counseling approach with this group of patients is to have family members observe a treatment session wherein the SLP demonstrates multimodal communication, repetition and rephrasing, reduced rate and increased intensity, and the use of a host of other facilitative techniques that can help the patient get a message across. One technique that has already been found to be effective in training non-aphasic spouses (Newhoff, Bugbee, & Ferriera, 1981) and, therefore, potentially instructive and helpful with the motor speech impaired population and their loved ones is to involve the entire family unit in *Promoting Aphasics Communicative Effectiveness* (PACE) therapy (Davis & Wilcox, 1985) wherein each participant is required to take turns giving and getting information. The opportunity to observe the effective use of drawing, gesture, tone of voice, facial expression, and so forth to convey a message in context is instructive to the "abled and disabled" and tends to allay the anxieties of all parties. The old dictum of "walk a mile in my shoes" is the right PACE.

## Cognitive Communicative Disorders Post Stroke

The person with a right hemisphere stroke may often present with euphoria, denial, and neglect behaviors that can confound the most patient family and the most patient-focused therapist. These are counseling issues that might typically arise with these patients (Beaumont, 1987):

Left neglect

Decreased judgment

Decreased understanding of limitations

Focus on irrelevant information

Decreased sequencing abilities

Decreased attention span

Impulsivity

Sensory deficits

Lability

Lack of midline awareness

Decreased recognition of humor

Decreased recognition of absurdities

Egocentric and demanding behaviors

Confabulation and confusion

Decreased problem solving skills

Decreased organizational skills

Changes in emotions and facial expressions

Writing errors

Reading comprehension problems

Decreased memory

Literal interpretation of information

Visual perceptual deficits

The underlying visual perceptual disturbance common in persons with right hemisphere injury is the phenomenon that sets this patient population apart from any other adult neuro-communication problem. Very often, family members are frankly at a loss when they see a family member neglect the left half of the universe or not recognize the face of a close friend. The sequelae of a right cerebrovascular accident (CVA) are sometimes scary and are never straightforward. There is very little that is "right" with this stroke population.

## Cognitive-Language Disorders Post-Traumatic Brain Injury

The person suffering from a traumatic brain injury may experience a plethora of staggering changes. The amount of change depends on the severity and the location of injury and these changes may be either temporary or permanent. Impairments in physical or cognitive ability, behavior problems, or personality changes may occur. Virtually any function of the brain can be either impaired or left unaffected. Tanner (1987) in his informational guide on TBI discusses a number of sequelae of TBI that have particularly devastating consequences for the patient and family:

Reduced or disordered awareness

Personality changes

The process of normal memory

Attention

Storage

Recall

Anterograde amnesia

Retrograde amnesia

Requirements to learn

Shallowness of emotions

Behavioral problems

Disorientation

Confused language

Stages of recovery

In his "What does it feel like to be brain-damaged?" Linge (1984), a clinical psychologist, who suffered a severe head injury in a motor vehicle accident, provides a consumer perspective on life with TBI. His discussion of coping needs is particularly germane:

> In learning to live with my brain damage, I have found through trial and error, that certain things help greatly and others hinder my coping. In order to learn and retain information best, I try to eliminate as many distractions as possible and concentrate all my energy on the task at hand. A structured routine, well-organized and serene atmosphere at home and as far as possible at work, is vital to me. In the past, I enjoyed a rather chaotic lifestyle, but now I find that I want 'a place for everything and everything in its place.' When remembering is difficult, order and habit make the minutia of daily living much easier.
>
> Coping is also easier in the milieu that is free of emotional tension, competitiveness, anxiety, and pressure. I see all of these as 'distractions' that lessen my ability to learn, just as surely as do noise, chaos, and change in the physical setting. I find it hard to absorb and retain new information in a meeting with people who are new to me and where there is a constant interchange of ideas and personalities. Yet, in a one-to-one situation with a familiar client, or working in my office with colleagues whom I know and trust, in an orderly and systematic fashion, I can retain far more and function far more effectively. In other words, simplification of the external situation, both physical and emotional, assists me to master new information. The more complexity around me, the less able am I to cope. I also find that physical fatigue cuts down my concentration and so I now try to tackle new tasks in the morning, when I am physically fresh. I resort to extensive note-taking on professional matters as well as carefully recording all appointments, financial details and so forth at home. In mastering new information, I go over the subject matter many times, using all possible sensory input channels; reading it, writing it down, repeating it aloud, and having someone re-read it to me. (p. 3)

Linge (1984) provided further insight to TBI by discussing understanding the brain-damaged person and regaining independence. Willer, Allen, Liss, and Zicht (1991) reported on the problems and coping strategies of 20 married men and 11 married women with TBI and their able-bodied spouses. All injured persons experienced severe head injury at least 18 months earlier. Those with TBI and their spouses identified problems in living as most important; loss of employment and restrictions on autonomy were reported as the most problematic. Men with TBI placed priority on controlling their anger, whereas women with TBI were concerned with their mood disorders, particularly depression. Women with TBI and able-bodied wives of men with TBI placed high priority on the use of support groups as a coping strategy. Men placed higher priority on individualistic approaches to adjustment, such as suppression of feelings. Further evidence that men are from Mars and women from Venus.

Kreutzer, Marwitz, and Kepler (1992) found in a review of the literature that family members of injured individuals are typically affected adversely for years after TBI. Increased stress levels, depression, anxiety, and diminished social adjustment have been reported routinely by researchers. Family members' reactions have been most influenced by the behavioral, personality, and emotional characteristics of patients. According to Kreutzer, Marwitz, and Kepler (1992), problems most disturbing to family members have included childishness, lability, adynamia, irritability, and aggression. Reportedly, family adjustment is less influenced by changes in intelligence and communication skills. In a two-year follow-up of 51 caregivers of TBI inpatients, Hall et al. (1994) found that although self-perceived measurements of stress did not increase over time, caregivers reported notable increases in medication and substance use and a decrease in employment and financial status over the two-year period. Clearly, counseling both the person with TBI and the family is a crucial component of a treatment regimen.

## Dementia

Dementia refers to an acquired syndrome characterized by persistent intellectual decline which is due to neurogenic causes (Shekim, 1990). Family members of persons with dementia are faced with an extremely different and difficult challenge than from those disorders described above. Persons with stroke or head injury suffer a sudden brain attack, but then generally proceed on a slow and steady course of recovery. Persons with dementia face a gradual onset followed by a slow and steady decline of intellectual functions. The counseling needs are therefore drastically different. Mace and Rabins (1991) in their classic *The Thirty Six Hour Day* provide a family guide to caring for persons with dementing illnesses and memory loss in later life. The issues discussed are:

Getting help for the impaired person

Characteristic problems of dementia

Problems in independent living

Problems arising in daily care

Medical problems

Problems of behavior

Problems of mood

Arrangements if you become ill

Getting outside help

You and the impaired person as part of a family

How caring for an impaired person affects you

Children and teenagers

Financial and legal issues

Nursing homes and other living arrangements

Brain disorders and causes of dementia

Research in dementia

The book is a treasure trove of useful information for the family member to become an educated consumer and a patient advocate. Family members who become conversant with this material will at the very least have the necessary tools to navigate the shoals of change that inexorably occur within the family coping with dementia. The SLP's role with persons with dementia and the family is threefold: (a) evaluate and conduct a differential diagnosis—dementia or not; (b) retest at medically indicated intervals to monitor change in status, particularly with regard to safety and judgment; and (c) provide counseling and support to the SO and family. Unlike persons with stroke and TBI, owing to the nature of the illness, the person with dementia is unfortunately not typically amenable to counseling, education, and support. For that very reason, family members are even more in need.

## WHENCE COUNSELING IN PERSONS WITH NEUROGENIC COMMUNICATION DISORDERS?

A consumer perspective was threaded throughout this chapter. Several theoretic models that are consonant with the disability model and match the needs of persons with adult neurogenic communication disorders were discussed. It was argued that counseling with this population IS treatment and, therefore, a functional and necessary ingredient to service delivery. A functional assessment is a prerequisite to treatment and therefore counseling. Several functional assessment tools were described as vehicles for eliciting family input and getting the clinical pulse of the patient and the family. Patients who have suffered brain crash and their family members are particularly vulnerable and at risk for a number of emotional problems such as depression, stress, substance abuse, and withdrawal. SLPs were advised of a number of counseling "caveats" and encouraged to request outside consultation when presented with a case that the SLP feels is beyond his or her expertise. In treating the adult population with neurogenic communication disorders, a menu of concerns, questions, and issues were listed for each disability category for the SLP to consider when counseling a given patient. The literature is just beginning to emerge in the area of outcomes research and family counseling. Does a person with aphasia have a more favorable long-term outcome when treatment is combined with regular counseling versus treatment alone? What role does gender play in the counseling dynamic? Cultural diversity? There are a number of variables that have not been controlled in counseling in SLP and the efficacy of SLP counseling efforts cannot be discussed until there is more systematic clinical research on counseling. There are data in the area of consumer satisfaction that complements the efforts of SLPs and speaks very favorably about consumer perception of SLP's professionalism, caring, preparation, advocacy, and service delivery (Rao, 1992b).

REFERENCES

Andrews, J., & Andrews, M. (1990). *Family based treatment in communicative disorders: A systemic approach.* Sandwich, IL: Janelle Publications.

American Speech-Language-Hearing Association. (1993). Preferred practice patterns for the professions of speech-language pathology and audiology. *ASHA, 35*(3), 1–102.

Beaumont. (1987). *Retraining of the right hemisphere: A team effort.* Royal Oak, MI: William Beaumont Hospital (1987).

Burns, M. S., Dong, K. Y., & Oehring, A. K. (1995). Family involvement in the treatment of aphasia. *Topics in Stroke Rehabilitation, 2*(1), 68–77.

Chaikin, J. (1989). Acceptance speech, National Aphasia Association Award, New York.

Christensen, J. M., & Anderson, J. D. (1989). Spouse adjustment to stroke: aphasic versus nonaphasic patients. *Journal of Communication Disorders, 22,* 225–231.

Davis, G. A., & Wilcox, M. J. (1985). *Adult aphasia rehabilitation: Applied pragmatics.* San Diego, CA: College-Hill Press.

Doyle, P., & Holland, A. (1984). Long term survival characteristics in stroke induced aphasia. In R. H. Brookshire (Ed.), *Clinical aphasiology conference proceedings.* Minneapolis, MN: BRK Publishers.

Frattali, C., Thompson, C. K., Holland, A. L., Wohl, C. B., & Ferketic, M. M. (1995). Functional assessment of communication skills for adults. Rockville, MD: American-Speech-Language-Hearing Association.

Hagen, C. (1981). Language disorders secondary to closed head injury: Diagnosis and treatment. *Topics in Language Disorders, 1,* 73–87.

Hall, K. M., Karzmark, P., Stevens, M., Englander, J., O'Hare, P., & Wright, J. (1994). Family stressors in traumatic brain injury: A two year follow-up. *Archives of Physical Medicine and Rehabilitation, 75,* 876–884.

Koppit, A. T. (1978). *Wings.* New York: Hill & Wang.

Kreutzer, J. S., Marwitz, J. H., & Kepler, K. (1992). Traumatic brain injury: Family response and outcome. *Archives of Physical Medicine and Rehabilitation, 73,* 771–778.

Linge, F. R. (1984). *What does it feel like to be brain damaged?* Framingham, MA: National Head Injury Foundation.

Lomas, J., Pickard, L., Bester, S., Elbard, H., Finlayson, A., & Zoghaib, C. (1989). The communicative effectiveness index: Development and psychometric evaluation of a functional communication measure for adult aphasia. *Journal of Speech and Hearing Disorders, 54,* 13–124.

Luterman, D. (1991). *Counseling the communicatively disordered and their families.* Austin, TX: Pro-Ed.

Mace, N. & Rabins, P. (1991). *The thirty six hour day.* Baltimore: Johns Hopkins University Press.

Malone, R. (1969). Expressed attitudes of families of aphasics. *Journal of Speech and Hearing Disorders, 34,* 140–150.

Maslow, A. (1968). *Toward a psychology of being.* New York: Van Nostrand Reinhold.

Medical Rehabilitation Education Foundation. (1993). *Medical rehabilitation: Restoring the quality of life.* Reston, VA: Medical Rehabilitation Education Foundation.

National Rehabilitation Hospital. (1986). Rehabilitation: Closing the gap. *NRH Newsletter,* Spring.

Newhoff, M., Bugbee, J., & Ferriera, A. (1981). A change of PACE: Spouses as treatment targets. In R. H. Brookshire (Ed.), *Clinical aphasiology conference proceedings.* Minneapolis, MN: BRK Publishers.

Rao, P. (1982). *Stroke ancillary programs: Stroke information, family counseling, and stroke club.* Mini-Seminar presented to the annual convention of the American Speech-Language-Hearing Association, San Francisco, CA.

Rao, P. (1992a) De senectute today: An SLP overview of aging in the 1990s. *Hearsay, 7*(2), 18–41.

Rao, P. (1992b). How to keep your customer satisfied: Consumer satisfaction survey. *Hearsay, 7*(1), 34–40.

Rao, P. (1994). Communication disorders. In M. Ozer, R. S. Materson, & L. R. Caplan (Eds.), *Management of persons with stroke.* St. Louis: Mosby.

Rao, P. (1995). Testimony presented to the agency for health care policy and research. *Topics in Stroke Rehabilitation, 2*(1), 80–81.

Sarno, M.T. (1993). Aphasia rehabilitation: Psychosocial and ethical considerations. *Aphasiology, 7*(4), 321–334.

Shekim, L. O. (1990). Dementia. In L. L. LaPointe (Ed.), *Aphasia and related neurogenic language disorders.* New York: Georg Thieme.

Simmons, N. (1990). Conduction aphasia. In L. L. LaPointe (Ed.), *Aphasia and related neurogenic language disorders.* New York: Georg Thieme.

Stone, J., & Alswang, L. (1989). The hidden challenge in counseling. *ASHA, 31,* 27–31.

Tanner, D. C. (1987). *The family's guide to stroke, head trauma and speech disorders.* Tulsa, OK: Modern Education Corporation.

Trieschman, R. (1987). *Aging with a disability.* New York: Demos Publications.

Webster, E. & Newhoff, M. (1981). Intervention with families of communicatively impaired adults. In D. S. Beasley & G. A. Davis (Eds.), *Aging communication processes and disorders.* Orlando, FL: Grune & Stratton.

Wertz, R. T. (1983). A philosophy of aphasia therapy: Some things that patients do not say but that you can see if you listen. *Communicative Disorders, 8*(1),1–17.

Willer, B. S., Allen, K. M., Liss, M., & Zicht, M. S. (1991). Problems and coping strategies of individuals with traumatic brain injury and their spouses. *Archives of Physical Medicine and Rehabilitation, 72,* 460–464.

World Health Organization. (1990). *International classification of impairments, disabilities, and handicaps.* Geneva, Switzerland: World Health Organization.

Ylvisaker, M., & Szekeres, S. F. (1994). Communication disorders associated with closed head injury. In R. Chapey (Ed.), *Language intervention strategies in adult aphasia* (3rd. ed.). Baltimore: Williams & Wilkins.

Yudkovitz, E. (1992). Going beyond where we are now: The need for a relational model in the clinical training of speech-language pathology graduate students. In E. F. Geller & J. J. Koller (Eds.), *Counseling: How to do it? How to teach it?*. Proceedings of the New York State Speech-Language-Hearing Association's Professional Preparation Conference, New York: New York Speech & Hearing Association.

RESOURCES

Alzheimer's Association, 70 East Lake Street, Suite 600, Chicago, IL. 60601; 800–621-0379.

American Heart Association, 7320 Greenville, Ave., Dallas, TX 75231; 214–373-6300.

National Aphasia Association, P.O. Box 1887, Murray Hill Station, New York, NY 10156–0611; 212–255-4329.

National Head Injury Foundation, 1140 Connecticut Ave., Suite 812, Washington, D.C. 20036; 800–444-6443.

National Stroke Association, 300 East Hampden Ave., Suite 240, Englewood, CO 80110–2622; 303–762-9922.

## Appendix 11.1: Rehabilitation: Closing the Gap

Superman leaps tall buildings in a single bound and Wonder Woman travels the skies at will, but the rest of us mere mortals must depend on stairs, elevators, airplanes, and a variety of other "assistive devices" to help us cope with environmental barriers.

Imagine an index of 0 to 100, from total dependence to total independence. Superman or Wonder Woman function at 100, and the person who functions at 0 is dead. Most of us fall between these two extremes and depend on various environmental supports (e.g., cars, escalators, eyeglasses, and so forth). Superman and Wonder Woman, of course, do not need any of these supports, and physically disabled individuals needs more of them to close the gap between their level of functioning and the level of environmental support

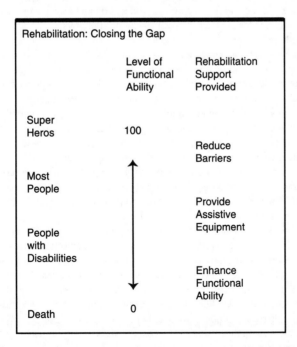

**Figure 11.A1.** Rehabilitation: Closing the gap. Illustrates the continuum from Ability to Disability to Inability. Also outlines strategies to "close" the rehabilitation gap. Adapted from *Newsletter of National Rehabilitation Hospital (NRH)* (1986). p.1. Reprinted with permission.

provided. There are three ways in which the gap can be narrowed (National Rehabilitation Hospital, 1986):

- Enhance the functional capacity of the disabled person through services such as occupational and physical therapy.

- Reduce the demands of the environment (wider doorways, ramps, elevators).

- Provide assistive devices (e.g., computerized wheelchairs, braces, artificial limbs, and so forth) to bridge the gap between the person's abilities and the environment.

The goal of rehabilitation is to remove as many barriers as possible, both physical and attitudinal, to help disabled people achieve maximal independence.

## Appendix 11.2:  Preparing for the Future of Poststroke Rehabilitation

The Agency for Health Care Policy and Research has as its mission to promote improvement in clinical practice and patient outcomes through more appropriate and effective healthcare services; to engender improvements in the financing, organization, and delivery of healthcare services; and to increase access to quality care. On June 12, 1992 its expert panel held a hearing on clinical practice guidelines on poststroke rehabilitation. The only consumer (person with stroke) to address the panel was C.R., whose poignant and prophetic testimony was as follows:

> My name is C.R. I am 37-years old and had a stroke in June of 1991, which left me with a right-sided paralysis and severe aphasia. I am here today during National Aphasia Awareness Week to talk about stroke after the fact, particularly for those folks with aphasia who might be unable to talk. The National Aphasia Association has asked me to talk to you about my stroke and continued recovery nearly one year later. Last year I could not say a word. Today, I'd like to say a word about stroke.
>
> The biggest problems for me after the stroke were not the physical, but the stroke's impact on me and my family, on me and my friends, on me and my job—it struck all of us and I'm still "recoiling." Stroke actually is a life-long recoiling, not a couple of weeks, or months, or years—a lifetime of recoiling with my family, friends, and co-workers. Everyday, I am trying to realign my relationship with all comers—my wife, my two boys, my friends, my employer. I will try to outline for you three of the major problems that have happened to me this past year and what I have learned from these experiences.
>
> First, the emotional and psychological toll stroke takes on me and my family is even more devastating than the financial toll. The fear, the anxiety, the anger, all weigh heavily in the equation of rehabilitation. The necessary support, understanding, and therapy is at best uneven for many people with stroke. United, we tell all, that this is a major concern—life daily requires persons with stroke to pay a penalty because of their handicap. Some stroke persons have more resources (rehabilitation team, family, community) than others. Policy must recognize these areas of need and not limit or ration therapy to weeks or months. Policy must regard potential for quality of life and the ripple effect this will have on the family and the community at large.
>
> The second problem was work re-entry. I am in my 30s and I want to work. As I see it, the person with stroke has four options: he can return to his old job; he can return to his old company in a different job; he can start a whole new job; or he can't or won't work. None of these options are easy or attractive. All except the latter may come after much work, money, and frustration have been expended. It seems that many roadblocks are in my way to becoming a gainfully employed taxpayer again. The Americans with Disabilities Act is not a solution but a tool. There must be a safety net that we can cling to in this regard. Hope is my only hope.
>
> The third problem is financial shock. The costs of stroke can be said to be the cause of another stroke. They are very high in terms of direct costs (healthcare dollars) and in terms of indirect cost (my not working). Typically, a stroke survivor does not have the financial resources to go it alone. To recoil from the stroke, government must provide additional spring—to cushion our fall and push us back into the mainstream. I'm told that a dollar spent on rehab saves $9.00. We must afford to invest

in the potential of 2 million stroke survivors—a million of whom have aphasia. The U.S. policy must be to strike back at stroke by supporting its survivors and preventing such a trauma from happening to others. Thank you for considering my testimony.

C.R. has not only returned to work, but as a result of his testimony, it is hoped he has helped to return the discussion of the clinical practice of poststroke rehabilitation to one with a face, a heart, and a vision. C.R. and his remarkable continuing recovery of his communication skills is certainly testimony to the resilience of the human spirit and the effectiveness of rehabilitation today.

Postscript: C.R. turns 40 next month. He has now been back to work full time as a customer service airline agent for nearly two years. His performance appraisals have been outstanding—he has resumed his leadership role in a complex and stressful work environment. He drives, parents, works, loves, and plays with renewed vigor. He has resumed his avocational loves, boating and golfing, with adapted equipment and attitude (Rao, 1995). (p. 80–81)

---

## Appendix 11.3: Suggestions to Aphasic Patients and Their Families

Prophylaxis: Includes all procedures that prevent development of maladaptive attitudes and response as the patient tries to come to grips with his or her altered abilities.

Procedures and Goals In Prophylaxis

Patient Counseling

1. Must understand what is wrong with his or her behavior.
2. Must understand what own future is.
3. Must understand treatment procedures and their rationale.
4. Must understand the difference between medical and nonmedical treatment.
5. Must understand the inevitability of "good times" and "bad times."
6. Must understand that time, if properly used, is the strongest ally.
7. Must learn to recognize productive and nonproductive attempts to cope.
8. Must learn to recognize and manage potentially dangerous influences on personal behavior.
9. Must prepare for independence, for an end to treatment.

Family Counseling

1. Must understand what is wrong with the patient, what can be done about it, and what the future holds.
2. Must learn patience.
3. Must learn to recognize when the patient's attempt is or promises to be successful.
4. Must learn a hierarchy of cues for helping the patient while preserving his or her independence.

Adapted from Wertz, R. T. (1983). A philosophy of aphasia therapy: Some things that patients do not say but that you can see if you listen. In R. T. Wertz (Ed.), *Communicative disorders, Vol 7, 1,* 6–8. Copyright 1983 by Grune & Stratton, Inc. Reprinted by permission.

# 12. Cleft Palate and Other Craniofacial Disorders

Betty Jane McWilliams

---

---

Successful treatment of the multiple and interactive problems associated with the various forms of cleft lip and palate and other orofacial and craniofacial anomalies depends on carefully organized interdisciplinary management teams, which include the patient and family. This was recognized by the Surgeon General of the United States (Koop, 1987) when he declared the need for (*a*) parent- professional collaboration; (*b*) providing parents with accurate and complete information; (*c*) making emotional and financial support available; (*d*) being sensitive to cultural attributes; (*e*) encouraging parent-to-parent support programs; (*f*) including the developmental needs of babies, children, and adolescents; (*g*) ensuring comprehensive care that includes appropriate social, emotional, and cognitive elements; and (*h*) carrying out treatment in interdisciplinary settings.

Using the Surgeon General's statement as a springboard, the American Cleft Palate-Craniofacial Association (ACPA) developed a document entitled *Parameters for Evaluation and Treatment of Patients with Cleft Lip/Palate or Other Craniofacial Anomalies* (ACPA, 1993). In the introduction, ten basic principles are stated. They include: (*a*) team management by (*b*) teams with adequate numbers of patients; (*c*) early initial evaluations; (*d*) attention to family adjustment; (*e*) provision of information to family and patients; (*f*) encouraging their participation in treatment planning; (*g*) executing treatment at convenient locations with complex diagnostic and surgical procedures restricted to major centers; (*h*) sensitivity to family characteristics that affect team-patient dynamics; (*i*) longitudinal assessment of patients and long-term outcome evaluations that (*j*) take into account both physical and psychosocial well-being.

The importance of counseling is explicit in four of these basic principles and implicit in the other six. Broder and Richman (1987), however, indicate that only 29 percent of the teams they surveyed screen developmental skills and that less than half of patients with clefts receive mental-health services. The result is that everyone on the team participates in this process with the primary responsibility often falling to the speech-language pathologist.

## PHILOSOPHY OF COUNSELING

This chapter is based on the philosophy that *all* clinical encounters involve counseling and that patient and family requirements for counseling are developmentally based (Speltz, Greenberg, Endriga & Galbreath, 1994), change over time, and are interactive from one developmental stage to another; and that there are no generalized formulas that can be applied equally to everyone. It is important to make no assumptions about counseling needs in specific cases (Pruzinsky, 1992) and to understand and reinforce patient and parent strengths as well as to modify weaknesses.

Counseling, in this philosophic context, includes the four major functions suggested by Webster (1977). These principles apply equally to counseling with patients. They are: (*a*) receiving and (*b*) giving information; (*c*) helping to clarify ideas, attitudes, and emotions; and (*d*) helping in the acquisition of new behaviors.

To perform these functions, the clinician must interact with patients and families in an atmosphere of mutual trust; must be sensitive and responsive to the cultural and developmental influences in all counseling encounters; be capable of "listening with the third ear" (Reik, 1948) to detect and understand the covert messages contained in overt content; be supportive without being judgmental; understand when to introduce specific information; and be open to seeking the assistance of others.

This approach assumes that the clinician is thoroughly grounded in human development, qualified to manage craniofacial problems, well trained and experienced, and intimately related to the responsible treatment team. Unfortunately, not all professional people and not all teams meet these criteria (Sidman, 1995).

The philosophy of counseling emphasized in this chapter leads to a natural organization of topics starting with the overall concerns of parents and moving into the problems associated with the prenatal period, infancy, early childhood, school age, teen years, and adulthood. In each category, discussion focuses on both parents and children, and various approaches to counseling are presented. Having said that, it is important that readers understand at the outset that, as in most systems of counseling, there is no sound theoretical foundation on which to build (Bennett & Stanton, 1993). Rather, empirical evidence, clinical experience, and clinical studies provide the support on which clinicians must rely.

## OVERALL CONCERNS

Interest in counseling is not a new feature in clinical care. As early as 1943, the University of Michigan published *The Child with a Cleft Palate* with Ollie Backus, a speech pathologist, as senior author (Backus, Clancy, Henry, & Kemper, 1943). Eugene McDonald, also a speech pathologist, wrote *Bright Promise* (McDonald, 1959) and *Understand Those Feelings*, which was described as a "guide for parents of handicapped children and everyone who counsels them" (McDonald, 1962). Although vocabulary, modes of treatment, and outcome have changed and improved over the years, parents remain much the same.

A number of older studies continue to provide valuable insights into the expressed concerns of parents. Weachter (1959) asked parents to list their major sources of worry.

Appearance ranked first, followed by (2) immediacy of surgery, (3) speech, (4) feeding, (5) reactions of the other parent, (6) responses of brothers and sisters, (7) reactions of family and friends, (8) mental development, (9) finances, and (10) the possibility of recurrence in future children. These concerns are still encountered, and most are addressed in three publications of the Cleft Palate Foundation (1987, 1989, 1992). Based on clinical experience, it is clear that parents also worry about what caused the cleft or other anomaly, what if anything they did wrong, the effects of hearing loss, and how their child will be accepted by peers. Because needs change with time and are not the same for all mothers and fathers, it is important to incorporate work with parents into the treatment plan so that it becomes an ongoing part of the child's care.

Parents often want information that they either have not been given or have not completely understood. Pannbacker and Scheuerle (1993) reported that over 90 percent of parents surveyed believed that they understood "a lot" about treatment, but 79 percent wanted more information. Communication between clinicians and parents remains a serious problem.

Poorly informed parents who do not understand the treatment program often do not comply fully with clinical recommendations, and this leads to less than ideal results for their children. Barriers to successful communication and the inability to integrate information also include feelings about the treatment team, whether positive or negative. Sometimes, positive feelings make parents or patients reluctant to express disagreement or concern about recommendations made by professional people whom they admire and respect. Negative attitudes, on the other hand, may lead to lack of confidence in the treatment plan and the inability to accept and comply with its demands. Also affecting treatment are underlying fear and unresolved conflicts about the potential dangers of treatment; the availability of resources; cultural differences between parents and care givers; acceptance of the child and his or her condition in relationship to treatment; or dysfunction within the marriage or family unit, often unrelated to but exacerbated by the cleft.

This array of possibilities points again to the need to work with parents so that they become an integral part of the treatment team and of the decision-making process. Otherwise, they may feel a significant loss of power and the real threat of external controls in their lives (Aspinall, 1995). Pannbacker and Scheurele (1993) reported that 91 percent of the 75 parents they surveyed indicated that they were participating in treatment decisions, but 36 percent wished for more participation. Careful listening to parents and responding to their concerns are essential parts of effective counseling.

Parents who are able to function as a part of the team are influential in extending their positive attitudes to their children, who, as they mature from infancy to adulthood, assume an increasing role in their own care. This outcome is possible only when enduring relationships are established between parents and care givers. That is a major function of effective counseling with ever-changing goals based on individual requirements.

The *probable* counseling needs that emerge as children with these birth anomalies develop will now be discussed.

## PRENATAL PERIOD

A new aspect of counseling for cleft palate-craniofacial teams results from the ability, in some cases, to diagnose facial malformations before the birth of the child. This early recognition of the defect presents both management and ethical dilemmas; and there is not professional unity about how these issues should be handled. Although intrauterine surgery is fast becoming a possibility, it is not yet a viable option in most cases. Thus, parents who learn that their unborn baby has a congenital defect may experience great emotional upheaval, and counseling is the only readily available source of assistance before the child's birth.

Clinical experience suggests that the basic stability of the mother and father plays a major role in their ability to seek the support they need and to plan ahead for the birth and care of their baby. This planning can result in trips to the library to read about the condition and in visits to and interviews with different teams and team members. This search may be reasonable and well thought out, or it may be frenetic and so desperate that the outcome is one of anger, confusion, and the inability to make use of the aid that is available.

Ideally, parents in this situation have an opportunity to sit in one-to-one sessions with a counselor who listens to their concerns and allows them to express their feelings. This sensitive situation requires the counselor to be compassionate and comforting and capable of reflecting on and interpreting both verbal and nonverbal cues. Direct questions are answered fully and honestly, but the highest priority is helping the parents over their initial pain so that they can act rationally and be supportive to each other. If there is guilt or assigned blame, that must be dealt with. Although the speech-language pathologist may successfully function in this regard, these problems may go well beyond his or her skills and require the services of a social worker, psychologist, or psychiatrist experienced in craniofacial problems. In some cases, referral for marriage counseling may be a wise choice.

As the parents are able to move away from their initial shock and grief, the counseling goal can be expanded to helping them ask substantive questions, begin to plan for their child's treatment, understand how care is delivered by the team, and acquire the knowledge and skills they will need after the baby is born. At this point, it is often useful for the parents to meet and become acquainted with the various team members so that they can ask more detailed questions of the different specialists. This is also a good time to introduce parent-to-parent contacts and to have the parents visit a clinic where they can meet children who have had treatment for similar birth defects.

For some parents, it is helpful to know that there are organizations concerned about them and their baby's well-being. While this applies to all patients and parents, the subject is introduced here because such information may be especially beneficial to parents who learn about their child's diagnosis prenatally. The packet of reading materials available free through the Cleft Palate Foundation (1218 Grandview Avenue, Pittsburgh, PA 15211) or by calling their Cleft Line (1–800-24-CLEFT) has been well received and deeply appreciated by both professional people and parents. After all, if an organization is devoted to problems associated with craniofacial malformations and publishes information about them, there must be others with similar concerns. This knowledge helps to alleviate parents' initial sense of loneliness and isolation.

Another source for parents (and patients as well) is AboutFace, a support and information network concerned with facial differences (P.O. BOX 93, Limekiln, PA 19535; 1–800-225–3223). This organization publishes a newsletter and sponsors an annual meeting for parents and patients in conjunction with the annual professional meeting of ACPA. Parents and patients participate in all aspects of the program.

Many communities have local support groups that are attractive to some parents, while others either are not ready for such participation or prefer to seek support through other mechanisms.

If programs of the type described here are to work, there must be ongoing and consistent coordination. The speech-language pathologist is often the person on the team to provide that structure.

## INFANCY

The birth of a child with a visible impairment presents immediate problems and has over-whelming ramifications in the lives of the parents and family. Most parents experience shock, disappointment, sadness, and, sometimes, guilt and must go through the grieving process as they come to terms with the reality of their child's life situation (Tisza & Gumpertz, 1962). We cannot predict the exact nature of these parental responses. Some parents are devastated, frightened, hopeless, and thrown into major crises, whereas others feel grief and shock but remain in control and are able to deal with their feelings with strength and compassion for their child. In short, parents bring to this experience all the strengths and weaknesses that make up their unique personalities, and they call on their previously used coping mechanisms to face this demanding situation (McWilliams, 1982; Mcwilliams, Morris, & Shelton, 1990).

The extent of the child's deformity is a factor in this process. These malformations vary in severity, and the newborn's "attractiveness" index is negatively affected as the facial dis-figurement increases (Slade, Bishop, & Jowett, 1995). However, there is not a one-to-one relationship between severity and parental distress. Very mild problems are sometimes ac-companied by high, unremitting anxiety brought about by other factors such as generally poor coping skills, prior marital problems, low self-esteem, guilt over past "sins," cultural influences, an unwanted infant, or a complicated amalgamation of these conditions. In the absence of these added stresses, parents of a more profoundly involved child may do much better.

Regardless of individual capacities for handling stress, most parents, in these early days, want and need assistance from a competent professional person early on. Early counseling is crucial; it helps the counselor, often the speech-language pathologist, learn the real needs of the parents. The earlier the parents are told about the anomaly or anom-alies and given an opportunity for discussion, the more quickly are they likely to accept the situation and to bond with their infant, who is remarkably different from the perfect child they had dreamed of. Early acceptance is not without difficulty for many parents (Brantly & Clifford, 1979; Clifford, 1969); and counseling in this regard has face validity if no real laboratory evidence of its effectiveness. It appears, however, that the way in which this early intervention is carried out has an impact on the parents' later feelings and on the ef-fectiveness with which they respond to their newborn (Spriestersbach, 1973). Speltz, Mor-ton, Goodell, and Clarren (1994) point out that the development of these important at-tachments in infancy may, in part, determine the nature of the child's psychological adjustment in later years. That view has long been held in the child-development and psy-chiatric literature.

The ideal counselor is compassionate but also matter of fact and optimistic without making promises that cannot be kept. For example, assuring parents that there will be no lip scar after surgery is always dishonest and unrealistic. The counselor must also be pre-pared to deal with the parents' specific questions as truthfully and honestly as possible and to refrain from overwhelming them with information that they may not be ready to hear or that is not relevant to this stage of their child's life.

It is desirable to see new parents several times in the first days after the baby's birth and to introduce another parent or parents who have successfully coped with similar prob-lems. Speech-language pathologists often join other professional team members as they provide training for parents to do this important work (Irwin & McWilliams, 1973).

Both professional and parent-to-parent counseling sessions are provided in order that new parents may gain a sense of support, seek answers to their most urgent questions, and begin to find solutions to the sometimes frightening events of this newborn period. It is crucial to realize that the counselor's ideal agenda may not coincide with the parents' needs at any particular time. It is for this reason that the counselor begins by listening.

Major considerations in these early days include bonding, other possible congenital abnormalities, feeding disturbances, ear disease, planning and executing surgical correction of the defect, and speech and language development. These matters must be addressed in order to ensure the infant a strong start in life and the parents the greatest security.

## Bonding

Of particular importance during the neonatal period are concerns about bonding or building the strong parent-infant attachments referred to above. This process begins at birth and can be enhanced by early intervention. It is especially helpful if the counselor, whether professional or parent, demonstrates positive responses to the new baby. Holding and looking at the infant while engaging in gentle talking and cuddling are encouraged as is commenting on the child's other features. This helps the parents see beyond the facial disfigurement and respond to their *baby* rather than to the birth defect. Encouraging parents to look at and appreciate their baby early on may lay the foundation for strong, positive parent-child relationships and prevent the kind of interaction described by Field and Vega-Lahr (1984) in which mothers of children with craniofacial defects smiled at and vocalized to their infants less frequently than did mothers of unimpaired babies. This seemed to result in reduced responsiveness from the children and, in turn, in less maternal imitative behavior and game playing. These breaks in the communication circuit represent a disruption that may never be overcome and that helps to explain later reductions in verbal output (Morris, 1962). The goal of counseling is to prevent this negative outcome.

Responsiveness to the infant also builds a bridge and helps the parents begin to deal with their fears about what other people will think. These anxieties are real and often reflect deeply entrenched cultural attitudes. For some parents with poor self images, a baby with a flaw is one more evidence that one or both of them never get anything right. The counselor, in these early encounters, can often pick up information helpful in later counseling sessions. Most importantly, however, the counselor's own acceptance and appreciation of the infant can help the parents realize that not everyone will have negative feelings about them and their newborn.

## Other Congenital Abnormalities

Children with clefts are at increased risk for other congenital abnormalities. This is especially true of infants with clefts of the palate only, well over half of whom are likely to have associated malformations or developmental deficits (McWilliams & Matthews, 1979; McWilliams et al., 1990). Of notable importance to speech-language pathologists are the data indicating that 76 percent of children with velopharyngeal insufficiency in the absence of palatal clefts have additional congenital anomalies (Jones, 1988). Many of these associated abnormalities include syndromes, some of which have major implications for future offspring (Jones, 1988; Jung, 1989; Siegel-Sadewitz & Shprintzen, 1982; Sparks, 1984; Witzel, 1983). By 1990, Cohen (1991) had identified 342 syndromes associated with clefting; and the number increases almost daily. Genetic counseling is a primary requirement in these cases.

While some of the additional anomalies may be mild, others may be life-threatening and take precedence over the cleft or other craniofacial defects (McWilliams et al., 1990). Thus, thorough pediatric and genetic evaluations and careful follow-along thereafter are essential for all infants with clefts. If other congenital defects are diagnosed, the appropriate counseling must be provided. The speech-language pathologist participates in the planning and execution of that aspect of care but usually does not carry it out independently.

It is stressed here that the counselor refrains from spreading before parents all the possibilities for additional abnormalities and related problems that may exist but, instead, quietly emphasizes the importance of good pediatric care for all children and takes steps to see that it is readily available. Counseling is then directed toward helping the parents cope with the situation as it exists rather than toward theoretical issues that may not apply to a specific case.

## Feeding

Babies with palatal clefts almost invariably experience feeding problems springing from the inability to impound intraoral pressure even though the sucking reflex is usually intact. The feeding difficulty is directly related to the lack of separation between the oral and nasal cavities. This is such a common problem that the Cleft Palate Foundation has published a booklet for parents entitled *Feeding an Infant with a Cleft* (Cleft Palate Foundation, 1992). It is important that parents understand that these feeding problems are usually the result of a mechanical failure and are not because of poor parenting. The best counseling in this connection is to demonstrate and teach the parents how to feed the baby as simply and normally as possible. This can often be accomplished quickly and without resorting to special equipment that calls attention to itself. The system recommended here is showing the parents how to hold the infant in a sitting position, using a cross-cut nipple rather than one with an enlarged hole that delivers the liquid too rapidly, and introducing a soft plastic bottle to which pressure can be gently applied to assist the baby in extracting the formula. The nipple should not be too short or so long that it stimulates gagging. It is usually necessary to experiment with positioning the nipple in the oral cavity in order to find the most efficient and comfortable place, often along the intact side of the palate.

Paradise and McWilliams (1974) have shown that, without feeding assistance, babies gain weight very slowly. With feeding instruction for the parents, weight gain assumes a more nearly normal profile but is likely to remain somewhat behind that of children who do not have clefts (Seth & McWilliams, 1988).

Successful feeding removes one important source of parental anxiety and makes mothers and fathers more confident of their parenting skills, freeing them to relate to their child in a more relaxed way. They are then able to make the soft, cooing, soothing sounds that are a normal part of infant feeding and that enhance bonding and stimulate early communicative development. The baby, in turn, no longer underfed and miserable, becomes more responsive to the parents' efforts to provide nurture and comfort. This type of counseling is educational in nature and is based on teaching skills and giving information so that parents can be effective in helping their baby with a difficult task. The success experienced by both the infant and the parents is likely to have positive effects on parental perceptions of the child and on themselves as "good" parents.

The educational approach to feeding is usually, but not always, successful. Some babies, particularly those with clefts of the palate only or in association with other congenital anomalies, may be more difficult to manage, and it may take longer to resolve their feeding problems. For some, more aggressive management, including nasogastric tubes, may be necessary. Parents require both professional and parent-to-parent support under these circumstances. It is always helpful to follow such babies closely to be sure that they get the required nourishment and that their parents do not have to resort to trial-and-error experiments. Such parents are in need of a good listener so that they can express their anxieties, have help in trying alternative feeding methods, receive reassurance when appropriate, and find compassion and support in facing the often painful realities about the severity of their child's condition.

A few infants fail to thrive because of poor nurture. Their parents require active intervention from the team and may need ongoing counseling with mental-health specialists. The speech-language pathologist can be a part of this effort but is only rarely equipped to serve as the primary counselor.

The issue of feeding is intensified for mothers who are eager to breast-feed, a difficult procedure in the presence of a cleft palate or other major deformities of the oral structures. However, given high motivation and determination, a few mothers breast-feed successfully, particularly if the baby has only a minor defect. Counseling is important in this regard as is careful documentation of the baby's weight gain. Some mothers have found the La Leche League to be helpful even though their feeding system is complex and time-consuming. Still other mothers are able to accept feeding breast milk by bottle. Such a compromise requires discussion and resolution of any conflicts that the mother may have about sacrificing this special closeness with her baby.

Feeding problems can be overwhelming and frightening to parents with the result that they may be tense and unspontaneous with their baby. Fortunately, with adequate help in the neonatal period, most parents and babies come through this crisis successfully and with no permanent repercussions.

## Ear Disease

There is general agreement that infants with palatal clefts have almost universal ear disease at birth (Stool & Randall, 1967; Paradise, Bluestone, & Felder, 1969). The ear disease is associated with mild conductive hearing losses and, if untreated, with more serious and complex losses. The evidence is that infants who are fed breast milk experience fewer episodes of otitis media than do babies fed formulas (Paradise, Elster, & Tan, 1994). This is important information for parents and suggests that counseling providing accurate and complete detail about the whole issue of ear disease and its treatment is essential.

The importance of compliance with the prescribed treatment program cannot be overemphasized. The speech-language pathologist is particularly concerned that treatment proceed on schedule because of the evidence that untreated ear disease may lead to a reduction in articulation skills by age six (Hubbard, Paradise, McWilliams, Elster, & Taylor, 1985) and to more serious language deficits if the loss escalates. The speech-language pathologist collaborates closely with the audiologist, pediatrician, and otolaryngologist in an effort to treat and control otitis media and to follow the baby longitudinally.

## Planning and Executing Surgery

Among the first questions that parents raise is whether or not the condition can be corrected. Underlying that question is usually the unexpressed wish to be told that all traces of the defect can be eliminated. Unfortunately, that reassurance can never be given. Although the entire team is involved at this stage, the surgeon usually has the primary responsibility for interpreting the recommendations, establishing the timing of surgical procedures, and explaining the details of the surgery and its aftermath. It may be the speech-language pathologist, however, who sees the parents on a regular basis and helps them with the many issues that arise and about which they need clarification and support.

It is important to realize that parents both want and dread surgery for their infant. They look forward to having the defect "fixed" but may be frightened that the child might die in the process or, in some way, be seriously damaged. They may fear feeding the baby after surgery, and they often have trouble accepting hospitalization. A few parents are so immobilized by their anxieties that they refuse to permit the surgery at all. Counseling about surgery may proceed on a one-to-one basis or in a group led by a well-informed speech-language pathologist. In either case, having the back-up assistance of parents who have been through the surgical experience with their own children can be helpful and is encouraged.

Another type of intervention that some counselors, including speech-language pathologists, use regularly is being available to parents during the actual surgery. Sitting quietly with them can mean the difference between an agonizing experience and one that is less traumatic. Again, the presence of another parent can be an added source of assistance. It should be understood, however, that the wishes of the parents are to be honored. Not everyone wants others present at this crucial time. That is one of the reasons that parent-to-parent intervention must be carefully monitored.

Parents have different counseling needs depending on the age of their baby when the surgery occurs. Lip repair is usually accomplished by three months of age and primary palatal repair some time prior to 18 months. Surgery is easier for a younger than an older child, and the parents have fewer difficulties with their infant than with their toddler, who experiences separation anxieties and fear of strange places. Fortunately, one or both parents can often stay with the child; and the period of hospitalization, while it varies, is relatively short.

The speech-language pathologist who serves a counseling role has a responsibility to explore with the parents their understanding of postoperative care. Although this care is usually not very complicated, the potential for misunderstanding is mammoth. An example of this is a five-year-old boy who ate nothing but baby food because the parents did not understand the instruction to keep him on a soft diet following surgery. Careful work with the parents prior to and immediately after surgery and routine evaluation of the child as he developed could have avoided what was an unnecessary major developmental deficit with repercussions in nutrition, speech production, and emotional well-being.

## Speech and Language Development

Some speech-language pathologists take the position that information about speech and language development and the possible effects of clefts or other craniofacial malformations should be introduced early in the child's life. One father, who has since published many research studies related to clefts, remembers that "everyone" wanted to talk about speech at a time when he and the baby's mother had many other more immediate concerns and saw speech as something well in the future.

Our view is that it is best not to raise issues that may not turn out to be matters of consequence for the approximately 75 percent of cleft children who do not develop permanent, significant speech problems (McWilliams, 1990). Rather, if the parents themselves raise questions about speech, discussion is appropriate; and they should be provided with whatever information is necessary to address their concerns. If, on the other hand, the issue is not raised, it may be best to avoid creating added anxieties and, instead, follow the infant closely and "gently guide the parents to be good language and speech stimulators" in a communicatively positive environment (McWilliams et al., 1990). This approach avoids the hazards of sounding what may be an unnecessary alarm. At the same time, it provides the surveillance necessary to ensure that the parents suffer no unpleasant shocks later on and that the child gets attention as indicated. Either method, wisely applied, is acceptable; and both point to the wisdom of the speech-language pathologist's early involvement with parents and child.

Readers who believe in intervening early with counseling and teaching parents to engage in prescribed speech activities may want to explore the work of Brookshire, Lynch, and Fox (1980); Hahn (1979); Lynch (1986); and Philips (1979, 1990).

## Approaches to Counseling in Infancy

During early infancy, the emphasis is on one-to-one encounters between parents and counselor, along with introducing parent-to-parent counseling aides. In addition, some parents want to read about their child's condition and will do so with varying degrees of success depending on the nature of the materials to which they have access and the extent to which they coincide with the child's particular set of problems and the treatment program that is in place. The educational status of the parents and the reading levels of the materials will also be factors. It is assumed that the counselor will recommend appropriate publications to interested parents and will be willing to discuss with them what they have read.

Parents who read independently may experience confusion and anxiety about what is best for their child. For instance, some clinicians recommend surgical repair of the lip and palate immediately after birth. Others prefer to wait for varying amounts of time thereafter. Surgeons usually prefer one operation over another, and the literature reflects the disagreement that abounds. Parents have limited backgrounds with which to assess the various positions and can easily become embroiled in uncertainty and find themselves in conflict with the treatment team. They may even travel hundreds of miles to get what they have concluded, perhaps erroneously, is the best treatment available in the world. Under these circumstances, parents require discussion with other team members. The counselor plays an important part in seeing that they get this additional assistance. Again, it is often the speech-language pathologist who assumes the coordinating role.

Later in infancy, after the acute anxieties associated with the birth, feeding, and provision of care have been alleviated and the baby is making progress, the task becomes one of following the infant's development, seeing that the parents are involved in the treatment program so that they are rigorous about keeping appointments, alerting the mother and father and the other team members to new clinical needs should they arise, and providing additional clinical services as they are indicated.

This is a time when an organized telephone counseling system can be helpful. Regular telephone calls to the family and encouraging them to call if they have questions are inexpensive, convenient, and effective means of maintaining a connection with parents between clinical visits.

As questions of child management arise, as they almost inevitably do, the speech-language pathologist has an opportunity to encourage discussion that sometimes provides crucial information and can lead to positive alterations in behavior. An example of this is an infant whose mother kept his face covered when she had him out in a stroller because she so feared the negative reactions of other people. Talking about those fears and helping her develop strategies for answering questions about his condition soon led her to realize that she could safely treat her baby as she would any other child, and she herself became more comfortable and relaxed when she did so. The baby was literally given eyes to see as a source of sensory deprivation was removed.

Bringing mothers, fathers, or both together with their babies in small groups is another approach that is often useful. The parents profit from meeting each other, engaging in both informal and directed conversations, and playing with their babies in ways suggested by the counselor and the parents themselves. Language and speech stimulation can occur in these play sessions so that indirectly the parents are taught new skills.

Although some parents require few or none of these activities, giving them the opportunity to participate is supportive and reinforces their awareness of the availability of assistance and of the interest of the professional team.

## EARLY CHILDHOOD

As the child matures and becomes more independent, the concerns of parents change. Problems of management and of child rearing may intensify. Questions about preparing this older child for hospitalization and surgery become important; developmental issues may be more apparent; expanding the child's world and helping in the transition from a restricted to a broader environment are necessary; and monitoring and sometimes assisting in the development of language and speech are crucial during this period.

When a child is developing well, it is important that the parents understand that and that they be reinforced for their positive role in their child's life. However, they still need to know that monitoring will continue to avoid hazards such as changes in the condition of the ears or in speech and language development that may require attention. They must also be reassured that they can expect to have help with any future concerns they may have.

If the child is experiencing developmental delays, language or speech problems, or disruptions in emotional well-being, the counselor's task is more complex; and additional sessions with parents and child will undoubtedly have to occur. This significant aspect of counseling is discussed in detail in a later section.

### Hospitalization and Surgery

A child old enough to recognize a threat to his or her person and to be frightened by the environment of the hospital but too young to understand or remember explanations can easily be traumatized by going to the hospital, undergoing surgery, and waking up in a strange place. Even though it is probable that the child has had previous surgery earlier in infancy parents are also likely to be uncomfortable. Yet, they play a sensitive role in easing their young child's burden. Parents who are effective in this regard are relaxed and confident and are able to communicate those attitudes to their child.

To ensure that sense of security, it is necessary that the mother and father have a clear understanding of what will happen before, during, and after the surgery and that they are informed ahead of time about such things as appearance and possible discomfort or other signs of distress. The plastic surgeon usually provides such information; and the speech-language pathologist serving in a counseling role follows up to be sure the parents understand what they have heard and that their subsequent questions are answered.

It is important, as always, for the counselor to listen carefully to what the parents say and to help them maximize their strengths and minimize their weaknesses. In allaying their anxieties, it is necessary to be realistic and to recognize that all surgery has some risk, even though today it is negligible. There can, however, be complications. Thus, it is not possible to assure parents that there will be a perfect outcome (McWilliams et al., 1990).

Most parents are neither overly optimistic nor overly pessimistic but fall between the extremes. They respond positively to talks with other parents who have already gone through similar surgical procedures with children in this age group, conferences with hospital staff, and help in arranging for one or both parents to stay with the child and to assist with feeding in an effort to minimize separation anxiety for both parents and child. Other ways to reduce trauma for the child may include, among other things, providing a favorite soft toy and much loved books, quiet talking, holding the child's hand, having a simple but pleasant surprise after the surgery, and anticipating going home. These techniques can be used as illustrations to stimulate the parents to develop their own ideas. As with infants, the speech-language pathologist will sometimes want to be with the parents during the surgery or, in some cases, arrange for the presence of an experienced parent.

After the child goes home, a telephone call to see how everyone is getting along brings some closure to the hospital events and also permits the parents to ask for additional help should they want it.

## Managing Developmental Deficits

As noted earlier, when developmental deficits are present, parents usually require special counseling. This is a major aspect of care because approximately 25 percent of children born with some form of clefting have concomitant developmental problems. Strauss and Broder (1993) found that 10.1 percent of their sample of 553 subjects with clefts of the lip and/or palate had various degrees of mental retardation, most commonly moderate in nature, whereas 13.9 percent had documented learning disabilities. These disorders occur across all classifications of clefts but are most prevalent in association with cleft palate alone, often accompanied by other anomalies or syndromes (McWilliams & Matthews, 1979; Strauss & Broder, 1993). In these cases, counseling cannot be focused on the cleft and other facial attributes to the exclusion of the often more far-reaching developmental differences. The speech-language pathologist cannot be effective in working with parents without the help of other developmental specialists or in the absence of valid information about the child's status.

Almost all teams recognize this clinical requirement, and ACPA considers developmental information to be essential. Yet, few teams actually provide for that aspect of care (Broder & Richman, 1987). That being the case, the speech-language pathologist often serves in a counseling capacity for the rest of the team to acquaint them with a child's special added deficits and to work with parents to accept referral for developmental assessment.

The ability to recognize and manage developmental lags is especially relevant to the speech-language pathologist, who must avoid the all too frequent decision to treat delayed onset of speech as a simple cleft-related delay or as an isolated expressive-language problem without reference to receptive-language abilities or to all other aspects of development. These additional and often significant deficits are difficult and painful for parents, who need time and help to understand and finally accept their child's limitations and the intervention required to ensure an optimal outcome.

Parents of developmentally delayed children can profit from one-on-one counseling from the speech-language pathologist and from experienced parents working with the speech-language pathologist. Group sessions with other parents with similar problems may also be beneficial. While the real strength of group sessions lies in the active participation of concerned parents, directing the sessions is best left to the professional counselor, again, often the speech-language pathologist. This structure is desirable so that:

- pertinent topics are not ignored
- sensitive issues are approached with insight and compassion
- emotionally charged experiences are diffused
- the best use is made of unexpected opportunities to help parents grow in their acceptance of reality
- accuracy is stressed in the interpretation of information

- parents are helped to understand the nature of developmental delay and its relationship to chronologic age

- activities appropriate to developmental age are encouraged

It usually takes a professional person to accomplish those goals in a group setting.

Some speech-language pathologists have created toy and book libraries so that they can help parents make wise selections appropriate to the developmental age of their child. In this way the parents learn about the advantages of capitalizing on capabilities and engaging in activities geared to strengthening weaknesses. This indirect approach to counseling uses example as a primary technique and depends on positive experiences to change parental behavior.

When children are very young, most counseling must obviously be directed to parents. However, actively involving the children by bringing them and their parents into directed group play can be an excellent way of counseling parents. The counselor has a well-planned program, usually multifaceted and designed to include motor, sensory, cognitive, social, language, and speech activities. Stimulus materials and procedures are presented and demonstrated for each parent to use with his or her own child as the counselor circulates and sometimes enters into the play to bring it into line with the child's interests and abilities, praises a particularly effective interaction, or demonstrates alternative ways of reinforcing the child's efforts.

Therapeutic, teaching, and counseling programs of this type prepare parents to accept more intensive developmental programs carried out at home, in the clinic, in home and clinic combined, or in a special facility designed for work with high-risk children. It is rarely enough simply to tell parents that their child ought to have such help. They must first overcome the threat that such a recommendation engenders (McWilliams et al., 1990).

### Counseling for Psychosocial and Language Development

The evidence is conclusive that children with clefts rarely exhibit major symptoms of mental illness (McWilliams et al., 1990; Tobiason, 1990). The evidence is equally persuasive, however, that they are often inhibited, shy, and withdrawn (Tobiason, 1990); socially immature (Goodstein, 1961; McWilliams & Matthews, 1979); reduced in creativity (Smith & McWilliams, 1966); immature in drawing the human figure (McWilliams et al. 1990); and somewhat delayed in verbal expression. They also encounter social malattitudes that are only rarely incorporated into counseling programs for young children. It is little wonder that verbal output is reduced in both quantity and quality and that their mean length of utterance in comparison with other children is reduced (Morris, 1962). It is clear that counseling in these areas must begin early for both parents and children.

### Work with Parents

Counseling about psychosocial development is especially amenable to group settings where parents can freely exchange feelings, observations, ideas for handling sensitive issues, concerns about child-rearing practices and behavior, questions about speech and language, issues of denial, and responses to various forms of intervention. The purpose is to stimulate parents to provide the environmental support necessary to ensure optimal psychosocial development. In this way, parents are helped to build on what they began during the infant period; to continue to talk about the anomaly freely; to seek answers to questions as they arise; to adopt and live by Mr. Rogers's motto, "I like you just the way you are"; to reflect interest in and approval of their children's verbal output; and to be so accepting of the situation themselves that their children grow up with strong self-images, positive attitudes, personal confidence, and objective information about the disorder and the necessary treatment.

Such groups can be made more dynamic by including experienced parents. The occasional addition of or reference to an older child, a teenager, or an adult with similar problems can also enrich these sessions. Patients of all ages are often able to express their feelings in ways that no one else can, and they may also share remarkably encouraging and supportive success stories. A psychiatrist, a nurse practitioner, a dentist, a director of religious education and family counselor, a financial counselor, an actor, a secretary, a mother, a speech-language pathologist with a doctorate, an award-winning scientist—all come to mind as real people whose stories can make a big difference.

Another approach is to provide intensive training for experienced parents, who then become group leaders. When this plan is used, it is important to have regular sessions with the leaders so that the dynamics of their parent groups can be explored and they can get needed assistance (Irwin & McWilliams, 1973).

Clinical evidence suggests that this type of counseling is an effective means of reaching out to parents and that they respond positively to it. As one mother put it, "I don't know what it is, but after these meetings I feel good all week. I look forward to coming to 'my group,' knowing that I can say what I think and you'll all understand." Well-adjusted parents can do more to encourage the development of outstanding social and communication skills in children than anything of a direct nature that speech-language pathologists have to offer. This view is supported by Campis, DeMaso, and Twente (1995) and by Krueckeberg and Kapp-Simon (1993), who found that parental stress was a predictor of the child's social skills.

## Work with Parents and Children

In these early years, outreach to parents with their children can be effective. They come together in play groups similar to the ones described for young children with developmental delays. Witzel and McWilliams (1977), concerned about the sometimes preponderance of negative statements from mothers to their children, initiated a 13-week group program in which each mother interacted with a child other than her own and later evaluated her verbal behavior from videotapes. For example, if a little boy reported that Bobby had hit him, a positive response would be, "You must have felt very bad, and maybe a little mad, when that happened." "What did you do to Bobby to make him hit you?" is an example of a negative answer. The participating mothers increased their positive responses in a range from 16 to 25 percent. They reported that they were listening to their own children more attentively and often discussed instances in which positive responses had either changed their children's behavior or stimulated them to increase the amount of speech used.

Play is the child's work and the foundation for early experimentation and learning. The parent who can enter into the play and respond positively while allowing the child freedom of direction with less emphasis on "correct performance" is providing an excellent foundation for a strong self-image in the future (Speltz, Morton, Goodell, & Clarren, 1993).

Parents can often alter attitudes and behavior when they experience success with new approaches. A case in point is a mother who had individual counseling about giving positive reinforcement to her determined little boy, who heard many "don'ts" and received much criticism all day long. When she actively sought ways to give him signals of approval, she found that he became less menacing and more cooperative. She was ecstatic and returned to the clinic with a question. "You know, that has worked so well with my little boy, do you think it would work with my husband?"

Still another technique is for the parents, singly or together, depending on the goal, to play with their child while the clinician observes through a one-way-vision mirror. Such sessions can be threatening to some parents and are not appropriate for everyone; but they can often provide more insights into parent-child relationships in a few minutes than can be discovered in hours of talking about issues.

An example of this is the mother who told her son to pick up the toys at the end of the session. He went on playing. She told him again. He ignored her. Then she yelled at him and he continued to go his own way. She wound up yanking him to his feet and literally pulling the now screaming child from the playroom. The toys were still scattered about; she was frustrated and angry; the day was ruined for them both.

The clinician and the mother discussed this episode, and the mother admitted to feelings of total failure. She also recognized that these tugs of war were typical of their life at home. The clinician asked her if she could think of other ways to elicit her son's cooperation. She thought of bribery, of spanking him on the spot, of using what she called "reverse psychology" by threatening to give away his favorite toy if he didn't shape up, or of telling him that she was leaving without him. She had no confidence, however, that these strategies would work and felt that the whole thing was hopeless.

The clinician then suggested that a different technique be tried in the next session. She helped by working for a short period with the child and then telling him that he had earned time for himself and his mother in the playroom. She gave him a timer and explained that, when his bell rang, he and his mother together would start to pick up the toys. She gave a second timer to the mother and told them both that the game was to see if they could get all the toys put away before the mother's bell went off. The child was fascinated, and the system worked like magic. The mother saw that there were simple ways to modify her son's behavior, and they left that day without tears and anger. The problems were not solved in this one encounter, but both mother and child were embarked on a new journey with a different road map.

## Work with Children

Because the goal of caring for children with these various congenital malformations is to have them grow up with the knowledge and the belief that their lives need not be dominated by their imperfections, it is the philosophy here that intervention occurs when it is necessary and that children who are doing well need not be subjected to special handling. It is helpful, however, to let children know that the problems they have are not shameful but are shared by many others. The introduction of a small cuddly teddy bear with a stitched lip has been useful in this regard. Karen Le Clair (Cleft Palate Foundation, undated) designed the bears when, as an adult, she saw a doll with a lip scar and wanted desperately to have one like it for herself. She made up the bears complete with stitched lips. Children and their parents were delighted with them. It was especially notable that a 25-year-old man wanted a teddy bear for himself. Information about buying the bears is available through the Cleft Palate Foundation.

These children, as with all children, need good early social experiences; and their parents sometimes need support in letting them move into the larger world. Enrollment in a normal preschool is an ideal way of enhancing development—social, motor, cognitive, creative, linguistic, and communicative—in a nonclinical environment that emphasizes strengths and normality and minimizes weaknesses and differences. The special toys, like the bear described above, can become a part of share-and-tell periods to acquaint other preschoolers about individual differences.

Even when there are mild developmental lags, especially in expressive language, this choice is often more effective than formal language therapy. Preschool is not a solution for children with substantial deficiencies requiring specialized management. However, many children with clefts and other deficits do not require special schools and may be harmed by attending them. Instead, the opportunity to identify with "just plain kids" is important and necessary.

Preparing parents for this experience may be in order because of their worry that other children will tease their son or daughter about the lip scar, distorted facial features, or aberrant speech. A joint session with the preschool staff, the parents, and the counselor can be most effective in this regard. The parents learn that other preschoolers also have speech variations and that teasing is something the teachers are well equipped to handle because it is so common among children who do not have special needs. The staff, on the other hand, can be informed about the nature of clefts and any necessary special considerations, including concern for strong social development. These sessions help to bring the school into the team as an extended member, thus avoiding the possibility of the staff members making conflicting problem-related recommendations.

If private preschools are not financially feasible, the counselor can sometimes help the parents find scholarship funds, which are available in a number of preschools, or can recommend an appropriate Head-Start program. It may be more difficult to arrange for staff orientation in Head-Start facilities, but the effort must be made. If all else fails, reading materials can be provided, along with a written report on the goals for a particular child.

Another approach to preschoolers that has been shown to be beneficial is creative dramatics. Irwin and McWilliams (1974) reported the results of 32 weekly sessions with children between three and six years of age. In the beginning, the children were reluctant to talk or even to move. To stimulate greater participation, the first ten sessions included dramatic play, rhythmic activities, and pantomime. In the next fourteen sessions, the children acted out structured stories. In the last eight encounters, they spontaneously began to verbalize fantasies, original stories, and fears.

During these sessions, there was often a rush of verbal output that was rich in psychodynamic information. An example follows:

> Brian had always refused to enter into any hospital play, but one day he suddenly became an ambulance driver and enlisted the aid of another boy to look after the "patient," whom he had also recruited. Suddenly, Brian brought his loud and wild "driving" to a halt and screamed at the aide, who was placing an oxygen mask on the patient, "Hey! You're not going to do that to him like they did to me!" In the discussion that followed, Brian explained, "That thing chokes you to death, and I didn't want that to happen to *him* like it did to *me*."

Brian's mother confirmed that he had had a frightening experience with a mask and that it had been difficult to get his cooperation in further surgery. He had never before verbalized any of these fears, but dramatic play helped him to do so, thus laying some of his anxieties to rest.

Observers rated various aspects of the children's participation in creative dramatics. They moved from no verbal behavior or the use of single words or short phrases to more frequent, complex, and spontaneous verbalizations. Behavior and speech output seemed to change together. Clinical observations later confirmed the lasting benefits of this enjoyable and emotionally invigorating activity. Because the children are likely to express sensitive, even threatening, material, it is essential that the counselor be well qualified to deal with delicate situations.

In a recent study of preschoolers with craniofacial anomalies, (Krueckeberg, Kapp-Simon, & Ribordy, 1993) showed that the ability to create varying facial expressions that accurately communicate emotion is an important predictor of social skills. Children appear to rely more on facial than situational cues in understanding their social environments (Hoffner & Badzinski, 1989). These authors also found that friendliness was a predictor of social skills. Facial expressions and friendliness are both specific attributes that can be taught and that can be incorporated into group programs, including creative dramatics, developed by speech-language pathologists.

## THE SCHOOL-AGED CHILD

If early treatment and counseling programs have gone well, the school years should not pose unexpected problems. However, school abounds with new experiences and enlarges the child's world in a number of different dimensions. Independence, sometimes difficult for children with clefts or other deficits, becomes an issue as does school progress and teacher evaluations, relationships with a larger number of peers, and adequacy of communication skills. During these years, the speech-language pathologist continues to work with parents and school personnel, including the school's speech-language pathologist who now begins to participate as a member of the extended team. A closer counseling relationship with the child may also emerge in response to needs for direct intervention.

In this context, it is necessary to understand the cooperative roles of the speech-language pathologist on the team and his or her counterpart in the school. Otherwise, serious conflicts in management may occur. For example, a school speech-language pathologist told a little girl and her parents that she should have an immediate lip revision in order to avoid negative evaluations of her appearance. This issue was being handled by the team, and plans had been made for a lip revision at a later date. The child was happy with that until she encountered the school speech-language pathologist. That event should not have taken place. Another poorly informed speech-language pathologist explained to a mother that her son's hypernasality should be treated by speech therapy instead of the surgery that had been scheduled. Although speech therapy was not a viable solution to this child's marked velopharyngeal incompetence, the mother could not accept the necessary surgery until additional counseling had taken place. The patient is always best served when there is cooperation and exchange of information between clinic and school.

Discussions of independence, school adjustment, relationships with peers, and communication skills follow. Many of the techniques already presented are useful as well in working with the school-aged child.

## Independence

Children who do not have congenital defects often find the transition from preschool to elementary school a difficult one because of demands for independence. Riding on a bus, eating in the cafeteria, beginning to assume responsibility for homework, having to respond verbally in class, and managing and keeping track of boots and other outdoor clothing all constitute hurdles. This aspect of school life may be particularly difficult for children with clefts and other facial problems. They tend to see themselves as less acceptable than their peers, as more likely to require assistance, and as more frequently sad and angry. They often identify with passive and isolated children, behavior that is consistent with evidences of their own social inhibition (Kapp-Simon, 1986), and have reduced personal and social self-concepts in comparison with their non-involved peers (Broder & Strauss, 1989).

In focusing on social inhibition, it would be unwise to ignore the group of cleft children, often with articulation problems unrelated to the cleft, who evidence bad temper and act out against others even while they prefer to spend time alone and are frequently enuretic (McWilliams & Musgrave, 1972). This combination of symptoms suggests children who are crying out for help. The speech-language pathologist will do well to consider individual counseling with such children in an effort to address their specific needs, including possible referral for psychological or psychiatric treatment.

It is hoped that the developmental counseling beginning at birth will have minimized these tendencies and that few children will fall into these classifications. However, it is advisable to be alert to those who are into trouble at this important period of life. A useful technique in this regard is to ask about friends, their names, and the kinds of things they do together (Cohn, personal communication, 1995). Children who are developing solid relationships answer readily and with enthusiasm, while others may be tentative and hesitant in their replies. A word of warning is in order here. Broder, Smith, and Strauss (1994) note that children with orofacial defects often report that they have more friends than do their non-involved peers. These authors stress the importance of verifying self-report data with independent observations. It is for this reason that it is necessary to ask for specific information about friends.

When problems with independence are identified, it is desirable to expand individual counseling and to introduce informal group activities that encourage independence and stimulate social interaction. These include, among others, creative dramatics, Cub Scouts and Brownies, church organizations, school social clubs and interest groups, and sports.

Finding something the child does well and encouraging that activity can pay large dividends. A little girl with a bilateral cleft found satisfaction, ego support, and recognition in dancing another in drawing and painting. Counseling can assist children in discovering and developing their special talents.

## School Adjustment

Richman (1976) explored school behavior and achievement in 44 cleft children between nine and fourteen years of age. Both boys and girls were rated by their teachers as having significantly more internalizing behavior and more inhibition (personality disorder) than control subjects. However, they did not differ on measures of conduct disorder as revealed by the Behavior Problem Checklist. Both boys and girls had significantly lower achievement scores than their peers, but the differences were greater for boys. Richman concluded that the children were not emotionally maladjusted but that they used questionable adaptive behaviors to avoid negative responses from others. These findings may be somewhat skewed by the inclusion of 29 children with clefts of the palate only as opposed to only 15 with clefts of the lip and palate. The evidence strongly supports a greater preponderance of problems in association with isolated clefts, and it would be unwise to generalize these findings to a broader population of cleft subjects.

Richman and Harper (1978) and Harper, Richman, and Snider (1980) added information suggesting that children with clefts are not emotionally disturbed but that even a mild handicap leads to modification in classroom behavior. These behavioral differences may be explained in part by teacher attitudes. Richman (1978) investigated the influence of facial disfigurement on teachers' perceptions of mental abilities. The teachers were more accurate in their ratings of children with only minimal facial disfigurement than they were in their assessments of children with marked facial disfigurement. In the latter group, those with above-average abilities were underestimated, whereas those with below-average abilities were overestimated. Such inaccurate assessments can create despair in children.

Although teachers are probably not different from the rest of society in regard to inaccurate assessment of children with facial anomalies, they are more influential in the lives of their students because they set the tone of their classrooms and communicate their attitudes toward individual children. An example of this is the teacher who referred a "retarded" child with a bilateral cleft of the lip and palate and a serious speech problem springing from velopharyngeal incompetence. She was not hopeful that anything could be done for him because she thought he was too slow to profit. However, this little boy was in reality a gifted child who suffered silently and was further penalized because of his un-intelligible speech. He required surgery to create a competent mechanism—not speech therapy—and extensive counseling to help him believe in his own remarkable abilities. The teacher was in need of counseling too.

It is little wonder that Spriestersbach (1973) found that fewer subjects with clefts than their controls liked school, volunteered in class, liked their schoolmates, or had aspirations for education after high school. Mothers of the clinical subjects knew that their children's class participation was below average, but they reported fewer teacher-initiated confer-ences about school progress. Again, counseling with teachers is indicated as is counseling with parents to stimulate them to take the initiative if the teacher does not. The well-informed speech-language pathologist can arrange and chair joint meetings with teachers and parents and can be in regular contact with teachers thereafter.

These studies, along with patient histories, all send a clear message. Speech-language pathologists counseling school-aged children with clefts and other forms of facial disfig-urement will want to explore school experiences and take appropriate steps to modify the classroom environment to the extent possible. This may mean individual work with in-volved teachers, continuing education for all teachers, and programming for children who do not have clefts.

### Relationships with Peers

An important aspect of school adjustment is relationships among peers. Getting valid in-formation on this matter is difficult because both parents and children tend to put a posi-tive spin on the extent to which true friendships exist. As with younger children, it is use-ful to ask a child to talk about friends and the things they do together. Probing beneath the surface often reveals loneliness and many solitary activities. As we shall see later, these ways of coping with social problems frequently extend into adulthood, thus limiting full participation in life.

The developmental approach recommended here should minimize this limited life participation, but it is important to be ever watchful and to continue to act to modify any tendencies in this direction. The types of activities recommended for younger children, up-graded to an age-appropriate level, can be used in this age group as well. In addition, this is a time when it is possible to have meaningful discussions with children and to enter into more direct counseling. In some cases, the speech-language pathologist may be most helpful by preparing the parents and child for referral to a mental-health specialist. In spite of the evidence of pain in the lives of some children, there has long been resistance to putting them into psychiatric treatment. Thus, some significant emotional disorders are never addressed (Wylie & McWilliams, 1966). Interviews with adults often reveal the hopelessness they experienced as children and continue to feel as adults (MacGregor, 1958). One talented woman remembered how she always hung back and took a place at the end of the line, feeling unworthy to be included in the midst of the other children. Counseling could have saved her years of anxiety.

### Communication Skills

Many children with clefts do not have disordered speech that is the direct result of the cleft. This percentage decreases as the anatomical deficits increase in severity and involve more structures. For those who do have speech problems, counseling is mandatory on a num-ber of fronts.

First of all, children, parents, and teachers are often too optimistic about the ability of the speech-language pathologist to bring about positive changes in speech patterns. Speech that is defective because of velopharyngeal incompetence or aberrant oral structures is unlikely to be modified by behavioral therapy, and the speech-language pathologist has an ethical responsibility to refuse to undertake it until there is objective information on the status of those all-important structures. This means working closely with the team and using therapy time to help the child, the family, and school personnel understand the limitations of behavioral techniques in the modification of anatomical and physiological deficits.

It is better to help a child understand why there are speech differences and to attempt to correct the underlying defects than to impose an endless regimen of useless therapy. There are too many children enrolled year after year in therapy programs even though they are ineffective. The cost of such intervention is high indeed. The constant failure leads to frustration, reduced self-esteem, guilt, and anger. More importantly, therapy may prevent diagnosis and treatment of the underlying defects that are responsible for the speech problem and, thus, delay correction beyond the time when it can have the greatest benefit for the child. The older a child is at the time of treatment, the less likely it is to be successful. The speech-language pathologist must know when to say "no" to speech therapy and "yes" to counseling directed toward finding better solutions to speech problems.

Speech that is marked by hypernasality seems to be a particular problem for those who have it because it is not acceptable to other children as early as kindergarten (Blood & Hyman, 1977). In fact, kindergarten children respond globally to the hypernasal speaker and provide negative responses to questions about attributes that have nothing to do with the speech characteristics.

The same general statements may be made about facial appearance (Schneiderman & Harding, 1984; Tobiason, 1987). Faces with clefts were rated by other children as less friendly, less popular, less likely to be chosen as friends, less intelligent, and less good looking. These ratings were not related to age or gender. Tobiason suggests that facial deformity may be a central cue for social stereotyping, because facial deformity may be seen as ugly and ugly as bad.

These responses on the part of other children to speech and appearance obviously influence communication attempts and skills. If a child senses personal rejection, the child is not likely be motivated to communicate with the rejecters. Under these circumstances, inhibition is intensified; and social withdrawal becomes the least painful way to cope.

Even children who speak well and are not facially disfigured but have deviations of which they alone are painfully aware may have such reduced self-esteem that they too shy away from communicating with others. Communication is more than language, articulation, voice, resonance, and fluency. We too often forget that perfect speech production is not always equated with high communicative skills. The speech-language pathologist may make a major contribution by intervening to provide counseling designed to enhance the desire to communicate and to help non-impaired classmates understand and accept differences in others.

## Counseling Techniques

Approaches already mentioned, modified to make them age-appropriate, can be useful with school-aged children. Of special value to the speech-language pathologist-counselor is creative dramatics. It relies on groups and the children in the group need not share common problems. Creative dramatics is useful when the speech-language pathologist is attempting to make newly acquired behaviors habitual in ordinary conversation or is stimulating increased verbal output, encouraging problem solving, and providing for the expression of children's concerns and anxieties. In fact, children who do not have traditional speech disorders but are low communicators may also be included along with interested peers who are not candidates for any form of therapy.

Creative dramatics can be used successfully as a classroom activity when the counselor's goal is to increase understanding and compassion and provide a positive environment for children with differences. Acting out stories and talking about the experience can open new opportunities for positive interaction among all children, especially those who have been sitting on the sidelines.

Another particularly valuable classroom plan is for the counselor and the teacher, together, to develop an assignment in which all the children are asked to give a short report on some unique feature in their lives. The counselor can then work with a specific child to create a presentation about his or her special problem, the experience of being in the hospital, and how it feels to worry about speech or appearance. Some treatment centers even have audio-visual aids that can be used to advantage in this context. Several children known to the author have undertaken such projects on their own without any special help. The results were truly amazing. This is an excellent way to combat teasing and to discover new friends.

In extreme circumstances, when a child has speech that is too seriously impaired to make classroom presentations feasible, it is sometimes advisable to enlist the aid of the other children by explaining to them why Johnny or Becky has to miss school to attend clinics, visit specialists, or go to the hospital for additional surgery. Asking them to help ease their classmate's very heavy burdens may lead to positive changes in their attitudes. The old cliche that "children can be cruel" is often more accurate when modified to "children can be thoughtless." When they understand a situation and what they can do to help, they often become caring and supportive.

## THE TEEN YEARS

Leonard, Brust, Abrahams, and Sielaff (1991) reported that children and adolescents with clefts did at least as well as a normal population on global self-concept as measured by the Piers-Harris Self-Concept Scale. Such results are not unusual when scales of this type are used, but the responses often do not match the children's actual behavior or the feelings they express when they are able to open up to an understanding counselor or to a group of their peers.

Clinical experience suggests that adolescence is a crucial age, as it is for all children, and that we may easily make wrong counseling decisions in these years. Some teenagers have had superb care, including necessary counseling, from birth onward; and they have no special needs beyond those that are common to most adolescents. If that is the case, speech-language pathologists must be wise enough to accept success and refrain from meddling.

Unfortunately, of the 110 adolescents whose speech was evaluated by Peterson-Falzone (1995), only 12 (10.9 percent) had had consistent team management from birth, and speech fell within normal limits in only 25 (22.7 percent). Another 32.7 percent had non-compensatory articulation errors. As the author points out, patients seen in the facility from which these subjects were drawn are often referred after previous treatment has failed. Thus, these statistics are not representative of outcome in large centers with intensive programs of care and follow-up, where a successful speech outcome occurs in most cases (McWilliams, 1990; McWilliams et al., in press).

Other children have had excellent physical management with no cleft-related speech or physical defects but have not yet dealt with their psychosocial inadequacies. These adolescents may still be able to achieve a positive outlook if counseling can be introduced either by the speech-language pathologist or by another psychological or psychiatric therapist, whichever is most appropriate. If referral is indicated, the speech-language pathologist serving in a counseling role will provide the support necessary to make the transition.

Still other young people may have had only marginal care from birth, and they retain an array of continuing deficits such as ear disease, compromised appearance, dental inadequacies, disordered speech, and psychosocial difficulties that have been inadequately addressed. These children require a combination of physical and emotional care over the time necessary to complete treatment, the results of which may not be ideal.

Children who are even more profoundly impaired are those whose treatment has been a complete failure, sometimes resulting in deviations of greater magnitude than those of the original deformity. These adolescents, if they are to improve even minimally, will need many different procedures over time and special counseling to help them deal with perhaps lasting limitations and disappointment.

## Awakening Teenage Concerns

Some teenagers must face remaining and perhaps increasing concerns about speech and appearance and the need for additional surgical and dental procedures. In addition, they must, along with their peers, accommodate to the rapid changes that are occurring within themselves, which they often find as difficult to understand as do their parents. Their social worlds are expanding; parental influence is decreasing, while there is an increasing awareness of peer relationships and peer pressures and the desire to be like everyone else. Boy-girl interactions become important as the arousal of sexual identity comes into focus. Interest in the nature and causes of their birth defects and questions about their chances of having similarly affected offspring may cause anxiety in this age group. Making decisions about and planning for education beyond high school and considering career options are all areas in which counseling may be required.

Leonard et al. (1991) concluded that all children with clefts are socially and interpersonally vulnerable. Thus, all could "benefit from professional guidance and support as well as peer group interactions to serve as a hedge against social isolation, estrangement, and feelings of marginality experienced by some of those children." We concur in that view. Reference to the section that follows on the adult confirms the impression that attention to counseling in the teen years is necessary for patients whose problems have not been resolved by that age. It is equally important, however, to recognize that adolescents with clefts and other orofacial anomalies are a heterogeneous group about whom it is unwise to make individual judgments based on assumptions that apply to only a few.

## Appearance and Speech

One major aspect of life for these teenagers is the reality of their differences and the realization that there may be few remaining treatment options. Surgical procedures with the possibility of only limited gains may be needed to improve either appearance or speech. Although a number of studies have shown that teenagers and young adults are generally satisfied with their appearance and speech, they also show the tendency to be less pleased with cleft-related characteristics such as noses, lips, profiles, teeth, and speech (Noar, 1991). This is especially true of patients whose outcome is not satisfactory. In spite of that, they may be unwilling to consider further surgery or other forms of intervention or may want inappropriate treatment. Parents and adolescents may be in disagreement on this issue (Kapp-Simon, 1995), as they are likely to be on many subjects at this age; and a significant investment in time and patience may be required to bring about a resolution (Canady, 1995; Riski, 1995).

One young man whose speech was normal and whose appearance, although not perfect, was acceptable had always expressed delight with everything until one day, when talking to a speech-language-pathologist counselor, he began to question the lip result and to wonder if anything more could be done to improve it. When asked why he had not previously inquired about his lip, he said that he liked all the doctors, that they had been good to him, and that he hadn't wanted to hurt their feelings. However, his lip was not the unscarred version he dreamed of and he wanted improvement. In his case, it was possible to do minor revisions and to help him realize and accept the fact that a perfect result was not possible. Had there not been an opportunity for him to talk with a counselor, he would never have been at peace with his appearance.

In cases like this, makeup artists are sometimes used to teach make-up skills designed to minimize remaining defects. Kapp-Simon (1995) also recommends the use of makeup. Sometimes, a particularly adept teenager, usually a girl, becomes so proficient in applying cosmetics that she can serve as an instructor for her peers. There is usually pleasure with the results achieved with makeup but an unwillingness to devote the time necessary to apply it on a regular basis. Just knowing that the possibility exists, however, can be a source of comfort and a resource for special occasions.

Giving adolescents many opportunities to meet with a counselor who is willing to listen and to take the time necessary to uncover hidden concerns can be an important ingredient in routine clinical care.

## Support Groups

Because there is such variability in treatment results, understanding of and information about existing problems, personal strengths and weaknesses, and teenage concerns, it is probably unwise to try to design a topical counseling program to serve all comers. With infants, feeding, ear disease, and surgery are universal considerations; but there is far less certainty with teenagers. Although group data suggest that they are likely to feel more unpopular than other kids and to have the concerns noted earlier in this section, it is not possible at any one time to predict what they want and need and are ready and able to explore in depth. For this reason, it is strongly recommended that there be support groups for teens and that the participants establish their own agendas. This approach encourages independence and allows them to move from subject to subject as they are able to do so. The counselor is an active participant in the groups and guides members as they select subjects for exploration.

One group at the University of Pittsburgh made a documentary videotape of their cleft-related life experiences and used it to educate others about the needs and the strengths of cleft kids, who kept reiterating that they were "just like everyone else" and wanted to be treated that way—a clear indicator that they felt they had often been treated differently in the past. These feelings, frankly expressed, were explored and worked out in the counseling sessions. Genetic counseling and career and educational planning are topics that lend themselves naturally to group work.

These are ideal years for teenagers to finish working out some of their remaining anxieties and to begin to look with hope beyond their birth defects. It is a good time for them to meet and get to know successful adults with clefts and other deficits. These role models are living proof that there is life beyond the clinic and that it can be good. Experiences of this type fit well into the support-group format.

## Social Learning

Support groups can evolve into educational sessions designed to teach special skills. Of particular interest is the introduction of opportunities for social learning as suggested by Kapp-Simon (1995). She described a program stressing (*a*) social initiation, (*b*) conversational skills, (*c*) assertion or direct communication, (*d*) empathy or active listening, and (*e*) conflict resolution and problem solving. This approach flows naturally from the counseling and programming recommended from early childhood onward. These skills can be directly taught, used as topics in group discussions, or approached in a more adult version of creative dramatics. Dramatic improvisation is an almost perfect tool for experimenting with various solutions to problems and trying new skills in a variety of contexts. The value of this technique is greatly enhanced by follow-up discussions and then again working through the situations in different ways.

Teenagers struggle for independence and recognition of their uniqueness. Giving them many opportunities to explore the dimensions of their lives and to learn skills and make relevant decisions can have major implications in the adult years.

## ADULTHOOD

The goal of treatment for children with clefts and other types of oro- and craniofacial defects is to make it possible for them to grow into well-adjusted, productive adults capable of reaching their full human potential. We know from anecdotal information that this is the outcome for many but certainly not for all, especially for those whose treatment occurred many years ago (MacGregor, 1951). It is difficult to generate data from a representative sample of adults because they tend to be lost to follow-up and only infrequently to seek clinical assistance. Thus, there are few studies available. Those that are in the literature, of necessity, reflect outcome of treatment initiated long ago, when technology was less sophisticated than it is today and the counseling recommended here was usually not available.

## Education and Occupation

In spite of the negative factors that interfere with drawing strong conclusions, the evidence is that those with clefts attended college as frequently as their noncleft peers (McWilliams & Paradise, 1973; Peter & Chinsky, 1974b). However, males with clefts were not upwardly mobile in their occupations as were their siblings and random controls (Peter, Chinsky, & Fisher 1975a); and they reported more feelings of job insecurity and more often felt that their jobs were unsuitable. This may be explained in part by the findings of Van Demark and Van Demark (1970) to the effect that subjects with clefts had somewhat unrealistic vocational goals even though Peter, Chinsky, and Fisher (1975a) reported that they had lower income aspirations than control subjects. These findings, tentative though they are, point to the need for careful vocational counseling in the teen years in order to alleviate these sources of dissatisfaction in later life.

## Marriage

Concern about relationships with the opposite sex was noted as an important aspect of counseling during the teen years. The need for that is borne out by several studies of adults. Van Demark and Van Demark (1970) noted that their subjects appeared to date less frequently than their peers, and this is a frequent clinical observation as well. The evidence also suggests that cleft subjects marry less frequently and somewhat later than control subjects (McWilliams & Paradise, 1973; Peter & Chinsky, 1974a; Heller, Tidumarsh, & Pless, 1981; Bjornsson & Agustsdottir, 1987).

## Social Integration

Van Demark and Van Demark (1970) reported that the young adults they studied seemed to be observers of life rather than participants. They were unsure of their social skills and, thus, preferred individual as opposed to group activities.

Peter, Chinsky, and Fisher (1975b) drew similar conclusions. Their subjects with clefts more frequently lived with or visited other family members than did their controls. Heller et al. (1981) supported this finding and also found that 56 percent of their cleft subjects expressed dissatisfaction with their social lives. Nearly half of the subjects studied by Peter et al. (1975b) had few leisure activities, and those they did have were likely to be of a passive nature.

## Proposed Sources of Help

This limited information about adults treated many years ago lends support to the developmental approach to counseling and clearly emphasizes the need from birth forward to work consistently to develop independence, personal confidence, and self-reliance. Studies completed in the future should provide evidence of the validity of early intervention.

Adults who may not have had access to assistance from birth through the teen years only rarely request additional help as they grow older. They seem most likely to do so when they encounter special, cleft-related problems, such as ear disease, dental difficulties, sinusitis, speech that may not be quite good enough to match career aspirations, need for genetic counseling, questions about the availability of additional corrective surgery, or dissatisfaction with the way in which life is unfolding. It is not unusual for these life concerns to be shrouded in some physical need. Thus, when adults seek clinical care, it is always wise to spend some time listening to what they have to say and to seek clues to a hidden agenda.

One highly creative and successful professional woman wisely sought improvement in her appearance, speech, and outlook. In her mid-thirties, she exchanged a prosthetic appliance for surgical closure of the palate combined with a pharyngeal flap and had massive dental restorations including implants. In the process of completing this lengthy treatment, she began to talk about her painful childhood, the divorce of her parents for which she felt responsible, and the awful sense of rejection with which she had lived.

She examined her marriage and her career and made changes in both. As she faced and dealt with problem after problem, she expressed the wish to talk with others who had had the cleft experience. The result was that she organized a support group that continued to meet regularly until the participants gradually realized that they were strong enough to do well on their own. Any member of such a group could be effective in working with future groups or individuals. They could be especially helpful to teenagers.

Some adults are unable to seek solutions directly. Instead, they may elect to write letters to people in the field, often a great distance from their own homes. One man indicated that he was a writer who wanted to do an article about the marital and child-rearing experiences of adults with clefts and needed "expert" advice. As time passed, he wrote additional letters, each more disorganized and distressed than the last, until a story of great unhappiness and life-long troubled relationships emerged. This man, in late middle age, had deep psychiatric disturbances that were too massive and too deeply entrenched for a speech-language pathologist to treat independently. The goal of counseling was to lead him to seek necessary psychiatric help. Many adults who come to the attention of the speech-language pathologist fall into that category. Counseling designed to make additional help a viable option is an important mission for speech-language pathologists working in this area.

## CONCLUSION

It is important to remember always that the best management programs that can be devised will not be acceptable to everyone and that there will always be a few who do not profit by what is offered. However, there is little doubt that babies who begin life with strong support and guidance and have that extra assistance throughout adolescence enter adulthood with fewer life deficits than those who struggle alone. Treatment is unsuccessful if a patient looks good and speaks well but has little desire to communicate and finds life more bitter than sweet. Speech-language pathologists have a major role in this vital aspect of care.

## REFERENCES

American Cleft Palate-Craniofacial Association. (1993). *Parameters for evaluation and treatment of patients with cleft lip/palate or other craniofacial anomalies.*

Aspinall, C. L. (1995). Family focused ethics. *Cleft Palate Journal, 32*, 507–509.

Backus, O., Clancy, J., Henry, L., & Kemper, J. (1943). *The child with a cleft palate.* Ann Arbor: University of Michigan Press.

Bennett, M. E., & Stanton, M. (1993). Psychotherapy for persons with craniofacial deformities: Can we treat without theory? *Cleft Palate-Craniofacial Journal, 30,* 406–410.

Bjornsson, A., & Agustsdottir, S. (1987). A psychological study of Icelandic individuals with cleft lip or cleft lip and palate. *Cleft Palate Journal, 24,* 152–157.

Blood, G., & Hyman, M. (1977). Children's perception of nasal resonance. *Journal of Speech and Hearing Disorders, 42,* 446–448.

Brantly, H., & Clifford, E. (1979). Maternal and child locus of control and field-dependence in cleft palate children. *Cleft Palate Journal, 16,* 183–187.

Broder, H., & Richman, L. (1987). An examination of mental health services offered by cleft/craniofacial teams. *Cleft Palate Journal, 24,* 158–162.

Broder, H., & Strauss, R. (1989). Self-concept of early primary school age children with visible or invisible defects. *Cleft Palate Journal, 26,* 114–118.

Broder, H., Smith, F., & Strauss, R. (1994). Effects of visible and invisible orofacial defects on self-perception and adjustment across developmental eras and gender. *Cleft Palate-Craniofacial Journal, 31,* 429–436.

Brookshire, B., Lynch, J., & Fox, D. (1980). *A parent-child cleft palate curriculum, developing speech and language,* Tigard, OR: CC Publications.

Campis, L., DeMaso, D., & Twente, A. (1995). The role of maternal factors in the adaptation of children with craniofacial disfigurement. *Cleft Palate-Craniofacial Journal, 32,* 55–61.

Canady, J. (1995). Emotional effects of plastic surgery on the adolescent with a cleft. *Cleft Palate-Craniofacial Journal, 32,* 120–124.

Cleft Palate Foundation. (1992). *Feeding an infant with a cleft.*

Cleft Palate Foundation. (Undated). *Bears for the Kids.*

Cleft Palate Foundation (rev. ed.). (1989). *The first four years of life.*

Cleft Palate Foundation (1987). *The genetics of cleft lip and palate: Information for families.*

Clifford, E. (1969). Parental ratings of cleft palate infants, *Cleft Palate Journal 6,* 235–243.

Cohen, M. M., Jr. (1991). Syndrome delineation involving orofacial clefting. *Cleft Palate-Craniofacial Journal, 28,* 119–120.

Field, T., & Vega-Lahr, N. (1984). Early interactions between infants with cranio-facial anomalies and their mothers. *Infant Behavior, 7,* 527–530.

Goodstein, L. (1961). Intellectual impairment in children with cleft palates. *Journal of Speech and Hearing Research, 4,* 287–294.

Hahn, E. (1979). Directed home programs for infants with cleft lip and palate. In K. R. Bzoch (Ed.), *Communicative disorders related to cleft lip and palate.* Boston: Little, Brown & Co.

Harper, D., Richman, L., & Snider, B. (1980). School adjustment and degree of physical impairment. *Journal of Pediatric Psychology, 5,* 377–383.

Heller, A., Tidumarsh, W., & Pless, I. (1981). The psychological functioning of young adults born with cleft lip or palate. *Clinical Pediatrics, 20,* 459–465.

Hoffner, C., & Badzinski, C. (1989). Children's integration of facial and situation cues to emotion, *Child Development, 60,* 411–422.

Hubbard, T., Paradise, J., McWilliams, B. J., Elster, B. A., & Taylor, F. (1985). Consequences of unremitting middle-ear disease in early life: Otologic, audiologic, and developmental findings in children with cleft palate, *New England Journal of Medicine, 312,* 1529–1534.

Irwin, E. C., & McWilliams, B. J. (1973). Parents working with parents: The cleft palate program. *Cleft Palate Journal, 10,* 360–366.

Irwin, E. C., & McWilliams, B. J. (1974). Play therapy for children with cleft palates. *Children Today, 3,* 18.

Jones, K. (1988). *Smith's recognizable patterns of human malformation.* Philadelphia: WB Saunders.

Jung, J. (1989). *Genetic syndromes in communication disorders.* Boston: Little, Brown & Co.

Kapp-Simon, K. (1986). Self concept of primary-school-age children with cleft lip, cleft palate, or both. *Cleft Palate-Craniofacial Journal, 23,* 24–27.

Kapp-Simon, K. (1995). Psychological interventions for the adolescent with cleft lip and palate. *Cleft Palate-Craniofacial Journal, 32,* 104–108.

Koop, E. (1987). *Surgeon General's report: Children with special health care needs.* Washington, DC: Office of Maternal and Child Health, U. S. Department of Health and Human Services, Public Health Service.

Krueckeberg, S., & Kapp-Simon, K. (1993). Effect of parental factors on social skills of preschool children with craniofacial anomalies. *Cleft Palate-Craniofacial Journal, 30,* 490–496.

Krueckeberg, S., Kapp-Simon, K., & Ribordy, S. (1993). Social skills of preschoolers with and without craniofacial anomalies. *Cleft Palate-Craniofacial Journal, 30,* 475–481.

Leonard, B., Brust, J., Abrahams, G., & Sielaff, B. (1991). Self-concept of children and adolescents with cleft lip and/or palate, *Cleft Palate Journal, 28,* 347–353.

Lynch, J. (1986). Language of cleft infants: Lessening the risk of delay through programming. In B. J. McWilliams (Guest Ed.), *Seminars in speech and language.* New York: Thieme, 255–268.

MacGregor, F. (1958). Some psychosocial problems associated with facial deformities. *American Sociological Review, 16,* 629–638.

McDonald, E. (1959). *Bright promise.* The National Society for Crippled Children and Adults, Inc.

McDonald, E. (1962). *Understand those feelings.* Pittsburgh: Stanwix House.

McWilliams, B. J. (1982). Social and psychological problems associated with cleft palate. In F. C. Macgregor (Guest Ed.), *Clinics in plastic surgery: Social and psychological considerations, 18,* 317.

McWilliams, B. J. (1990). The long-term results of primary and secondary surgical correction of palatal clefts. In J. Bardach & H. L. Morris (Eds.), *Multidisciplinary management of cleft lip andpalate.* Philadelphia: WB Saunders, 815–819.

McWilliams, B. J., & Matthews, H. (1979). A comparison of intelligence and social maturity in children with unilateral complete clefts and those with isolated cleft palates. *Cleft Palate Journal, 16,* 363–372.

McWilliams, B. J., Morris, H. L., & Shelton, R. L. (1990). *Cleft palate speech.* Philadelphia: BC Decker.

McWilliams, B. J., & Musgrave, R. (1972). Psychological implications of articulation disorders in cleft palate children. *Cleft palate Journal, 9,* 294–303.

McWilliams, B. J. & Paradise, L.P. (1973)., Educational, occupational, and marital status of cleft palate adults, *Cleft Palate Journal, 30,* 223–229.

McWilliams, B. J., Randall, P., La Rossa, D., Cohen, S., Yu, J., Cohen, M., & Solot, C. (In press). Speech characteristics associated with the Furlow palatoplasty as compared to other surgical techniques. *Plastic and Reconstructive Surgery.*

Morris, H. (1962). Communication skills of children with cleft lips and palates. *Journal of Speech and Hearing Research, 6,* 79–90.

Noar, J. (1991). Questionnaire survey of attitudes and concerns of patients with cleft lip and palate and their parents. *Cleft Palate-Craniofacial Journal, 28,* 279–284.

Pannbacker, M., & Scheuerle, J. (1993). Parents' attitudes toward family involvement in cleft palate treatment. *Cleft Palate-Craniofacial Journal, 30,* 87–89.

Paradise, J., Bluestone, C., & Felder, H. (1969). The universality of otitis media in 50 infants with cleft palate. *Pediatrics, 44,* 35–42.

Paradise, J., Elster, B., & Tan, L. (1994). Evidences in infants with cleft palate that breast milk protects against otitis media. *Pediatrics, 94,* 853–860.

Paradise, J., & McWilliams, B. J. (1974). Simplified feeder for infants with cleft palate. *Pediatrics, 54,* 566–568.

Peter, J., & Chinsky, R. (1974a). Sociological aspects of cleft palate adults. I. Marriage. *Cleft Palate Journal, 11,* 295–309.

Peter, J., & Chinsky, R. (1974b). Sociological aspects of cleft palate adults. II. Education. *Cleft Palate Journal, 11,* 443–449.

Peter, J., Chinsky, R., & Fisher, M. (1975a). Sociological aspects of cleft palate adults. III. Vocational and economic aspects. *Cleft Palate Journal, 12,* 193–199.

Peter, J., Chinsky, E., & Fisher, M. (1975b). Sociological aspects of cleft palate adults. IV. Social integration. *Cleft Palate Journal, 12,* 304–310.

Peterson-Falzone, S. (1995). Speech outcomes in adolescents with cleft lip and palate. *Cleft Palate-Craniofacial Journal, 32,* 125–128.

Philips, B. J. (1979). Stimulating syntactic and phonological development in infants with cleft palate. In K. R. Bzoch (Ed.), *Communicative disorders related to cleft lip and palate.* Boston: Little, Brown & Co.

Philips, B. J. (1990). Early speech management. In J. Bardach & H. Morris (Eds.), *Multidisciplinary management of cleft lip and palate.* Philadelphia: WB Saunders, 732–736.

Pruzinsky, T. (1992). Social and psychological effects of major craniofacial deformity. *Cleft Palate-Craniofacial Journal, 29,* 578–584.

Reik, T. (1948). *Listening with the third ear.* New York: Farrar-Strauss & Co.

Richman, L. (1976). Behavior and achievement of cleft palate children. *Cleft Palate Journal, 13,* 4–10.

Richman, L. (1978). The effects of facial disfigurement on teachers' perceptions of abilities in cleft palate children, *Cleft Palate Journal, 13,* 4–10.

Richman, L., & Harper, D. (1978). Observable stigmata and perceived maternal behavior. *Cleft Palate Journal, 25,* 215–219.

Riski, J. (1995). Speech assessment of adolescents. *Cleft Palate-Craniofacial Journal, 32,* 109–113.

Schneiderman, C., & Harding, J. (1984). Social ratings of children with cleft lip by school peers. *Cleft Palate Journal, 21,* 219–223.

Seth, A., & McWilliams, B. J. (1988). Weight gain in children with cleft palate from birth to two years. *Cleft Palate Journal, 25,* 146–150.

Sidman, J. D. (1995). The team approach to cleft and craniofacial disorders—the down side [Editorial]. *Cleft Palate-Craniofacial Journal, 32,* unnumbered.

Siegel-Sadewitz, V., & Shprintzen, R. (1982). The relationship of communication disorders to syndrome identification. *Journal of Speech and Hearing Disorders, 47,* 338–354.

Slade, P., Bishop, P., & Jowett, R. (1995). Relationships between cleft severity and attractiveness of newborns with unrepaired clefts. *Cleft Palate-Craniofacial Journal, 32,* 318–322.

Smith, R., & McWilliams, B. J. (1966). Creative thinking abilities of cleft palate children. *Cleft Palate Journal, 3,* 275–283.

Sparks, S. (1984). *Birth defects and speech-language disorders.* Boston: Little, Brown & Co.

Speltz, M., Greenberg, M., Endriga, M., & Galbreath, H. (1994). Developmental approach to the psychology of craniofacial anomalies. *Cleft Palate-Craniofacial Journal, 31,* 61–67.

Speltz, M. L., Morton, K., Goodell, E. W., & Clarren, S. K. (1993). Psychological functioning of children with craniofacial anomalies and their mothers: A follow-up from late infancy to school entry. *Cleft Palate-Craniofacial Journal, 30,* 482–489.

Spriestersbach, D. C. (1973). *Psychosocial aspects of the cleft palate problem.* Vol. l. Iowa City: University of Iowa Press.

Stool, S., & Randall, P. (1967). Unexpected ear disease in infants with cleft palate. *Cleft Palate Journal, 4,* 99–103.

Strauss, R., & Broder, H. (1993). Children with cleft lip/palate and mental retardation: A subpopulation of cleft-craniofacial team patients. *Cleft Palate-Craniofacial Journal, 30,* 548–556.

Tisza, V., & Gumpertz, E. (1962). The parents' reaction to the birth and early care of children with cleft palate. *Pediatrics, 30,* 83–90.

Tobiason, J. (1987). Social judgments of facial deformity. *Cleft Palate Journal, 24,* 323–327.

Tobiason, J. (1990). Psychosocial adjustment to cleft lip and palate. In J. Bardach & H. Morris (Eds.), *Multidisciplinary management of cleft lip and palate.* Philadelphia: WB Saunders, 820–825.

Van Demark, D., & Van Demark, A. (1970). Speech and socio-vocational aspects of individuals with cleft palate. *Cleft Palate Journal, 7,* 284–299.

Weachter, E. (1959). Concerns of parents related to the birth of a child with a cleft of the lip and palate with implications for nurses. Unpublished master's thesis, University of Chicago, Chicago, IL.

Webster, E. J. (1977). *Counseling with parents of handicapped children: Guidelines for improving communication.* Orlando, FL: Grune & Stratton.

Witzel, M. A. (1983). Speech problems in craniofacial anomalies. *Communication Disorders, 8,* 45–59.

Witzel, M. A., & McWilliams, B. J. (1977). The effect of training procedures on mother-to-child verbal statements, *Canadian Speech Journal Human Communication,* Spring, 7–13.

Wylie, H.L., & McWilliams, B. J. (1966). Mental health aspects of cleft palate: A review of literature intended for parents. *ASHA, 8,* 31–34.

# 13. Children and Adolescents with Hearing Impairment and Their Parents

Lisa Lucks Mendel

Audiologists are challenged continually throughout their careers to review their effectiveness as professionals in helping individuals who have hearing loss. This is particularly true in the area of counseling. Although the audiology profession developed originally as a rehabilitative field because of the many World War II veterans suffering from hearing loss, technologic advances have moved the focus of the field more toward diagnosis. Unfortunately, this shift has moved audiologists' thinking and training further from the client, and in so doing has de-emphasized the importance and relevance of counseling in helping people and their families adjust to the effects of hearing impairment.

Moving back to a (re)habilitative perspective helps to focus audiology more on the individual and family with hearing loss by following patient care well beyond diagnosis into appropriate treatment and management. It is in the realm of management that counseling becomes an integral component of intervention with hearing impairment, as it is truly the cornerstone for (re)habilitative audiology. Shifting emphasis back to the individual and family and providing successful counseling improves the quality of life for clients with hearing impairment. Thus, the effectiveness of counseling determines the extent to which all other (re)habilitative measures succeed or fail (Clark, 1994). Moreover, if audiologists are to serve as the entry point to service delivery and assume the role of autonomous hearing care professionals, they must look at hearing loss and its causes and effects from many different viewpoints and assume responsibility for total care of the patient and family. Of course, total care includes many aspects of counseling, including knowing when to make appropriate referrals to more specialized professionals.

## AUDIOLOGISTS' ROLE AS COUNSELOR

The role of audiologist as counselor is one that is foreign to many audiologists. This is true at least partially to the lack of emphasis counseling receives during our academic and practical education. McCarthy, Culpepper, and Lucks (1986) surveyed Educational Standards Board (ESB)-accredited programs regarding their requirements in counseling course work and practicum specific to communicative disorders. Their findings indicated that most programs did not offer courses or practicum in counseling specific to communicative disorders and those that did provided them on an elective basis. Eight years later, Culpepper, Mendel, and McCarthy (1994) repeated this survey and found similar results indicating that very little has changed in the way audiologists are educated with regard to counseling and their role as counselors. Although in concept respondents appeared supportive of the need for more training and education in counseling, very little is happening to improve the situation.

Audiologists also may be uncomfortable with their role as counselors because many medical settings do not allow audiologists the opportunity to provide counseling. In some medical settings, the audiologist performs appropriate testing and sends the client to the physician for interpretation and counseling of both the audiologic and medical test results. In essence, the audiologist's role as counselor is often overshadowed by medical personnel.

Despite having limited course work and practical experience in counseling, audiologists are in a position to provide counseling to parents of children and adolescents with hearing impairment and to the children and adolescents themselves. Therefore, they must learn how to become more comfortable with their role as counselor and be sensitive and caring to the needs of the individuals with whom they work. Audiologists must develop successful patient-professional relationships by responding sensitively to the needs and experiences of parents and patients. Lowering audiologists' level of expectation will relieve some of the uncertainty of their role as counselors. If audiologists recognize that they are not expected to solve all emotional conflicts each parent and child has, they can focus on what they are capable of doing. With this mind set, the rest will fall into place (Clark, 1994).

As counselors, audiologists should provide information both regarding the child's potential for communicative and academic achievement and developing realistic and supportive educational plans. Audiologists also must provide emotional support for parents, and enhance parents' understanding of the impact of the hearing disorder on their child's development and adjustment. In so doing, audiologists and parents together will work toward greater acceptance of the child's hearing impairment (Clark, 1994; Kricos, 1993).

### Competence of Audiologists as Counselors

Sweetow and Barrager (1980) reported results of a survey of parents' perspectives on the competence of audiologists in counseling. Their findings indicated that parents were happy with the audiologic services they received but reported weaknesses in audiologists' counseling skills. This weakness was perceived by parents as having been particularly true when audiologists described aspects of hearing loss using terms that were too technical. The parents surveyed in this study indicated that they wanted suggestions from audiologists regarding how to communicate with their child, how to contact other parents who had children with hearing impairment, what resources were available for emotional and financial support, and where to obtain educational information. These findings should be useful for the audiologist who works with parents of children with hearing impairment.

Haas and Crowley (1982) also surveyed parents of children with hearing loss and found that parents felt that educators, not audiologists, provided the most meaningful input regarding the implications of their children's handicaps. Their findings were in agreement with Sweetow and Barrager (1980) in that audiologists were found not to be successful in providing supportive counseling necessary for parents to understand the ramifications of their child's hearing loss. Given the findings of these two studies, it is clear that effective management during and after diagnosis is critical to the acceptance of permanent hearing loss and subsequent involvement in (re)habilitative training (Williams & Darbyshire, 1982).

## TERMINOLOGY

### The Process of Counseling

The term counseling as used here refers to a process where audiologists facilitate an individual's adjustment to the auditory and nonauditory consequences of hearing loss. This definition applies both to the parent of a child who is hearing impaired as well as to the child or adolescent him- or herself. The process of counseling is designed to facilitate resolution of problems by enabling individuals to find appropriate solutions for their difficulties (Sanders, 1993).

The counseling process consists of two components: *informational counseling* and *personal-adjustment counseling*. Informational counseling provides information about aspects of the hearing impairment, such as the audiogram, the consequences of the hearing loss, and the use of amplification. Personal-adjustment counseling refers to the emotional aspects of adjusting to the hearing loss and assists the parent and child in finding solutions to their problems and ways of achieving independence (Luterman, 1979).

### Definitions of Hearing Loss

The terminology used to describe different conditions of hearing loss is very important because there needs to be commonality in the understanding of terms. The term *hearing impairment* is an all-inclusive term referring to all types and degrees of hearing loss (Sanders, 1993). There are generally two categories of hearing impairment: *hard-of-hearing* and *deaf.*

The term *hard-of-hearing* categorizes the child in terms of how he or she functions communicatively. Typically, children who are hard-of-hearing use their residual hearing and amplification as their primary mode of communication. Although most hard-of-hearing children learn speech and language to some degree, many even learn sign language to help them relate to the deaf and deaf culture.

The term *deaf* generally refers to profound hearing loss that prevents the child from using hearing as a primary mode of communication. This degree of hearing loss evokes distinction in culture as well as in audiometric designation (Sanders, 1993).

Finally, some terminology refers to the functional effects of an individual's hearing impairment. It is important to view all children with hearing impairment individually, as many have the same degree and configuration of hearing loss, but behave or function quite differently in terms of language, communication, and learning situations. For example, a child with a 70-dB sensory loss who uses hearing aids could function as a deaf child or a hearing child depending on success with amplification, speech and language development, psychosocial development, and so forth.

## APPROACHES TO COUNSELING

### Counseling Theories and Methods

There are several counseling approaches for parents of children and adolescents who are hearing impaired, as well as for children and adolescents themselves. These approaches/methods fall into four main categories: (*a*) cognitive/rational, (*b*) behavioral, (*c*) affective/humanistic, and (*d*) eclectic. The following brief discussion of each of these approaches is provided to expose the audiologist to the options available when counseling these individuals.

#### COGNITIVE/RATIONAL APPROACH

The cognitive or rational approach to counseling focuses primarily on thought processes and logic by emphasizing intellectual or logical means of resolving problems. In this approach, the counselor attempts to modify the individual's cognitions (i.e., his or her thoughts, ideas, beliefs, opinions, interpretations, values, and perceptions) using both active and passive means. The counselor helps explore the inappropriateness of a client's perceptions by persuading and arguing in an accepting yet at times confrontational manner. This approach is based on one's ability to control personal feelings by controlling his or her thoughts (Beck, 1976; Erdman, 1993).

#### BEHAVIORAL APPROACH

The behavioral approach emphasizes the body and physical actions as opposed to the mind and intellect. It is based on learning theory, which employs learning principles (e.g., classical conditioning) to change inappropriate behaviors and teach adaptive behavior. The behavioral approach is analytic and empiric in nature and provides measurable results (Erdman, 1993). The behavioral approach has been useful with individuals who are hearing impaired in a number of settings (DiMichael, 1985; Erdman, 1980). It also has been combined with cognitive approaches for the benefit of clients (Meichenbaum, 1974, 1977).

#### AFFECTIVE/HUMANISTIC APPROACH

In this approach, the counselor focuses on modifying clients' feelings and emotions to facilitate adjustment rather than on their behavior or thought processes. The premise behind this approach is that clients can redirect their lives given a healthy, beneficial climate conducive to allowing them to explore themselves. Unfortunately, an inherent problem with this approach is that emotions can be dealt with only indirectly (Erdman, 1993).

Generally, there are two ways in which counselors can approach their clients using the affective or humanistic method. Person-centered therapy is based on the work of Carl Rogers (Rogers, 1942; 1951) and on the self-theory views of personality and behavior. Individuals are viewed as innately good, constructive, and growth oriented. In person-centered therapy, the counselor's role is nondirective because focus is on self-actualization by the client. The other approach in the affective or humanistic method to counseling is Gestalt therapy (Perls, 1973). This is a phenomenologic-existential approach that is similar to person-centered therapy because it is holistic and integrates individuals to the point that they are self-directive. However, the counselor's role in this process is different from that in person-centered therapy in that the focus is on the here-and-now and on awareness of all elements that configure one's entire being (gestalt). This approach enables one to remain in contact with the current situation (Erdman, 1993).

ECLECTIC APPROACH

The eclectic approach is a combination of different aspects of several of the approaches discussed. There is considerable overlap among approaches, making it difficult to adhere completely to only one. Thus, by including factors from cognitive, behavioral, and affective methods, the eclectic approach incorporates different mechanisms of change that come together for the benefit of the client (Erdman, 1993; Meier, 1989).

## General Counseling Process

Regardless which counseling approach is chosen, the counseling process undoubtedly will have at least some aspects from each of the methods discussed. The counseling process certainly has a humanistic factor that allows the counselor and client to focus on emotions and feelings to facilitate adjustment and enhance quality of life.

Sanders (1993) outlines some objectives for audiologists to consider when counseling parents of children with hearing impairment and the children and adolescents themselves. These include (a) creating a climate of trust, (b) establishing a partnership between the audiologist and parent and child; (c) assisting the parent and child in describing the problems they face; (d) helping the parent and child translate their feelings into needs; and (e) determining appropriate referrals for professional counseling as needed. Sanders (1993) discusses some general counseling strategies that can be useful to the audiologist in providing services to this population. Using these strategies in the context of counseling can be quite beneficial to the client.

Sanders' (1993) strategies direct the audiologist to ask the parent or child to describe problems as they see them at the time and then to restate the problems just described to ensure complete understanding. Restating the problem ensures that the audiologist as counselor understands the problem as described by the parent or child. Restatement also allows the parents and child to hear someone else articulate their feelings. It is important for audiologists as counselors to ask for clarification on points that are unclear and to focus the discussion on areas of central concern. Sanders suggests being reflective—that is, offering impressions of what the parent or child seems to be experiencing.

Listening is one of the most important aspects of being a successful counselor (Sanders, 1993). Improved listening skills strengthen the counselor-client relationship as clients will feel that the audiologist/counselor truly cares about them and their concerns and feelings. Improving listening skills requires that audiologists resist distractions and suspend all judgment while listening to the client. Good listeners wait to respond to clients' comments or questions until their complete thoughts have been expressed. It is often helpful to repeat verbatim what the client says to clarify the concern as well as to allow the client to hear what he or she has just articulated. Good listeners also are well prepared so that during the counselor-client interaction, full attention is on the client, not on the previous test results or other issues. Setting aside time specifically for counseling in an environment void of distractions also paves the way for good listening.

A final key to good listening is paying attention to the types of questions asked by parents. Sanders (1993) classifies these questions into three groups: content, confirmation, and affect. Content questions are those that seek specific information about something. Content questions include inquiries about hearing test results, hearing aids, educational programming, and so forth. Confirmation questions are those asking an opinion or position from the audiologist but are phrased as content questions. For example, parents may ask about whether it would be appropriate for them to learn sign language, which may be a cover to ask the audiologist's opinion about sign language in general. Finally, affect questions contain emotional overtones that may have little to do with the content, but more to do with the way parents are feeling about the fact that their child is hearing impaired or deaf. Affect questions may be an indication that clients are in need of personal-adjustment counseling.

Sensitive clinicians listen carefully to all types of questions posed by their clients to assess the true meaning of their queries. Because counseling is an integral part of the audiologic process, it is important to remember that the abnormality is in the ear, not within the individual. Establishing a sense of trust and a good working relationship with the individual enhances the adjustment process.

## Multidisciplinary Approach to Counseling

The identification of hearing loss in children has ramifications that reach well beyond the need for amplification and intensive speech and language training. The child may have other problems or limitations that require the expertise of and referral to many other professionals. Also, parents are often at a loss regarding how to pay for the multitude of services that the child needs immediately and in the future. Therefore, to be truly effective for parents and their children with hearing loss, professionals must work together as a team to aid in (re)habilitation and counseling. The multidisciplinary approach consists of formulating a team of professionals with expertise in several areas that have an impact on parents and their children with hearing impairment.

A *physician* is one of the professionals that should be considered for the team. The physician can be of great assistance if the child has other medical problems in addition to hearing loss. If the medical problems are ear-related, the physician serves as the key to diagnosis and treatment of the hearing impairment or ear anomalies. It is therefore essential that the physician and audiologist have a strong working relationship that includes understanding and respecting each other's skills in order to work together to habilitate the child's hearing.

Another team member to be considered is a *psychologist.* At times, parents of children and adolescents who are hearing impaired as well as the children and adolescents themselves may be unable to work through all of the feelings and emotions they have regarding the hearing loss and its effects. A psychologist on the team provides a strong referral source for the audiologist who feels that the client's emotional problems exceed his or her ability to treat. The psychologist can also be helpful in group counseling sessions for parents and children.

A *social worker* is another professional who might serve on the team. Social workers interact with a combination of social, economic, environmental, and personal problems. They can help determine whether the parents of children with hearing impairment are capable of accomplishing their life tasks. A social worker can respond to the family's needs and its social difficulty because social workers are usually very aware of community resources (e.g., educational, financial, religious, social, consumer groups) to help them.

Another individual who can be supportive of counseling needs and financial resources is a *vocational rehabilitation counselor.* The United States Office of Vocational Rehabilitation is an agency that provides services to individuals of employment age who are unable to earn a living because of a disability such as hearing impairment. The Office of Vocational Rehabilitation may be an excellent resource when dealing with adolescents or young adults who are hearing impaired.

The *family* of a hearing-impaired child and the parents play a major role in (re)habilitation and counseling. It is very important for the audiologist to welcome family members to the team because family support is so critical to successful management. Having the family involved at all times also helps the audiologist identify family members, other than the parents and the child with the hearing impairment, who may be in need of counseling and support.

Of course, the *speech-language pathologist* and *audiologist* are integral members of this multidisciplinary team. The speech-language pathologist will provide intensive speech and language training for the child making full use of any residual hearing. The speech-language pathologist also works closely with the audiologist regarding the speech, language, and auditory development of the child. The audiologist often coordinates the management of the child with hearing impairment by making the other members of the team aware of the hearing testing procedures, the proposed management plan, and the role needed by them.

## Counseling Referrals

Although audiologists do serve as counselors, there are times when parents and their children may need more counseling than an audiologist can provide. This is particularly true when clients stop moving forward and seem to be unable or unwilling to confront the emotions experienced from hearing loss (Clark, 1994). When this situation exists, the audiologist must recognize that this client should be referred to a specialized counselor, clinical psychologist, or psychiatrist.

Making appropriate counseling referrals is an important activity that the audiologist should not take lightly. Parents and children will have established a strong relationship with the audiologist early on and may be dependent on the audiologist for more than audiologic services. Consequently, clients may be skeptical about a referral made to an unknown therapist. Audiologists should refer their clients with confidence and make them realize that they are not abandoning them, but that they are getting additional resources and help for them. If a good relationship has been established with clients, they should respond well to this referral (Clark, 1994).

To make appropriate referrals, audiologists should be fully aware of local resources for psychological and social intervention. Mental health professionals who have some awareness and preferably some experience with hearing impairment are ideal referral sources. Many schools for the deaf are a useful resource of such professionals. In some cases, it will be the parents who need further treatment or family therapy; in others, it may be the child with the hearing impairment who needs to be referred for psychological counseling. Audiologists should not hesitate to seek the advice of other professionals in the field of counseling to assist them in making such referrals.

## INFLUENCE OF HEARING IMPAIRMENT ON FAMILY LIFE

### Parental Reactions to Children with Hearing Impairment

When parents learn that their child has a significant hearing impairment, they experience a multitude of reactions. For some, there is a sense of relief and confirmation that the behaviors they have been observing in their child have some justification. When parents suspect that their child may have a problem hearing, they often seek help from their physician who hopefully will make a referral to an audiologist for evaluation. If the audiologic test results indicate a significant hearing loss, parents may experience relief that the problem finally has been identified. However, many other reactions follow this sense of relief and confirmation.

Parental reactions to hearing impairment in their children is similar to those experienced when a loved one has died (Luterman, 1979). In a sense, parents have lost the hopes, dreams, and aspirations that they may have had for their child. Their once "perfect" child is now not so perfect; these parents tend to go through a grieving process in dealing with such knowledge about their child. The grief parents experience is understandable, but it can have negative effects on habilitation. Thus, it is critical that professionals respond to the grieving process in a manner that facilitates acceptance of the loss (Luterman, 1979).

Shontz (1965) describes the psychological reactions to crisis as a useful model for understanding the reaction of parents who have deaf children. Immediately after parents receive the diagnosis of deafness, they often experience a crisis. The psychological reactions to crisis are also similar to the stages of grief described by Kubler-Ross (1969).

In crisis reactions, Shontz suggests that parents initially experience *shock.* During this relatively short stage, parents may divorce themselves from the crisis situation as a defensive reaction. They may be present physically but may not be emotionally or intellectually attentive. It is important for the audiologist to recognize that the initial reaction (the first stage) is when the audiologist explains to the parents that their child is deaf. Because of the shock parents experience, they often do not hear much of what the audiologist says after they hear that their child is deaf. Audiologists therefore should be aware that they may need to repeat many times the important information about the child's deafness and intervention until they are sure parents are emotionally and intellectually attentive.

The second stage in crisis reaction according to Shontz (1965) is *recognition.* In this short-term stage, parents begin to realize the awfulness of the situation and begin to acknowledge it emotionally. Parents may ask, "Why me?" as they recognize what is really happening. They may be totally overwhelmed in this stage and have feelings of inadequacy, confusion, anger, frustration, depression, and guilt. Parents may experience total confusion over new terms and treatments that are being recommended for their child. They may experience *anger* because their expectations have been violated. Their anger may stem from disappointment and frustration. This anger may be expressed toward the audiologist so it is important to depersonalize this anger as a clinician. *Guilt* is the parents' way of searching for the cause for the deafness. Parents often express their guilt by saying things like, "If I had only . . . , maybe this would not have happened." Feelings of guilt can lead to resentment and overprotection of the child and a loss of trust. Finally, in this stage parents try to *bargain*—that is, they will "do anything" as long as the child's deafness is alleviated. All of these feelings are natural responses to deafness, so clinicians should be very supportive during this stage and try to provide nonverbal consolation by using good listening skills.

During the recognition stage, parents may expect that the audiologist will take care of them by repairing the damaged ear or assuming all responsibility for education of the deaf child. They may have unrealistic expectations for hearing aids and expect to conquer the deafness without any feelings of despair (Luterman, 1979).

The third stage, *denial,* can be a long-term stage. In this stage, parents may go back to their defensive retreat as a coping mechanism with wishful thinking that their child is not deaf. They may reject the diagnosis of the hearing loss and get other opinions; or they may accept the diagnosis but reject the permanence of it. When parents react in this way, it may appear to the clinician that they are blocking attempts at intervention. What is actually happening, however, may be that parents are building inner strength to deal with what lies ahead. If parents stay in the denial stage too long and avoid recommendations for early intervention, the child may be slighted. Audiologists should accept parental denial and continue to provide appropriate information for the child's habilitation.

The fourth stage, *acknowledgment,* is a life-long stage. In this stage parents begin the acceptance process. As Luterman (1979) so aptly describes it, parents begin to accept their child's hearing impairment in this way:

> I have a deaf child and he will always be deaf, and although there is nothing I can do about changing the hearing impairment, there are things I can do to help this child grow into a responsible human being. (p. 13)

It is a sign of acceptance when parents begin to take good care of hearing aids and follow through on recommendations made for the child.

Shontz (1965) suggests that the final stage and ultimate goal of crisis reaction is *constructive action*. This is also a life-long stage in which evidence that the grief is resolved first occurs. During constructive action, parents adapt more easily to changes and are more positive about their child and management of the impairment.

Awareness of the stages of crisis reaction and grief is important for audiologists as they provide both informational and personal-adjustment counseling to parents of deaf children. The length of each stage may vary from parent to parent. However, if parents experience acute reactions that last beyond six months, they may need psychological help from other professionals. Audiologists also should recognize that parental grief may reappear at a later time even after they appear to have moved into the acknowledgment and constructive action stages.

## Impact of Deafness on the Family

A deaf child born into the family may disrupt the delicate family structure and can have a significant impact on family dynamics. Audiologists must consider the entire family (i.e., grandparents, siblings, and other family members or close friends) and make appropriate adjustments to changing family needs. Over the years, the family structure has changed significantly with increases in the number of two-career, single-parent, and low-income families. These changes affect the options available for intervention and management of children with hearing impairment. Many women with young children work outside the home, which makes it difficult for home instruction to occur (Luterman, 1979). Therefore, audiologists and other professionals must be sensitive to these changes and try to be flexible in the management options provided to parents.

The child who is deaf may impact on the relationships between husband and wife, parents and grandparents, and siblings. The emotional needs of both the husband and wife must be considered as additional stress is placed on them during the intervention process. Grandparents often remained fixed in the denial stage because they lack an understanding of the problem. They are not only experiencing the impact of a grandchild who is deaf, but are also hurting because their own child is suffering. The parents of the child who is deaf may seek support from their parents, but it may not be there. Audiologists might recommend support groups for parents and grandparents to help deal with these issues. Grandparents can be very helpful to parents by being available for respite care and babysitting so parents can have some time out. Grandparents can also be helpful in parenting older siblings and providing a surrogate-parent role (Luterman, 1979).

Siblings of children who are deaf also can have emotional problems. Siblings may get less attention from their parents because of the increased demands on their time in dealing with the child who is deaf. Some siblings attempt to get their parents' attention by developing pseudosensory deficits. Others may appear to be good, uncomplaining children who are asked to assume more responsibilities at young ages, but still may be experiencing emotional problems as a result of their sibling's deafness. It is important, therefore, to keep siblings incorporated into family activities and decisions (Kricos, 1993; Luterman, 1979).

The parent-child interaction is of course the most important one. Even though parents are dealing with their grief and crisis reactions, they cannot put their lives on hold until the grieving process is over. They still must love and care for their rapidly growing child who is deaf as well as other family members and deal with life's responsibilities.

In Erickson's discussion of the life cycle (Erickson, 1959), he identifies several stages that people experience in development. The first stage, which occurs during the first eighteen months of life, he calls "Trust versus Mistrust." It is during this stage that the child develops a sense of hope and trust about the world. The normally hearing child is raised in the home having a warm relationship with the mother and varied cognitive input. However, when the child is deaf, there is often difficulty with the parent-child relationship because the birth of a child who is deaf puts stress on parents. Optimal attachment may not develop if the parent is still experiencing grief. Further, if the child is deaf, parents may not know how to communicate with their child, which will limit vocal play and parent-child interactions.

Parents are less likely to provide verbal praise for the child who is deaf. Many nonverbal communication attempts by preschoolers who are hearing impaired may be ignored or misunderstood by parents. Also, parents may respond inappropriately to their child's communication attempts and fail to request clarification of their utterances. All of these behaviors may affect the child's psychosocial development, which may lead to the need for counseling throughout their lives.

## COUNSELING PROCESS: THE PARENT

### General Model of Intervention Management

Sanders (1993) proposes a general model for intervention management that contains eight steps: (*a*) providing emotional and informational support, (*b*) reviewing and interpreting available test results, (*c*) ascertaining present situation and needs, (*d*) supplementing interview and test results, (*e*) determining primary and secondary goals, (*f*) identifying appropriate resources, (*g*) developing a management plan, and (*h*) monitoring effectiveness of intervention strategies. Because early intervention is critical to the successful habilitation of children who are deaf, parents should be aware of the general management plan proposed for their child. The following discussion considers the steps in Sanders' (1993) model as they relate to counseling in the habilitation process for deaf children and their parents.

PROVIDING EMOTIONAL AND INFORMATIONAL SUPPORT

This initial step in intervention is the most critical one with regard to the counseling needs of parents of children who are deaf. During this intervention step, audiologists must provide reassurance to parents who are seeking their help by assisting them in understanding the problem and reassuring them that many management options are available that can address the problem directly. To do this successfully, audiologists must recognize that parents' immediate fear and anxiety is based on the unknown; thus, this fear and anxiety must be addressed so that parents are maximally attentive and cooperative in the habilitation process.

Audiologists should acknowledge and legitimize parents' feelings and make them aware that they are experiencing a natural and normal reaction. Audiologists should also attempt to reduce parents' stress by helping them acknowledge and accept their feelings as they go through the stages of crisis reaction and grief as discussed. Developing trust between parents and professionals is a critical element needed to reduce stress. The development of trust is based on experience and must be earned, so audiologists must establish a comfortable relationship with parents. As parents begin to accept their feelings, trust will soon follow (Sanders, 1993).

In addition to dealing with the personal adjustment of parents during this initial stage of habilitation, audiologists should impart information to parents continually. Sufficient information limits the degree of the unknown and, therefore, minimizes parents' fears and anxieties. Informational counseling makes the problem easier to deal with and more tangible for parents. It is helpful at this stage for counselors to provide an outline of a plan to proceed with therapy including any additional testing needed and information to be obtained. Determining the intervention plan together with parents builds their confidence in the plan and reduces their anxiety about their child's future.

## REVIEWING AND INTERPRETING AVAILABLE TEST RESULTS

In this stage of intervention, Sanders indicates that audiologic test information is evaluated and used as a guide to determine the child's present situation and needs. At this time, expectations concerning auditory behavior with hearing aids are shaped; predictions are made regarding the probability of speech and language development and the use of supplemental sensory avenues in communication stimulation. Both informational and personal-adjustment counseling are utilized at this stage.

## ASCERTAINING PRESENT SITUATION AND NEEDS

During this phase of intervention, audiologists attempt to establish a positive relationship with parents while gaining a general picture of their perception of their child's problem. The personal-adjustment counseling done in this stage emphasizes the importance of parents' perceptions of their child's difficulties and needs and encourages parents to describe their feelings and perceptions. In this way, audiologists can establish a partnership role and make parents comfortable within the management setting. Focusing on what the parents perceive as reality encourages them to trust in the professional who shows respect for them.

## SUPPLEMENTING INTERVIEW AND TEST RESULTS

This is an informational step in intervention as the audiologist obtains information from parents, other audiologists, schools, preschools, and speech-language pathologists. This information is used to diagnose problem situations, assess side effects of communication difficulty (educational, social, and emotional), and explore resources (client, family, school setting, other professionals, and technology).

## DETERMINING PRIMARY AND SECONDARY GOALS

Although many of the goals developed for the child who is deaf are habilitative in nature, this intervention stage should also include some goals specific to counseling. The personal adjustment of parents, grandparents, siblings, and the child who is deaf is of paramount importance if habilitation is to be successful and if other goals are to be achieved.

## IDENTIFYING APPROPRIATE RESOURCES

In this stage of intervention, supplemental support and services should be explored, including different types of amplification and assistive devices, assistance from other professionals, and modifications of the child's environment that enhance the development of auditory, speech, and language skills. Access to additional counseling resources also should be explored in the event that a referral is needed beyond the realm of audiology.

## DEVELOPING A MANAGEMENT PLAN

The actual intervention plan is developed and implemented in this stage, and habilitation is well under way. It is important to keep in mind that counseling is an ongoing process and should always be available as children and their families evolve.

MONITORING EFFECTIVENESS OF INTERVENTION STRATEGIES

In Sanders' final step, the effectiveness of the intervention is assessed. Objective and subjective evaluation criteria should be programmed into the habilitation plan to monitor the effectiveness of all aspects of intervention. Personal-adjustment and informational counseling should be reviewed periodically to ensure that parents and their children are progressing well emotionally and psychosocially.

## Family-Centered Counseling

One of the goals of counseling in the habilitation of children who are hearing impaired is parents' achievement of confidence in their ability to cope with situations that are affected by their child's hearing impairment (Sanders, 1993). Achieving this goal results in improvement of the quality of life for parents and children by reducing the negative physical and psychological influences of hearing loss (Sanders, 1993). The counseling relationship established between audiologist and parent should be a partnership where the two parties coordinate their resources to reduce the actual or potential negative impact of hearing impairment. The audiologist combines expertise regarding communication, hearing loss, and hearing aids with first-hand knowledge of the parents regarding the total impact of deafness on the family as well as financial, social, and emotional burdens. A successful counseling relationship, then, is one that allows both parties to work together on all aspects of intervention and which allocates time throughout habilitation for counseling (Sanders, 1993).

In recent years, the target of intervention services has shifted from child to family partially owing to the mandate given by PL 99–457, Part H. This legislation has dramatically increased family involvement in intervention services for handicapped infants and toddlers and has increased awareness among the profession and the community regarding the family's role in their child's overall development (Kricos, 1993). Consequently, these changes also have increased the emphasis on a family-centered approach to counseling.

Family-centered counseling utilizes family resources and strengths and allows for an active role for families in the habilitation of their children. Family-centered counseling also emphasizes the need for families to be intimately and directly involved in the decisions made for their children throughout their habilitation.

Audiologists should be aware of certain multicultural aspects of family-centered counseling. Cultural diversity has a significant impact on family dynamics and the counseling process (Kricos, 1993). With significant changes occurring in the demographics of the world's population, audiologists are already working with individuals who may have different values and cultures than their own. These differences are critical to the success of a healthy counseling relationship between parents and professionals. Therefore, audiologists must take time to learn about different cultural perspectives so that they can work effectively with families whose views may be different from their own (Kricos, 1993). (See also, Chapter 5 in this text.)

## Genetic Counseling for Parents

Another aspect of the counseling process for parents is the need for genetic counseling. If the parents have normal hearing and their children are hearing impaired, they need to be made aware of the potential risk for having more children who may be hearing impaired. Audiologists often should make referrals to genetic counselors who can discuss the percentage of risk that another child may be hearing impaired. Because the majority of children who are deaf are born to parents who have normal hearing, parents must increase their knowledge of risks to their future children through genetic counseling.

## Counseling Parents Regarding Habilitation Methodology

When habilitation begins for the infant who is deaf, audiologists must consider what method of habilitation will be followed for the child. There is considerable controversy regarding which type of methodology is most appropriate for individual children; consequently, making the decision regarding communication philosophies is not a simple process. Audiologists should recognize that when this decision is made, parents are still experiencing emotional reactions to hearing loss and may be well into the grieving process. Therefore, audiologists must be sure that parents are well informed about the options available regarding habilitation methodologies so that they can contribute to the decision-making process as well.

There are three general methodologies available to children who are deaf: (*a*) auditory/verbal, (*b*) manual communication, and (*c*) total communication. The *auditory/verbal* method attempts to maximize the child's use of his or her residual hearing through amplification so that he or she can communicate using oral speech and language. Auditory/verbal training focuses on enhancing lip reading and audition skills and excludes the use of any natural signs or gestures. Children must have some usable and aidable hearing to be successful with this method. This method often appeals to parents who have normal hearing as they will be able to communicate with their child using their natural mode of communication.

*Manual communication* refers to the use of a sign system and/or sign language as the primary mode of communication. Children who have little residual hearing or receive minimal benefit from amplification often succeed using this methodology. The use of American Sign Language (ASL), which is a unique natural language, provides a method of communication for individuals who are deaf. ASL is often considered the most important attribute of deaf culture.

The third option, *total communication,* is a philosophy that incorporates any mode of communication that can help get the message across to the individual. Total communication uses aural, oral, tactile, and manual methods to ensure effective communication. Children who benefit from amplification but do not receive significant enhancement in audition, often benefit from total communication using both oral and manual cues.

Regardless of which methodology is chosen for a particular child, parents should be counseled regarding the advantages and disadvantages of each method. Audiologists also should offer their experience and clinical opinions regarding the child's prognosis with each method. However, because the selection of methodology can affect whether the child communicates in the hearing world or in the deaf world, there are many cultural aspects that must be considered in this decision as well. The following brief discussion regarding deaf culture is provided to make audiologists aware of some of the views of deaf individuals that may affect decisions regarding communication philosophy.

DEAF CULTURE

Many individuals who are deaf prefer to be referred to as "The Deaf." These individuals live in communities with other people who are deaf and use ASL as their primary mode of communication, which is often seen as a critical aspect of deaf culture. The Deaf feel that deafness is not a disorder; it is a biologic and cultural difference. They do not view their deafness as a negative factor or a disability; they view themselves as different only in the way that they communicate. Individuals who are part of the Deaf culture make up a diverse group of people who have varying degrees of hearing loss and differing viewpoints about hearing impairment, communication methods, and lifestyles. They feel that although they have limited ability to hear, they are not handicapped because they can communicate successfully with other Deaf via ASL. Therefore, their primary difference from a society that hears is cultural.

In contrast, audiologists often view deafness as a disability or disease that needs to be cured by the hearing community. Researchers continue to look for a cure for genetic deafness. Deaf culture sees audiologists as hearing people attempting to change children who are deaf by advocating that they use hearing aids or cochlear implants, learn speech production, and learn the auditory/verbal mode of communication. The Deaf perceive these actions as inappropriate attempts to change or restrict their culture. In fact, they see cochlear implants as a threat to the very existence of Deaf culture (Tyler, 1993).

Audiologists should appreciate and respect the philosophic differences between the hearing world and the Deaf community when selecting an appropriate communication method for children. As counselors, they must understand and accept Deaf culture and learn how to interact successfully with the Deaf. Audiologists must provide fair and accurate counseling by stressing a positive view of Deaf culture and by being honest regarding predictions of successful management of deafness. They also must recognize that there is diversity in both hearing and Deaf cultures and that some individuals within the Deaf culture have benefited from hearing aids and cochlear implants (Tyler, 1993).

## Summary: Counseling the Parent

The counseling process for parents who have children who are deaf is ongoing throughout the child's life, although it is most critical in the early years. If audiologists follow a management model that provides both informational and personal-adjustment counseling while the child's habilitation is being planned and carried out, they will be successful in developing a partnership between themselves and parents. Such a successful counseling relationship makes the family-centered approach beneficial to both the parents and the child. Parents should be involved in all decisions made for their children, especially with regard to the habilitation methodology chosen. Parents are often the key to the success of such methodologies. Finally, audiologists should make parents aware of the influence that Deaf culture may have throughout the child's life.

### COUNSELING PROCESS: THE CHILD WHO IS HEARING IMPAIRED

When the child reaches the age of about three years, the focus of habilitation and counseling begins to shift from parent to child. At this age, it is important to focus on the child to encourage independence; enhance cognitive, social, and linguistic skills; and prepare the child for school. Despite this shift in focus, however, it is critical that the family maintain its role in habilitation. The parents' role should not be diminished because the child will still be receiving significant input from parents at home (Sanders, 1993).

Because counseling is an ongoing process, it is important for the audiologist to remain in contact with both the parent and child to provide the necessary personal-adjustment and informational counseling as needed. Even though the shift in habilitation focuses more on the child, counseling the young child may not yet be necessary. However, as children with hearing impairment grow and mature and begin to achieve more independence in their lives, they begin to notice differences between themselves and other children their age. At this point, it is important for the audiologist to begin to teach the child about his or her hearing impairment. Some children reach this stage at an earlier age than others; the audiologist must be aware of aspects of the child's behavior and overall development that may indicate when the child is ready to take on more responsibility regarding hearing loss.

When the child is at the point where informational counseling can be effective, the audiologist should teach the child about the hearing loss. Audiologists should create instructional techniques that are appropriate for the child's level of understanding and explain the audiogram, the effects of the hearing loss on speech understanding, the importance of hearing aids, and how to use and take care of hearing aids. A child about eight or nine years old should have enough independence to take on the responsibility of the hearing aids. Counseling should ensure that the child knows how to insert the hearing aids properly, how to adjust them, when to wear them, and how to take care of them. Early in intervention, parents take on these responsibilities. When the child achieves such a level of independence, the parents should step back and allow the child to take on these responsibilities.

### Hearing-Impaired Adolescent

As the child continues to develop, personal-adjustment counseling may be needed in addition to informational counseling. This is particularly true during adolescence. Adolescence is a normal adjustment process where the child moves from the relative stability and protection of childhood through a period of intense biologic, psychological, and social change (Sanders, 1993). Adolescents strive for independence as the responsibility of adulthood looms in the near future. The adolescent who is hearing impaired goes through these normal changes, but also deals with some additional adjustments because of the hearing loss. It is during this time that there is an increased need for counseling. Adolescents who are hearing impaired need an avenue through which they can express their aspirations, verbalize their fears, assess their strengths, and identify and test their personal limitations.

Counselors of adolescents who are hearing impaired should define their role broadly at first to establish cooperative interaction with the adolescent. The goal of such counseling is to define problem areas and explore solutions together. It is important not to minimize the significance of the feelings expressed by the adolescents, but to stimulate self-exploration of their feelings and attitudes. The counseling intervention plan should grow out of an understanding of the way the adolescent perceives difficulties related to his or her hearing loss (Kricos, 1993; Sanders, 1993).

### Adjustments for the Adolescent

Adolescents often have difficulties in four main areas by the time they reach high school: (a) peer relationships and social experiences, (b) relationships with the opposite sex, (c) acceptance by teachers, and (d) academic limitations (Sanders, 1993).

Adolescents have difficulty with *peer relationships and social experiences* because of the intense desire to conform and be like everybody else. An adolescent who is hearing impaired is already considered different. Further, if the adolescent wears hearing aids, they can be perceived as a deviation which makes adolescents wearing them feel less like their peers. When adolescents who are hearing impaired experience these feelings, audiologists often have to deal with the adolescent's rejection of the hearing aids. Many adolescents, therefore, refuse to wear hearing aids during this time because they make them feel different from their peers. Audiologists or counselors should focus on the feelings the adolescent is having that are leading to this rejection rather than on reasons why the hearing aid should be worn.

Adolescents who are hearing impaired often have difficulty using the telephone, which can be a major limitation in trying to communicate with peers and achieve acceptance from them. Audiologists should explore modifications to traditional telephone use (e.g., assistive listening devices) so that these adolescents can use the telephone successfully. Adolescents who are hearing impaired thrive for acceptance by their peer group. This acceptance is often influenced by the image they project of themselves. Thus, counseling should focus on ways that the adolescent can show success and competence and avoid a negative projection (Sanders, 1993).

It is also very important that parents recognize that adolescence is the time to begin letting go of their children and allow them more independence than ever before. Parents must learn the delicate balance between giving freedom to their children who are hearing impaired and still being available to them when needed. Parents often underestimate their children's abilities and are very overprotective, so it is important for parents to recognize what their children need during this time of maturation (Luterman, 1979).

*Relationships with the opposite sex* are often difficult for teenagers, especially the hearing impaired. The adolescent's self-concept needs to be strong and healthy before he or she can feel comfortable in a relationship. The counselor can help the adolescent better evaluate him-or herself by considering the teenager as a whole person. Also, the adolescent's communication skills and sociolinguistic competence should be assessed to be sure they are adequate (Sanders, 1993). Relationships with peers may even help motivate the hearing-impaired adolescent to work on speech production, voice quality, and so forth.

High school students who are hearing impaired often have difficulty being *accepted by teachers.* Most postsecondary teachers do not get as much education about hearing impairment as primary teachers do. Therefore, these educators may not fully understand the problems that postprimary students with hearing loss experience. Audiologists and counselors may need to educate these teachers so they can help students with hearing impairment adjust.

Finally, the high school student who is hearing impaired may have some *academic limitations* to be considered especially if the hearing impairment is significant enough to affect the development of normal speech and language skills. These students may have difficulty with certain courses because of the complexity of the language used in the class. They also may have difficulty because of the environment in which the courses are taught or because of the teaching method used. In this situation, the audiologist or counselor should identify the primary support services needed to enhance the student's learning in the course and continue to monitor needs as the student matures through adolescence and young adulthood.

## Personal Adjustment for the Adolescent

Deafness often has a *stigma* associated with it as many individuals who are deaf are viewed as different from normal. This *difference* is often manifested while the Deaf are communicating using ASL, because the act of signing often sets these individuals apart from society. Consequently, society often labels these individuals first as being deaf, which makes deafness their chief defining characteristic.

Deaf adolescents also may experience a feeling of *marginality*, i.e., not being completely part of either the hearing world or the deaf world. These individuals often belong to two cultural worlds and have considerable difficulty with psychological identification and emotional well-being. This is particularly true for adolescents who are deaf and live with families who have normal hearing. In some cases, the deafness itself may be less of a problem than the feelings of marginality across the two different cultures.

Audiologists can help these adolescents determine their roles in society. Deafness can be considered a social handicap because it tends to isolate the individual from the rest of the group. This may lead to low self-esteem in the adolescent who is hearing impaired. Thus, it is important for the audiologist to nurture a positive self-concept in children who are hearing impaired by acknowledging their feelings, reinforcing their strengths and achievements, and encouraging them to set goals (Kricos, 1993).

## CONCLUSION

Counseling children with hearing impairment and their parents is a challenging task for audiologists. They must become comfortable in the role of counselor to facilitate the adjustment of individuals with hearing impairment. With training and experience, audiologists can be successful counselors and provide both informational and personal-adjustment support throughout the (re)habilitation process.

## REFERENCES

Beck, A. T. (1976). *Cognitive therapy and emotional disorders.* New York: International Universities Press.

Clark, J. G. (1994). Audiologists' counseling purview. In J. G. Clark & F. N. Martin (Eds.), *Effective counseling in audiology: Perspectives and practice* (pp. 1–15). Englewood Cliffs, NJ: Prentice-Hall.

Culpepper, N. B., Mendel, L. L., & McCarthy, P. A. (1994). Counseling experience and training offered by ESB-accredited programs: An update. *ASHA, 36* (6), 55–58.

DiMichael, S. G. (1985). *Assertiveness training for persons who are hard of hearing.* Rockville, MD: SHHH Publications.

Erdman, S. A. (1980). The use of assertiveness training in adult aural rehabilitation. *Audiology Journal of Continuing Education, 5* (12).

Erdman, S. A. (1993). Counseling hearing-impaired adults. In J. G. Alpiner & P. A. McCarthy (Eds.), *Rehabilitative audiology: Children and adults* (pp. 374–413). Baltimore: Williams & Wilkins.

Erickson, E. (1959). Identity and the life cycle. *Psychological Issues, Monograph 1.* New York: International Universities Press.

Haas, W. H., & Crowley, D. J. (1982). Professional information dissemination to parents of pre-school hearing-impaired children. *Volta Review, 84* (1), 17–23.

Kricos, P. B. (1993). The counseling process: Children and parents. In J. G. Alpiner & P. A. McCarthy (Eds.), *Rehabilitative audiology: Children and adults* (pp. 211–223). Baltimore, MD: Williams & Wilkins.

Kubler-Ross, E. (1979). *On death and dying.* New York: Macmillan.

Luterman, D. (1979). *Counseling parents of hearing-impaired children.* Boston: Little, Brown, & Co.

McCarthy, P. A., Culpepper, N. B., & Lucks, L. E. (1986). Variability in counseling experiences and training among ESB-accredited programs. *ASHA, 28* (9), 49–52.

Meichenbaum, D. (1974). *Cognitive behavior modification.* Morristown, NJ: General Learning Press.

Meichenbaum, D. (1977). *Cognitive behavior modification: An integrative approach.* New York: Plenum.

Meier, S. T. (1989). *The elements of counseling.* Pacific Grove, CA: Brooks/Cole.

Perls, F. S. (1973). *The Gestalt approach.* Palo Alto: Science and Behavior Books.

Rogers, C.R. (1942). *Counseling and psychotherapy.* Boston: Houghton Mifflin.

Rogers, C. R. (1951). *Client-centered therapy.* Boston: Houghton Mifflin.

Sanders, D. A. (1993). *Management of hearing handicap: Infants to elderly* (3rd ed.). Englewood Cliffs, NJ: Prentice-Hall.

Shontz, F. (1965). Reactions to crisis. *Volta Review, 67* (5), 364–370.

Sweetow, R. W., & Barrager, D. (1980). Quality of comprehensive audiological care: A survey of parents of hearing-impaired children. *ASHA, 22* (10), 841–847.

Tyler, R. (1993). Cochlear implants and the deaf culture. *American Journal of Audiology, 2* (1), 26–32.

Williams, D. M., & Darbyshire, J. O. (1982). Diagnosis of deafness: A study of family responses and needs. *Volta Review, 84* (1), 24–30.

# 14. Hearing Impairment: Adults and Seniors

Jerome G. Alpiner

---

---

The past several years have seen increased awareness in health care reform in the United States. Varying philosophies have been introduced regarding ways in which all individuals may be served for health care needs. Regardless of philosophy, there is consensus that patient outcomes must result in improved quality of life. Hearing loss can impair quality of life. The two most common causes of adult hearing loss are presbycusis and noise exposure. There are approximately 28 million adults with significant hearing loss in this country. Their ability to communicate adequately in everyday living situations may be limited. Hearing loss is one of those disorders that often "sneaks up" on individuals; hearing loss usually does not just happen all at once. For example, the "typical high frequency loss" results in a person thinking that there is no problem because low frequency sounds are heard well, giving a false notion that all is well auditorily. The person may not realize that high frequency sounds, such as /s/ and /f/, are not heard.

The primary mission of the audiologist is to provide both diagnostic and rehabilitative audiology for those with hearing loss. Health care proponents suggest that services provided by all professionals must be effective and cost efficient. The routine audiologic protocol is to conduct a diagnostic hearing evaluation with follow-up recommendations for hearing help. The recommendation most often made is for hearing aids and counseling. Other types of assistance may include telephone amplifiers, infrared TV listening systems, conference pocket talkers, or other devices.

Hearing aid technology has seen considerable advances and improvements during the past five years. Included are K-Amps, Complete in the Canal Aids (CICs), Class D amplifiers, nonlinear circuits, and more. Hearing aid users, therefore, may find significant improvement in hearing. Subsequently, some health care providers tend to believe that counseling is not essential now due to the advances in amplification. It is assumed that

307

amplification fulfills the complete need for improved communication. It is true that some individuals' communication may be significantly improved with hearing aids. This situation, however, is not completely true and will be discussed later.

This chapter, therefore, discusses counseling needs for adults and provides procedures and techniques that can be used to help persons with hearing loss be better communicators in family, social, and vocational roles in everyday living situations. Counseling includes hearing aid orientation at the time of fitting, hearing aid follow-up, informational counseling, and audiologic rehabilitation. It is important to recognize that the audiologic diagnostic process is essential, but we also need to consider statements by Lowe (1992):

> While the equipment gets more complex and next year's screen will be in six colors instead of four, we must ensure that tomorrow's audiologists will be people oriented and skilled at personal interaction with their clients. To do that requires rigorous training in the art of rehabilitation. Such a concept does not appear to be a high priority issue in our training programs, however, and has not been for far too long. Perhaps it is time for the pendulum to swing a bit. (p. 21)

Martin, Barr, and Bernstein (1992) reported on professional attitudes regarding counseling by otologists, otolaryngologists, and clinical audiologists. This study provides a baseline for current practices and beliefs of professionals who diagnose hearing impairments in the adult population. The authors indicate that professionals may gain some new insights into greater provision for emotional and informational support desired by hearing-impaired adults. It is emphasized that information regarding techniques used in counseling hearing-impaired adults may provide diagnosticians a guide by which to better evaluate their own procedures.

## AUDIOLOGIC REHABILITATION EVALUATION

It simply is not a matter of stating that we need to counsel clients. It must be known whether or not counseling is indicated and what problem areas exist for the client. Problems should be identified and quantified. Jinks (1991) addressed this issue as it relates to continuing education for nursing staff involved in counseling older adults with hearing loss. Of importance to audiologists is the staging of the counseling environment in order for communication to be accomplished appropriately. Suggestions include:

1. Be positioned as physically close to the client as is comfortable.
2. Face the client and speak directly to him/her.
3. Do not stand when the client is sitting, or vice versa.
4. Avoid pacing or turning the head.
5. Maintain eye contact to hold the client's attention.
6. Make sure the client knows when you are ready to speak.
7. Minimize background noise.
8. Select a well-illuminated area for conversation.

These suggestions establish ground rules for the audiologist to follow throughout the counseling session. At the Veterans Administration (VA) Medical Center in Denver, a protocol is used to gather basic client information. This preliminary information affords a better understanding of the client's status regarding hearing loss and associated feelings caused by the loss (Appendix 14.1).

### Tinnitus

Tinnitus is included in the counseling process for hearing loss because it frequently accompanies hearing loss. It is not uncommon for clients to request audiology appointments solely because of tinnitus annoyance. Tinnitus is defined as "head noise, conscious sound that originates in one's head" (Sullivan, Katon, Dobie, et al., 1988) or the perception of sound when there is not environmental noise. Tinnitus can occur in a variety of forms: tonal or noise, steady or pulsing, intermittent or continuous. It can be unilateral or bilateral. Tinnitus can sound like high pitch ringing, crickets, rushing water, buzzing, and so forth. Questionnaires may be used to identify the nature of tinnitus (Appendix 14.2). The impact of tinnitus on an individual's well-being needs to be determined. Medically treatable tinnitus must first be ruled out in the evaluation process. In the majority of situations, tinnitus is not reversible, and efforts need to be directed toward managing the problem. Several of the factors associated with tinnitus are aging, noise-induced hearing loss, ototoxicity, stress, acoustic neuroma, Meniere's disease, and hypertension. Tinnitus counseling has long been ignored. With increased interest in this problem, it should be included in the counseling process.

## Audiologic Rehabilitation and Outcome Measures

The overall goal of adult audiologic rehabilitation is to increase the likelihood that mutually satisfactory communication will occur between the client and people in his or her everyday communication (Montgomery, 1994).

Establishing outcome measures permits audiologists to quantify the success of procedures used in rehabilitation. It also focuses direction for setting client goals. For example, a goal may be to improve telephone communication using a new hearing aid. The goal may simply be to understand telephone conversations without feedback when the handset is placed near the ear. The client is taught how to rotate the handset until feedback is eliminated. The desired outcome is successful telephone conversation with the hearing aid.

## Determination of Audiologic Rehabilitation Goals

A variety of self-assessment procedures are available to aid the audiologist in determining problem areas so that audiologic rehabilitation plans can be developed. Once the problems have been identified, goals can be established and desired outcomes stated.

Montgomery (1994) has compiled a list of components that may contribute to communication difficulties for adult clients:

1. *Speech presence and quality.* Level and signal-to-noise ratio of auditory and visual speech signals reaching the client's sensory cells.
2. *Speech processing capability.* Signal transmission through auditory and visual channels.
3. *Speech recognition behavior.* (Amplified) auditory (A) and visual (V) and combined auditory-visual (A-V) recognition of speech (including client's knowledge base as well as cognitive and linguistic correlates of speech understanding).
4. *Situation management.* (*a*) Awareness of difficulty in various situations, ability to analyze a communication setting and identify components that contribute to difficulty or breakdown; and (*b*) ability to change or prevent negative components in communication settings.
5. *Emotional reactions.* Attitudes toward communication handicaps, reactions to breakdown, and general personality structure of the individual.

## HEARING AID COUNSELING

The need for and degree of counseling hearing aid users often depends on whether or not the client is a first time wearer. It is important not to take for granted the amount of information a client has about hearing aids. In a practice that dispenses large numbers of hearing aids, audiologists sometimes feel that they become redundant about presentation of counseling information because many of the basic principles are presented "over and over . again" with many clients. It is best to assume, especially for first time users, that very little is known about hearing aids.

In the Denver VA Medical Center practice, it has been found helpful to provide pre-counseling information after the hearing aid evaluation has been completed and the earmold impressions taken. Each client is given a brochure, *Getting Ready for Hearing Aids*, and asked to read it prior to the hearing aid fitting, which usually takes place in about two to four weeks. This orientation provides the opportunity for the client to develop some insight into the concept of amplification. The brochure also serves as an outline for individual or group audiologic rehabilitation counseling:

1. Why do you need hearing aids?
2. Individuals have communication difficulties in various environments because of hearing problems:
   a. With family and friends
   b. At work
   c. In social gatherings
   d. At recreational events
   e. Other situations
3. There may be difficulties such as:
   a. Loudness
   b. Clarity
   c. Frustration
4. Different things may happen, such as:
   a. You may think people mumble
   b. You may think people avoid you
   c. You don't understand all of the words
   d. It may be easier to stay home and avoid people

The above outline permits the audiologist to stimulate conversation regarding individual difficulties. It is common for clients to begin to understand their particular situations more fully and how problems may be minimized and communication improved. The program then sequences to a discussion of hearing aids:

1. What are hearing aids and how can they help?
2. What are the different kinds of hearing aids?
   a. Behind-the-ear
   b. In-the-ear
   c. Eyeglass
   d. Body-type
   e. Cros-bicros
   f. Programmable
   g. Complete in-the-canal (CIC)
   h. Implantable
   i. Other
3. What kind of hearing aids are you going to get?
4. Why are you getting this type?
5. Are you getting one or two hearing aids?
6. What make and model are you getting?

The prefitting protocol is a learning process that helps to create a realistic expectation level for clients waiting for the actual hearing aid fitting. Alpiner and Hansen (1995) developed pre-and postexpectation questionnaires in a pilot study of CIC hearing aid fittings for first-time hearing aid users (Appendix 14.3). Items include, for example, "conversation over the telephone will be easy to understand," and "in background noise, I will be able to understand speech." Client information affords an opportunity for the audiologist to personalize the hearing aid fitting process by better understanding individual expectations prior to hearing aid fitting as well as feelings which may emerge. Our experience has revealed that clients' adjustment is enhanced with this input.

## Counseling and Hearing Aid Fitting

Prior to placing the new hearing aids in the ear, an explanation is provided regarding the various components of the hearing aid such as the location of the microphone, receiver, battery drawer, gain control, and so forth. The aspects of adjusting to amplification are discussed at this time. If the client has a severe loss and is not wearing an aid, a pocket talker device may be used so that the information presented can be heard. It is highly recommended that a family member or significant other attend the hearing aid fitting and orientation. If help is needed at home, these persons can be of considerable help. Further, a better understanding of communication between client and significant others occurs. For example, a spouse may be told not to speak from another room or turn on the dishwasher when engaging in conversation.

Palmer and Hedges (1993) have devised an excellent hearing aid check list (Palmer Index) for use in counseling clients regarding the logistic aspects of hearing aids (Table 14.1).

**TABLE 14.1**
**Hearing Aid Use, Care and Maintenance: Palmer Index**

| PATIENT: | HEARING AID MAKE: |
|---|---|
| SSN: | MODEL: |
| DATE: | EAR(S) FIT: |
| AUDIOLOGIST: | BATTERY SIZE: |

ATTITUDE ABOUT HEARING AID USE:  ☐ SELF-MOTIVATED   ☐ NEEDS ENCOURAGEMENT

| HEARING AID (HA) SELF-USE INDEX | "Can accomplish without supervision" | | "Can accomplish with some supervision" | | "Cannot accomplish even with supervision" | | COMMENTS/SUGGESTIONS: |
|---|---|---|---|---|---|---|---|
| Insert HA into correct ear | R | L | R | L | R | L | |
| Adjust volume level | R | L | R | L | R | L | |
| Remove HA | R | L | R | L | R | L | |
| Remove battery from pkg | R | L | R | L | R | L | |
| Open battery door | R | L | R | L | R | L | |
| Insert battery into HA | R | L | R | L | R | L | |
| Remove battery from HA | R | L | R | L | R | L | |
| Adjust HA for phone use | R | L | R | L | R | L | |
| | R | L | R | L | R | L | |

| CARE AND MAINTENANCE INDEX | "Can accomplish without supervision" | | "Can accomplish with some supervision" | | "Cannot accomplish even with supervision" | | COMMENTS/SUGGESTIONS: |
|---|---|---|---|---|---|---|---|
| Keep HA clean using brush and/or tissue | R | L | R | L | R | L | |
| Clear wax from receiver opening using wax loop | R | L | R | L | R | L | |
| Place HA in storage case | R | L | R | L | R | L | |
| Dispose of spent batteries | R | L | R | L | R | L | |
| Turn HA off if not in use | R | L | R | L | R | L | |
| | R | L | R | L | R | L | |

Reprinted by permission from Palmer, C.T., & Hedges, A.M. Department of Veterans Affairs, Audiology and Speech Pathology Services, Little Rock (1993).

The index consists of two areas: Hearing Aid Self-Use, and Care and Maintenance. It can be used during the initial fitting as well as for follow-up hearing aid orientation sessions. The use of this index complements the fitting procedure.

There are general guidelines which may be used in hearing aid counseling. The client is presented with several techniques for hearing aid use (Alpiner & Hansen, 1995). These guidelines are intended to provide the audiologist with some suggestions that can be presented and discussed with clients:

1. Practice putting your hearing aids in your ears and adjusting the volume controls. For brief periods of time, wear the hearing aids in a quiet room. Read aloud to yourself. Speak naturally and listen for pitch changes in your voice.
2. Talk with one person at a time from a distance of no greater than six feet. Watch the speaker's face attentively while listening. Ask the person to speak in a clear, natural voice—not too fast nor too slow. Watch the person's face all of the time; you can put together what you see and what you hear to make speech more meaningful.
3. Try to reduce or avoid background noise during your listening situations. Television, air conditioners, dishwashers, or other noisy appliances can make communication much more difficult.
4. Listen to radio or television. Try to identify voices and music. Ask a family member to adjust the volume on the television set to a reasonable level. Sit six feet away and adjust your hearing aids carefully. At first, you may want to sit closer, then gradually move back.
5. Increase the time you wear your hearing aids. Rest if the aids tire you or makes you nervous. However, you should wear the hearing aids as long as you can tolerate them. When you are completely comfortable with your hearing aids, you may choose to put them on when you get up in the morning and take them off when you go to bed at night.

Informational counseling concludes with some hearing aid basics outlines in Table 14.2.

Traditional hearing aid orientation is essentially informational in nature. It is that time in which the audiologist fits hearing aids, instructs clients about them, and answers questions.

Erdman (1994a, 1994b) states that the assumption underlying the continued perception of hearing aid orientations as adequate rehabilitative intervention is that hearing aids resolve the disabling handicapping consequences of hearing impairment for most hearing-impaired clients. Erdman continues that this assumption is false by indicating that (a) hearing aids may alleviate the communicative disabilities experienced secondary to hear-

**Table 14.2.**
**Do's and Don'ts**

DO
1. Clean your hearing aids every night.
2. Remove the battery or open the battery door when not wearing the hearing aids.
3. Remove your hearing aids before bathing, showering, shaving, or swimming.
4. Remove your hearing aids while fixing your hair, using hair spray, or if undergoing diathermy or other electrical treatment.

DON'T:
1. Expose your hearing aids to intense heat or cold.
2. Leave your hearing aids where they may be picked up by animals or small children.
3. Attempt to repair the hearing aids yourself.
4. Subject your hearing aids to excessive humidity.
5. Use alcohol or any other cleaning fluids on the plastic case of your hearing aids.

From Alpiner J. G., & Hansen E. M. (1995). Expectation questionnaire (p. 25). *Project Acoustic Module:* Hear Now. Copyright by J. G. Alpiner and E. M. Hansen. Reprinted by permission.

ing impairment but they do not eliminate them, and (b) hearing aid use cannot, in and of itself, resolve the psychosocial handicap experienced secondary to hearing impairment and hearing disability. The audiologist, therefore, needs to make decisions about whether or not to counsel because no agreement exists on the relationship of amplification to personal adjustment for everyday living. In assessing and evaluating hearing there are two major areas that need to be considered: one is *hearing impairment* and the other is *hearing disability (hearing handicap)*. Impairment refers to the loss of hearing as measured by pure-tone and speech thresholds. Disability refers to the effect or impact of the loss on everyday life. The effects of hearing loss may be of a social, emotional, or occupational nature.

## Counseling Indications

The rationale for informational counseling has been discussed and guidelines for its use have been provided. Clark and Martin (1994) suggest counseling services that may be used in audiologic rehabilitation. These services, in addition to informational counseling, include assessment of counseling needs, use of strategies to modify behavior and/or the client's environment, and development of coping mechanisms and systems for emotional support.

## Self-Assessment and Counseling

Management of persons with hearing loss typically has been based on audiometric results. Erdman (1994a, 1994b), however, states that audiometric tests are direct measurement procedures involving physiologic or behavioral recordings or observations; they provide a basis for an assessment of hearing impairment. Swan and Gatehouse (1990) emphasize that hearing-impaired persons pursue assistance because disability may not always correspond to the loss of hearing.

Interest in the use of self-assessment procedures has increased significantly during the past several years. Numerous articles have been written on the subject and significant research appears on an increasingly frequent basis. Communication evaluation efforts have not resulted in the perfect instrument but there are a variety of self- assessment questionnaires that can be used at the discretion of the audiologist. Giolas (1990) states that a self-assessment tool can be a valuable part of the audiologist's rehabilitation procedures by indicating how an individual feels about hearing loss. In addition to determining attitudes and feelings, questionnaires can be used to determine specific communication breakdowns. This information can be extremely helpful in enabling audiologists to plan a counseling program for clients. Contrast this approach to earlier times when rehabilitation, if any, was based only on audiometric data. Erdman (1994a, 1994b) comments that for both research and clinical purposes, self-assessment instruments are easy and inexpensive to administer and can be used with a wide range of populations and for a wide variety of purposes. They are noninvasive and nonthreatening, and this flexibility and efficiency account for the general popularity of self-assessment among clinicians and researchers alike. Alpiner and Schow (1993), Schow and Gatehouse (1990), and Skinner (1988) report on the wide range of assessment tools available for use with a broad range of populations. Whitcomb (1982) reports that a 1980 survey of American Speech-Language-Hearing Association (ASHA) audiologists revealed that only 18 percent were using self-assessment procedures. A 1990 survey of ASHA audiologists indicated that 33 percent were using such procedures. Alpiner (1992) surveyed Department of Veterans Affairs Medical Centers regarding assessment procedures used by audiologists. Of 65 responses, 16 centers (25%) were using self-assessment scales. The assessment scales most often used in the above studies were *Hearing Handicap Inventory for the Elderly* (HHIE); *Hearing Handicap Scale*

(HHS); *Denver Scale of Communication Function* (DSCF); *Hearing Performance Inventory* (HPI); *Self-Assessment of Communication* (SAC); *Significant Other Assessment of Communication* (SOAC); and *Communication Profile for the Hearing Impaired* (CPI). Although these are the tools reported, there are numerous other assessment procedures available. The purpose of this chapter is audiologic rehabilitation oriented rather than research. As research efforts continue, audiologists still need to work with their clients using the best tools and techniques available.

## REHABILITATION EVALUATION

Preparation for audiologic rehabilitation requires identification of client problems related to hearing loss, a plan of action, and selection of outcome measures. The selection of the self-assessment procedure is the choice of the audiologist. As previously indicated, a number of procedures are available from which to choose. Audiologists should keep in mind that health care reform focus calls for cost-effectiveness. Another factor deals with the reality that most audiologic rehabilitation is not covered by third party payments. Finally, many medical offices and hospital clinics stress diagnostic evaluations to the exclusion of rehabilitation; time is of the essence. When one considers which tools to use, key words should be appropriate, quick to administer, and easy to interpret.

It is a good idea to commence the rehabilitation evaluation with a screening scale that can quickly identify if problems exist. Schow and Nerbonne (1982) emphasize the need for a screening tool for this purpose. They developed the *Self Assessment of Communication* (SAC) and the *Significant Other Assessment of Communication (SOAC)* evaluation tools. Both are ten-item questionnaires (Appendices 14.4 and 14.5). The items examine communication difficulties and general feelings about hearing handicap. When assessing client problems, there should be awareness of specific communication breakdowns such as those that might occur watching TV, speaking on the telephone, listening to a speaker at a lecture, and so forth. Feelings about these communication breakdowns may emerge, for example, frustration and anger. A comparison of responses between client and significant others can provide insight for the audiologist in planning rehabilitation designed to eliminate or reduce communication difficulties.

## Audiologic Rehabilitation Screening Scale

The *Alpiner-Meline Aural Rehabilitation (AMAR) Screening Scale* (Appendix 14.6) is designed to identify individuals who may be in need of audiologic rehabilitation. The AMAR takes only a few minutes to administer and score; it is consistent with the need for a tool which is quick and efficient, allowing the audiologist to rule out rehabilitation or to consider more comprehensive assessment procedures. The AMAR allows audiologists to identify problems related to hearing loss in three categories: (*a*) self-assessment, (*b*) visual aptitude, and (*c*) auditory aptitude. Further, the AMAR identifies the effects of hearing loss that cannot be identified on the basis of diagnostic audiometric data. To measure hearing handicap behavior, nine items were selected from the *McCarthy-Alpiner Scale of Hearing Handicap (M-A Scale)* (McCarthy & Alpiner, 1983). This test provides (*a*) an index of whether the organic hearing loss has manifested itself as a handicap; (*b*) diagnostic data with rehabilitative implications; and (*c*) for detailed analysis of psychological, social, and vocational problem areas. To measure visual aptitude for speechreading, five items were selected from the *Denver Quick Test of Lipreading Ability* (Alpiner, 1978). This test correlated ($r = 0.90$) (McNeill & Alpiner, 1975) with the *Utley Sentence Test of Speechreading Ability* (Jeffers & Barley, 1971). The Larsen *Sound Discrimination Test* (Larson, 1950) was selected to represent auditory aptitude. This test was designed to provide information about particular consonant sounds that present discrimination difficulties for listeners. A collection of six word-pair items was selected for use on the basis of pilot data. The word pairs emphasize high-frequency consonants, which tend to be confused in sensorineural hearing loss.

The AMAR scores were calculated as the total number of "minuses" or problems indicated on the AMAR form. The total test time for administration and scoring is only a few minutes. It should be kept in mind that it is a *screening scale.* Analysis indicates that individuals who score within the 85th percentile or above for the number of errors on the scale are identified as those with absolute need for audiologic rehabilitation. Those whose percentile rankings are between 70 and 84 are in questionable need of rehabilitation. Questionable need is defined as those individuals who demonstrate moderate difficulty in psychological, social, or vocational adjustment to hearing loss, and/or limited aptitude in using auditory or visual cues to enhance communication ability. Those persons in the 1st to 69th percentile are considered unlikely to be in need of aural rehabilitation. Additional data continues to be evaluative regarding the predictive value of the AMAR. The experience of the audiologist is relevant in interpretation, particularly for those clients in the 70th to 84th percentile range.

## Beyond the Screening Procedure

Screening scales are primarily designed to identify potential problems that require additional audiologic rehabilitative evaluation. At this point it becomes necessary to engage in further, more specific evaluation. There is no one comprehensive evaluation that addresses all problem areas. Schow and Gatehouse (1990) point to the need to agree on important hearing domains and concepts relative to self-assessment procedures. Areas of confusion relate to definition of terms as audiologists attempt to evaluate the problems encountered by clients due to hearing loss. As stated, hearing impairment refers to the loss of hearing measured by pure-tone and speech thresholds. Hearing disability refers to the impact of hearing loss on everyday living. From screening we move to assessing the handicapping factors involved in hearing loss. Selection of self-assessment instruments, therefore, needs to satisfy specific evaluation interests for audiologic rehabilitation. Numerous instruments are available to evaluate specific domains. Audiologists may be interested in measuring hearing aid benefit, pre- and postfitting; measurement may focus on communication breakdowns such as on the telephone, in a restaurant, attendance at a religious service, or proficiency of job performance. Other interests may address themselves toward feelings caused by loss of hearing such as frustration, inferiority, avoidance, and withdrawal. There may be a need to assess clients in a specific population such as working middle-age adults, retired seniors, or those persons who may now be residents of a nursing home. No one instrument can satisfy all rehabilitative needs. The instruments selected, however, must be directed toward information to assist in the counseling process. Brammer (1973) has discussed seven states of the helping relationship that delineate the stages of the counseling process and which may help in the selection of an evaluation instrument.

The *entry* state opens the avenue for assistance from the audiologist and enables the patient to define his or her problems related to hearing loss. *Clarification* is the second state in which the client defines specific problems, allowing the audiologist to observe the effects of hearing loss on general life situations. The information obtained should enable the audiologist to (*a*) determine if the necessary counseling tools available to the audiologist can meet the client's needs, and (*b*) identify agencies or types of help which may be needed and for which the audiologist is not qualified to provide. At this point, the audiologist and client continue the *counseling relationship* and determine whether or not it should be continued. If the relationship continues, then the next state of *exploration* occurs in which strategies for intervention are determined, the client's feelings are clarified, and action procedures are outlined. In the *Consolidation* stage, the client decides on a course of action, feelings are further clarified, and the client engages in new strategies to reduce or eliminate problems. *Planning* for termination or other referrals are considered. Finally at *termination,* the relationship ends along with a promise of follow-up, if necessary, and the audiologist's willingness to be available. Several evaluation instruments are now presented, each relating to a specific domain of hearing handicap.

## Evaluation of Hearing Aid Benefit

Hearing aid evaluation is the major component of audiologic rehabilitation and the need to evaluate successful fittings is mandatory. The *Abbreviated Profile of Hearing Aid Benefit* (APHAB) is a clinical rehabilitative instrument that may be used for quantifying both the disability associated with a hearing loss and the reduction of the disability that is achieved with a hearing aid (Cox & Alexander, 1995). All statements deal with communication ability; clients' responses indicate how frequently a statement is true (Appendix 14.7). Four categories of the APHAB are *ease of communication* (EC), *reverberation* (RV), *background noise* (BN), and *aversiveness* (AV). There are six items each with the instrument consisting of 24 items. Seven levels of response are used for each item: Always, Almost Always, Generally, Half-the-Time, Occasionally, Seldom, and Never. Cox and Alexander (1995) state that clinical applications include: (*a*) prediction of likely success with amplification based on prefitting unaided responses, (*b*) comparison of aided performance of an individual with that of a reference group such as successful hearing aid wearers; or (*c*) documentation of benefit in various environments either for accountability purposes, to troubleshoot an unsuccessful fitting, or to compare the profit derived from different instruments.

## Evaluation of Hearing Handicap: Adults

The *Hearing Handicap Inventory for Adults* (HHIA) (Newman, Weinstein, Jacobson, & Hug, 1991) is a modification of the *Hearing Handicap Inventory for the Elderly* (HHIE) (Ventry & Weinstein, 1982). It was modified for use with younger adults.

The HHIA is a self-assessment scale designed to measure client perception of hearing handicap; it can be used to assess outcomes for both hearing aid benefit and rehabilitative audiology. It is used pre- and postamplification or rehabilitation. The inventory consists of 25 items to assess both social and emotional aspects of clients (Appendix 14.8). For example, one item (emotional) is, "Does a hearing problem make you irritable?" Response would be either, "Yes," "Sometimes," or "No." A numerical score is obtained for each response: 4 for yes, 2 for sometimes, and 0 for no. The greater the problem, the higher the score. A score of 100 would indicate serious problems related to the client's hearing loss. It is hoped that a low score would result after a time owing to hearing aid use or rehabilitative audiology counseling. Both specific situations and feelings are assessed in this inventory.

## Evaluation of Hearing Handicap: Retirement Centers

For individuals living in nursing homes or retirement centers, it is feasible to use assessment procedures designed for this population. Zarnoch and Alpiner (1977) modified the *Denver Scale of Communication* (Alpiner, Chevrette, Glascoe, Metz, & Olsen, 1974) to devise the *Denver Scale of Communication Function for Senior Citizens Living in Retirement Centers (DSCF)* (Appendix 14.9). The purpose of this scale is to account for the environment in which older persons live and function. It is entirely possible that some persons live in retirement centers and still work full- or part-time. Audiologists may have to use combinations of assessment procedures and make professional judgment regarding a client's varying roles in everyday living. As stated, "there is no one scale that meets all assessment needs."

The DSCF is designed for an interview presentation. This procedure consists of seven major questions including topics of family, emotions, other persons, general communication, self-concept, group situations, and rehabilitation. Scoring is either "Yes" (-) or "No" (-). Each major question has a *probe effect* and an *exploration effect.* The probe effect attempts to specify the problem areas for each question. The exploration effect determines how applicable the question is to the individual. This aspect of the procedure helps to eliminate questions that are irrelevant for the client, thereby negating their consideration for rehabilitation. The scoring form helps in interpreting the responses. The scale allows audiologists to evaluate performance prior to and following audiologic rehabilitation. Further, it is designed to compare each individual with him- or herself.

## COUNSELING AND THE ROLE OF THE AUDIOLOGIST

A considerable portion of this chapter has been devoted to gathering information so that rehabilitative action can be planned and outcome measures determined. It is not unusual for the audiologist to be asked the limits of his or her responsibility in the counseling process. After all, audiologists are not psychologists or psychiatrists. The question is legitimate and needs a response. Clark and Martin (1994) state that audiologists frequently take on the role of "nonprofessional" counselors. He states that counseling is often provided by professionals who are not trained counselors (e.g., educators, lawyers, physicians, and so forth). Further, rarely do those in need of counseling seek out social workers, psychologists, or psychiatrists. The critical issue is to keep in mind the emotional and physical safety of persons served. A contemporary responsibility issue, for example, is the removal of excessive cerumen from a client who needs impressions for hearing aids. The client may be referred to an otologist. Many audiologists are reluctant to refer because a majority of ear nose and throat physicians dispense hearing aids and the client may not be referred back to the audiologist. The dilemma is how this matter is discussed with the individual who is not aware of these professional situations. Audiologists have presented varying opinions on this subject. Certain thoughts and guidelines indicate that it is appropriate if the cerumen is not impacted and if the audiologist has had proper training for this procedure. At present there are no national guidelines regarding a credential for cerumen removal. The audiologist, therefore, has to decide whether the removal can be done in an appropriate and safe way, keeping in mind professional relationships and legal concerns. There is not always a definitive answer regarding the limits of audiologic counseling.

Audiologists engage in a considerable amount of informational counseling (i.e., how the hearing aid works, its controls, how batteries are changed, and how the hearing aid should be cleaned on a regular basis). The other aspects of hearing loss with which audiologists deal include acceptance of hearing loss; awareness of communication breakdowns with family, friends, co-workers, and others; feelings of vanity and aging, and so forth. It is helpful for audiologists to have some knowledge of the different psychological theories that may be used in the counseling process. The major aspects of these theories are discussed in Chapters 3 and 4.

Generally, audiologists will probably use concepts from people-centered counseling, behavioral counseling, and cognitive counseling. The first theory is basically client-centered counseling in which the individual with hearing handicap ultimately reaches his or her own solutions with the nondirective assistance of the audiologist. The second theory deals with an approach in which appropriate behavior is learned through positive re-

**TABLE 14.3.**
**Counseling Responsiblities of Audiologists**

| Informational | Rational Acceptance/Adjustment | Emotional Acceptance/Adjustment |
|---|---|---|
| Hearing loss | Hearing loss | Effect of hearing loss on self |
|   Description |   Permanency of |   Feelings |
|   Comparison with normal |   Need for treatment |   Attitude |
|   Cause |   Need for additional testing |   Image |
| Anatomy/function of ear |   Need for hearing aid(s) |   Ability to communicate |
| Availability of medical assitance |   Need to conserve residual hearing | Effect of hearing loss on relation- |
| Hearing aids | Aural Rehabilitation | ships |
|   Costs |   Need to learn new communi- |   Family |
|   Where to purchase |     cation skills |   Friends |
|   Advantages/disadvantages |   Need to improve communi- |   Associates |
|   Care/use/function |     cation habits | |
| Availability of other |   Family | |
|   technical devices |   Friends | |
| Availability of other services |   Work place | |

Reprinted by permission from Wylde, M. A. (1982). The remediation process: psychologic and counselling aspects. In J. G. Alpiner (Ed.), *Handbook of Rehabilitative Audiology*. Baltimore: Williams & Wilkins.

inforcement, which provides an acceptable solution to the problem. The third theory teaches the client ways in which behavior can be modified so that positive solutions may emerge, thereby minimizing or eliminating the handicap caused by hearing loss.

Wylde (1982) outlines specific counseling responsibilities of audiologists that are helpful in implementing the process. Three domains are presented: informational, rational acceptance/adjustment, and emotional acceptance/adjustment (Table 14.3).

## Informational Counseling

Consider an example of *informational counseling.* Mr. Smith comes to the audiology clinic because his wife complains that he "just doesn't hear her," and she is tired of shouting at him. Audiologic results indicate a moderate hearing loss in both ears with reduced speech recognition ability (76%). He has never worn hearing aids and he doesn't think he has much of a hearing loss, if any, because he hears. It is explained to this 55-year-old insurance agent that he does indeed hear, but primarily only low-frequency sounds owing to his high-frequency hearing loss. He hears parts of words but doesn't understand everything. A frequency display is used, which shows the sounds of language as related to frequency and intensity. Mr. Smith is told he hears the low frequency sounds like /m/ and /n/, and the vowel sounds but that he misses /s/, /f/, and /Θ/. An example to him is that he may not know if a word in a sentence is *see, free,* or *three.* His loss is sensorineural, which is explained to him it in terms of the outer, middle, and inner ears. (There is no medical treatment per the otologist's referral.) He asks about help and hearing aids; he says that he heard they can't help because he has a "nerve" loss. Amplification is explained to him so that he has a better understanding of hearing aids, both their advantages and limitations. He is told the cost of hearing aids as well as information that they may be purchased on a 30-day trial period. We also explain to him the persons who dispense hearing aids and the qualifications of both audiologists and hearing aid dispensers. He is informed that the hearing loss is permanent and that no medical treatment is available for it. It is explained to him that hearing aids will probably help and that he will function better in family, social, and vocational situations. Self-assessment procedures identify more specifically that he does feel frustrated, that he experiences frustration on the job with his insurance clients, and that he realizes that he argues quite a bit with his spouse about the volume on the TV and at restaurants. It is emphasized to him that it is more embarrassing to miss conversation than to admit hearing loss and to avoid amplification. The decision then must be made by the client regarding the trial use of amplification. Although this session included heavy use of informational counseling, it should be realized that, with the use of assessment procedures, his audiologist was engaged in additional counseling procedures in order to create understanding, awareness, and a willingness to seek help.

### Rational Acceptance/Adjustment

There is some overlap between informational and rational acceptance/adjustment aspects of counseling. The next step for the client is to accept amplification, even if for a trial period. Most individuals are willing to accept amplification, knowing that it is for a trial period. There are some audiologists who do not like the idea of a trial period, feeling that persons will not take the process seriously if they know "they can get their money back." Although controversial, the issue may be insignificant because the standard in this country is the 30-day trial period. When follow-up is used with clients after they are fitted and if audiologists work with them on adjustment to amplification during the trial period, success is possible in most cases. It is common for persons to come in for follow-up for a variety of reasons: adjustment of hearing aid controls, explanation of cleaning procedures, check of the fit if the aids hurt, and check of batteries. In a project at the VA Medical Center in Denver, Complete in-the-Canal (CIC) hearing aids are evaluated; and follow-up counseling provides adjustment of hearing aid controls and improvement of the fit. It should not be assumed that hearing aids work as easily as turning on a new television set.

*Communication Strategies Training* (Tye-Murray, 1994) is a necessary part of the counseling process. Communication strategies are categorized as either *facilitation* or *repair*. Facilitation strategies include (*a*) clients' speech recognition skills, (*b*) the communication environment, (*c*) communication partners' speaking of the messages, and (*d*) the messages themselves. From these strategies, ways can be suggested in which the individual with hearing loss can hear better:

1. Speech recognition skills
   a. Attend to the speaker of a message
   b. Don't be afraid to guess
   c. Know the topic of the conversation
2. Communication environment
   a. Select seating to observe speakers better
   b. Control background noise as best as possible
   c. Control lighting so speaker can be easily seen
3. Communication partner
   a. The partner should speak naturally
   b. Make sure person is watching before you speak
4. Message
   a. Consider using short/simple sentences
   b. Indicate when topic of message changes
   c. Use concrete language if possible

The second type of strategy in communication training is repair. This strategy is used when there is a breakdown in communication; that is, the individual is not able to hear or understand what is said. Clients use specific measures to reduce the communication breakdown. Some examples which individuals use are:

1. Please repeat what you said.
2. It will help if you speak more slowly.
3. I would like to know the topic.
4. Please write down what you said.

It is the audiologist who needs to assume responsibility in making sure that the talker knows what to do to improve communication, and to ensure that individuals are aware of both facilitation and repair strategies.

## Emotional Acceptance/Judgment

This aspect of counseling focuses on emotional attitudes and feelings. These feelings are also considered in terms of relationships with family and significant others as well as the ability to work productively. An example of a client response from the AMAR scale illustrates this point: "I feel like I am isolated from things because of my hearing loss." The person's pre-rehabilitation response was "yes." The reasons for the client's "yes" response was explored. This client, a 45-year-old woman, had a severe acquired hearing loss due to antibiotics of several month's duration. Isolation was reported due to an inability to communicate adequately with her two middle-school students and her husband. In addition, she was reluctant to shop, go to church, and meet socially with her friends. It was felt that it was urgent to schedule a session with family members, the client, and the audiologist. An initial session was scheduled. The client was not wearing a hearing aid and so a Pocket Talker was provided to permit adequate communication. Discussion tended to indicate feelings of inferiority and inadequacy due to the hearing handicap. All members of this family were able to express their feelings as well as their frustrations. Hearing loss was simulated for family members to help them better understand the client's problems.

Boundaries for the counseling process are outlined (Wylde, 1982, p. 358) as follows:

1. Should be related to assisting the client to improve communication and alleviating problems caused by the loss of hearing sensitivity.
2. Should be guided by the individual and family members.
3. Should be supportive of the individual and family members.
4. Should center on the course of action best suited for the individual.
5. Should not enter the realm of the clinical psychologist or psychiatrist.

## Considerations for Older Adults

Regardless of age, the goal for audiologic rehabilitation is the same for all adults. Success may vary depending on other existing physiologic and emotional problems, problems which are not a result of hearing loss. Alpiner (1978) developed a model to help audiologists better understand the attitudes that may emerge in older clients (Fig. 14.1). These attitudes ultimately result in the individual staying in the mainstream, withdrawing, or choosing isolation. Lipkin and Williams (1986) address this issue by reporting on the comments of a 79-year-old physician with hearing loss, who stated: "the degree of disability shown by hearing-impaired people varies greatly depending on factors intrinsic in the particular person . . . some older people simply withdraw . . . some demand that people around them modify their speech . . . some become frustrated and angry . . . some acknowledge the infirmity, others conceal or deny it . . . some accept the need to help themselves . . . some use every possible help to continue meaningful work . . . others just give up . . . some mourn the loss of a considerable part of life's pleasures . . . as with most

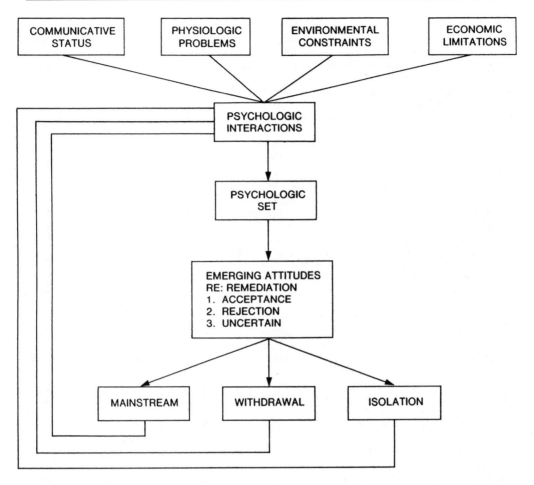

**Figure 14.1.** Emerging attitudes of geriatric patients. (From Alpiner, J. (1979). The psychology of aging. In M. Henoch (Ed.), *Aural rehabilitation for the elderly.* New York: Grune & Stratton.)

handicaps, attitudes are a major determinant of the degree of impairment of the quality of life."

Audiologists' responsibility as counselors is to eliminate hearing loss as a reason for the above situations, at least to minimize the effects of hearing loss. It is advisable, therefore, to consider each adult according to specific problems and the effects of these problems on everyday living.

## CONCLUSION

Counseling is an integral part of audiologic rehabilitation. It serves to complement amplification and enhance communication of those with hearing disability. Diagnostic audiology is only the beginning of the process. Hearing aid fitting and orientation are essential in rehabilitation. Various assessment procedures are available to help audiologists define hearing aid benefit and identify additional counseling needs. The goal, regardless of age, is similar, although special problems of aging should be considered as audiologists eliminate or minimize the difficulties in everyday living caused by loss of hearing.

## REFERENCES

Alpiner, J. G. (1993). Rehabilitative evaluation of adults. In J. Alpiner & P. McCarthy (Eds.), *Rehabilitative audiology: Children and adults* (p. 239). Baltimore: Williams & Wilkins.

Alpiner, J. G. (1978). Evaluation of adult communication function. In J. Alpiner (Ed.), *Handbook of adult rehabilitative audiology* (p. 29). Baltimore: Williams & Wilkins.

Alpiner, J. G., Chevrette, W., Glascoe, G., Metz, M., & Olsen, B. (1974). *The Denver scale of communication function.* Unpublished study, University of Denver, Denver, CO.

Alpiner, J. G., & Hansen, E. M. (1995). *Expectation questionnaire.* Project Acoustic Module. Hear Now, Denver, CO.

Alpiner, J. G., & Schow, R. L. (1993). Rehabilitative evaluation of hearing-impaired adults. In J. G. Alpiner & P. A. McCarthy (Eds.), *Rehabilitative audiology: Children and adults* (2nd ed.). Baltimore: Williams & Wilkins.

Brammer, L. (1973). *The helping relationship: Process and skills.* Englewood Cliffs, NJ: Prentice-Hall.

Clark, J. G., & Martin, F. N. (1994). Audiologists' counseling purview. In J. G. Clark & F. N. Martin (Eds.), *Effective counseling in audiology: Perspectives and practice.* Englewood Cliffs, NJ: Prentice-Hall.

Cox, R. M., & Alexander, G. C. (1995). The abbreviated profile of hearing aid benefit. *Ear and Hearing, 16,* 176–186.

Erdman, S. A. (1994a). Counseling hearing-impaired adults. In J. G. Alpiner & P. A. McCarthy (Eds.), *Rehabilitative audiology: Children and adults* (2nd ed.), Baltimore: Williams & Wilkins.

Erdman, S. (1994b). Self-assessment: From research focus to research tool. *Journal of the Academy of Rehabilitative Audiology, 27*(Monograph Supplement), 67–90.

Giolas, T. G. (1990). The measurement of hearing handicap revisited: A 20-year perspective. *Ear and Hearing, 11*(5), 28–58.

Jeffers, J., & Barley, M. (1971). Speechreading (lipreading). Springfield, IL: Charles C Thomas.

Jinks, M. J. (1991). Counseling older adults with hearing impairment. *Journal of Practical Nursing, 41,* 43–51.

Larson, L. L. (1950). *Consonant sound discrimination.* Bloomington, IN: Indiana University Press.

Lipkin, M., & Williams, M. E. (1986). Presbycusis and communication. *Journal of General Internal Medicine, 1,* 399–401.

Lowe, A. D. (1992). Trust me audiology: A threat to our future? *Audiology Today, 4,* 21.

Martin, F. N., Bar, M. M., & Bernstein, M. (1992). Professional attitudes regarding counseling of hearing-impaired adults. *American Journal of Otology, 13,* 279–287.

McCarthy, P., & Alpiner, J. (1993). An assessment scale of hearing handicap for use in family counseling. *Journal of the Academy of Rehabilitative Audiology, 16,* 256–270.

McNeil, M., & Alpiner, J. (1975). *A study of the reliability of the Denver Scale of communication function.* Unpublished study, University of Denver, Denver, CO.

Montgomery, A. A. (1994). Treatment efficacy in adult audiological rehabilitation. *Journal of Academy of Rehabilitative Audiology, 27*(Monograph Supplement), 317–336.

Newman, C. W., Weinstein, B. E., Jacobson, G. P., & Hug, G. A. (1991). Test-retest reliability of the hearing handicap inventory for adults. *Ear and Hearing, 10,* 355–357.

Palmer, C. T., & Hedges, A. M. (1993). *Hearing aid use, care and maintenance: Palmer index.* Little Rock, AR: Department of Veterans Affairs, Audiology and Speech Pathology Service.

Schow, R. L., & Gatehouse, S. (1990). Fundamental issues in self-assessment of hearing. *Ear and Hearing, 11*(5), 6–16.

Schow, R. L., & Nerbonne, M. A. (1992). Communication screening profile: Use with elderly clients. *Ear and Hearing, 13,* 135–147.

Skinner, M. W. (1988). *Hearing aid evaluation.* Englewood Cliffs, NJ: Prentice-Hall.

Sullivan, M., Katon, M., Dobie, W., Sakai, C., Krusso, J., & Harrip-Griffiths, J. (1988). Disabling tinnitus-association with affective disorders. *General Hospital Psychiatry, 10,* 258–291.

Swan, I. R.C., & Gatehouse, S. (1990). Factors influencing consultation for management of hearing disability. *British Journal of Audiology, 24,* 155–160.

Tye-Murray, N. (1994). Communication strategies training. *Journal of the Academy Rehabilitative Audiology, 27*(Monograph Supplement), 193–208.

Ventry, I., & Weinstein, B. (1982). The hearing handicap inventory for the elderly: A new tool. *Ear and Hearing, 3,* 128–134.

Whitcomb, C. J. (1982). *A survey of aural rehabilitation services among ASHA audiologists.* Unpublished manuscript, Idaho State University, Pocatello, ID.

Wylde, M. A. (1982). The remediation process: Psychologic and counseling aspects. In J. G. Alpiner (Ed.), *Handbook of adult rehabilitative audiology.* Baltimore:Williams & Wilkins.

Zarnoch, J. M., & Alpiner, J. G. (1977). *The Denver scale of communication function for senior citizens living in retirement centers.* Unpublished study. University of Denver, Denver, CO.

## Appendix 14.1  Case History Protocol

**VA MEDICAL CENTER—DENVER**
**AUDIOLOGY**

AUDIOLOGY BRIEF CASE HISTORY FORM

PATIENT NAME: _____  DATE:_____

BIRTHDATE: _____  SSN:_____  TEL:_____

ADDRESS: _____

_____

1. DURATION OF HEARING LOSS: ____YEARS ____GRADUAL ____SUDDEN

2. DIZZINESS:  ____YES ____NO  COMMENTS:_____

3. TINNITUS:  ____NONE ____YES ____RIGHT ____LEFT

   SOUNDS LIKE:  RIGHT: _____LEFT: _____

   FREQUENCY OF EPISODES (e.g., daily/weekly/monthly): _____

   _____

   DURATION OF EPISODES (e.g., min/hours/constant/): _____

   _____

4. EAR PAIN: ____BIL ____UNL ____DISCHARGE: ____RIGHT ____LEFT

5. EAR SURGERY: _____

6. MEDICATIONS: ____ASPIRIN ____MYCIN ____OTHER _____

   FOR: _____

7. FAMILY HISTORY: _____

8. NOISE EXPOSURE: ____MILITARY; TYPE: _____

   ____ CIVILIAN; TYPE: _____

9. HEARING AIDS: ____RIGHT ____LEFT ____TIME: ____YRS TYPE:_____

10. BETTER EAR:  ____RIGHT ____LEFT ____SAME  COMMENTS: _____

    _____

11. COMPLAINTS BY SIGNIFICANT OTHERS: _____

12. DESCRIBE YOUR HEARING PROBLEM: _____

13. SERVICE CONNECTED: ____YES ____NO  OTHER: _____

14. OTHER COMMENTS: _____

    _____

AUDIOLOGIST: _____        8/95

## Appendix 14.2  University of Iowa Tinnitus Questionnaire

### *UNIVERSITY OF IOWA TINNITUS*
### *QUESTIONNAIRE*

### Part A
(To be filled in by the patient)

1. Where is your tinnitus? (Please choose only *ONE* answer.)

   a. Left ear
   b. Right ear
   c. Both ears, equally
   d. Both ears, but worse in left ear
   e. Both ears, but worse in right ear

   f. In the head, but no exact place
   g. More in the right side of head
   h. More in the left side of head
   i. Outside of head
   j. Middle head

If you hear more than one sound or a different sound in each ear, answer the following questions with regard to the one most annoying sound.

2. Describe the most prominent *PITCH* of your tinnitus by circling *ONE* of the numbers below. Number 1 is like a *VERY LOW* pitched fog horn, and Number 10 is like a *VERY HIGH* pitched whistle.

PITCH

1        2        3        4        5        6        7        8        9        10
(VERY LOW)                                                                  (VERY HIGH)

3. When the tinnitus is there does it ever change *PITCH?*
   a. No
   b. Yes, suddenly
   c. Yes, gradually

4. Does the *PITCH* of the tinnitus vary from day to day?
   a. No
   b. Yes

5. Describe the *LOUDNESS* of your tinnitus by circling *ONE* of the numbers below. Number 1 is a *VERY FAINT* tinnitus, and Number 10 is a *VERY LOUD* tinnitus.

LOUDNESS

1        2        3        4        5        6        7        8        9        10
(VERY FAINT)                                                               (VERY LOUD)

6. When it is there, does the tinnitus ever change *LOUDNESS?*
   a. No
   b. Yes, suddenly
   c. Yes, gradually

7. Does the *LOUDNESS* of the tinnitus vary from day to day?
   a. No
   b. Yes

8. Which of all these qualities *BEST* describes your tinnitus? (Please circle only *ONE.*)
   a. Buzzing
   b. Clanging

   j. Pounding
   k. Pulsing

Reprinted by permission from Stouffer, J. L., and Tyler, R. S., Characterization of tinnitus patients. *J. Speech Hear. Dis.,* 55, 439–453 (1990).

c. Clicking
d. Crackling
e. Cricket-like
f. Hissing
g. Humming
h. Musical note
i. Popping
l. Ringing
m. Roaring
n. Rushing
o. Steam whistle
p. Throbbing
q. Whistling
r. Whooshing
s. OTHER, PLEASE SPECIFY_____

9. Does the tinnitus ever change to a completely different sound?
   a. No
   b. Yes, suddenly
   c. Yes, gradually

10. During the time you are awake, what percentage of the time is your tinnitus present?
    For example, 100% would indicate that your tinnitus was there all the time, and 25%
    would indicate that your tinnitus was there [1\4] of the time.
    _____% Please write in a single number between 1 and 100.

11. On the average, how many days per month are you bothered by your tinnitus?
    _____ days per month (maximum = 30 days)

Since your tinnitus began, is your tinnitus *NOW:*

12. a. higher      b. lower      c. same IN PITCH (circle a, b, or c)

13. a. louder      b. softer     c. same IN LOUDNESS (circle a, b, or c)

14. a. higher      b. lower      c. same IN SEVERITY (circle a, b, or c)

15. When your tinnitus first began, how many sounds was it composed of?
    _____ (number of sounds)

16. How many sounds is your tinnitus composed of *NOW?*

17. How many years have you had tinnitus?
    _____ years

18. How many years has your tinnitus really bothered you?
    _____ years

19. When you have your tinnitus, which of the following makes it *WORSE?*
    (CIRCLE ALL OF THESE THAT APPLY TO YOU.)
    a. Alcohol
    b. Being in a noisy place
    c. Being in a quiet place
    d. Changing head position
    e. Coffee/tea
    f. Constipation
    g. During your menstrual period
    h. Drugs/medicine
    i. Emotional or mental stress
    j. Food (please specify) _____
    k. Having just recently been in a noisy place
    l. Having just recently worn a hearing aid
    m. Lack of sleep
    n. Relaxation
    o. Shooting guns, rifles, etc.

    p. Smoking
    q. Sudden physical activity
    r. When you are excited
    s. When you are tired from doing physical work
    t. While you are wearing a hearing aid
    u. When you first wake up in the morning
    v. OTHER, PLEASE SPECIFY_____
    w. Nothing makes it worse.

20. Which of the following *REDUCES* your tinnitus?
    (CIRCLE ALL OF THE ANSWERS THAT APPLY TO YOU.)
    a. Alcohol
    b. Being in a noisy place
    c. Being in a quiet place
    d. Coffee/tea
    e. Drugs/medicine
    f. Food (please specify) _____
    g. Having just recently been in a noisy place
    h. Having just recently been in a quiet place
    i. Listening to television or radio
    j. Sleep
    k. Smoking
    l. Wearing a hearing aid
    m. OTHER, PLEASE SPECIFY_____
    n. Nothing reduces my tinnitus.

21. What do you think originally caused your tinnitus? Select *ONE* only.
    a. Accident (please specify)_____
    b. Alcohol
    c. Drugs/medicine
    d. Food (please specify) _____
    e. Hearing loss
    f. Illness (please specify) _____
    g. Noise
    h. Smoking
    i. Surgery
    j. OTHER, PLEASE SPECIFY_____
    k. I have no idea.

22. Please write a *single* number between 0 and 100 to indicate how *ANNOYING* you find your tinnitus—a "0" would indicate that it is not annoying at all, a "100" would indicate that it is extremely annoying.
    _____ (Please write a *single* number between 0 and 100.)

23. What percentage of the time does your tinnitus interfere with your getting to sleep (0% = does not interfere; 100% = interferes every night).
    _____ (Please write a *single* number between 0 and 100.)

24. To what degree are you *DEPRESSED* by your tinnitus? (0 indicates your tinnitus does not depress you; 100 indicates you are extremely depressed by your tinnitus.)
    _____ (Please write a *single* number between 0 and 100.)

25. Do you have trouble *CONCENTRATING* because of your tinnitus? (0 indicates your tinnitus does not affect concentration; 100 indicates that your tinnitus always interferes with concentration.)

_____ (Please write a *single* number between 0 and 100.)

26. Does your tinnitus interfere with your understanding speech? (0 indicates your tinnitus does not interfere with speech; 100 indicates your tinnitus interferes extremely with understanding speech.)

_____ (Please write a *single* number between 0 and 100.)

27. I am concerned that my tinnitus is a symptom of a much worse disease
    Yes / No

28. I am concerned that I might go deaf because of my tinnitus.
    Yes / No

29. Were you taking any medications just *BEFORE* your tinnitus began?
    a. No
    b. Yes

30. Are you taking any medications *NOW?*
    a. No
    b. Yes

### Part B
(To be filled in by the audiologist)

1. Primary Diagnosis (circle only *ONE*)
   1. Noise-induced hearing loss
   2. Presbycusis
   3. Ménière's
   4. Middle-ear disorder (please specify) _____
   5. Retrocochlear (please specify)_____
   6. Normal hearing (please specify)_____
   7. Other (please specify) _____
   8. Unknown

2. Primary Complaint (circle only *ONE*)
   1. Hearing loss
   2. Dizziness
   3. Tinnitus
   4. Pain or headaches
   5. Other (please specify) _____

3. Hearing Thresholds

| Left Ear | | Right Ear | |
|---|---|---|---|
| 1000 Hz | 4000 Hz | 1000 Hz | 4000 Hz |
| 1. _____ dB HL | 2. _____ dB HL | 3. _____ dB HL | 4. _____ dB HL |

## Appendix 14.3  Expectations Questionnaire

### EXPECTATIONS QUESTIONNAIRE

*Answer true or false to each question*

When I am using my hearing aids . . .

_____ 1.   Conversation over the telephone will be easy to understand.

_____ 2.   Watching people's lips and faces will always be a major part of my communication.

_____ 3. In background noise, I will be able to understand speech.

_____ 4. Most television programs will be easy to understand with hearing alone.

_____ 5. It will be possible for me to separate one word from another when listening to normal conversation.

_____ 6. I will be able to understand all speech when using my hearing aids.

_____ 7. I will be able to understand speech when at a theatre, church, etc.

_____ 8. It will be possible to hear my own voice.

_____ 9. I may have better job opportunities by using my hearing aids.

_____ 10. I will be able to hear and appreciate music with the hearing aids.

_____ 11. Others will not know that I have a hearing disability.

_____ 12. Speech will sound natural to me.

_____

Reprinted by permission from Alpiner, J. G., and Hansen, E. M., *Project Acoustic Module,* Hear Now, Denver, Co (1995).

## Appendix 14.4  Self-Assessment of Communication Function (SAC)

### SELF-ASSESSMENT OF COMMUNICATION (SAC)*

Name _____

Date _____    Raw Score _____ × 2 = _____ − 20 = _____ × 1.25 _____%

Please select the appropriate number ranging from 1 to 5 for the following questions.
Circle only one number for each question. If you have a hearing aid, please fill out the form according to how you communicate when the hearing aid <u>is not</u> in use.

Various Communication Situations

1. Do you experience communication difficulties in situations when speaking with one other person? (for example, at home, at work, in a social situation, with a waitress, a store clerk, with a spouse, boss, etc.)
   1) almost never (or   2) occasionally   3) about half of   4) frequently   5) practically
      never)                (about ¼ of the      the time          (about ¾ of      always (or
                            time)                                  the time)        always)

2. Do you experience communication difficulties in situations when conversing with a small group of several persons? (for example, with friends or family, co-workers, in meetings or casual conversations, over dinner or while playing cards, etc.)
   1) almost never (or   2) occasionally   3) about half of   4) frequently   5) practically
      never)                (about ¼ of the      the time          (about ¾ of      always (or
                            time)                                  the time)        always)

3. Do you experience communication difficulties while listening to someone speak to a large group? (for example, at a church or in a civic meeting, in a fraternal or women's club, at an educational lecture, etc.)
   1) almost never (or   2) occasionally   3) about half of   4) frequently   5) practically
      never)                (about ¼ of the      the time          (about ¾ of      always (or
                            time)                                  the time)        always)

4. Do you experience communication difficulties while participating in various types of entertainment? (for example, movies, TV, radio, plays, night clubs, musical entertainment, etc.)
   1) almost never (or   2) occasionally   3) about half of   4) frequently   5) practically
      never)                (about ¼ of the      the time          (about ¾ of      always (or
                            time)                                  the time)        always)

5. Do you experience communication difficulties when you are in an unfavorable listening environment? (for example, at a noisy party, where there is background music, when riding in an auto or bus, when someone whispers or talks from across the room, etc.)

   1) almost never (or   2) occasionally   3) about half of   4) frequently   5) practically
      never)              (about ¼ of the      the time         (about ¾ of      always (or
                          time)                                 the time)        always)

6. Do you experience communication difficulties when using or listening to various communication devices? (for example, telephone, telephone ring, doorbell, public address system, warning signals, alarms, etc.)

   1) almost never (or   2) occasionally   3) about half of   4) frequently   5) practically
      never)              (about ¼ of the      the time         (about ¾ of      always (or
                          time)                                 the time)        always)

Feelings About Communication

7. Do you feel that any difficulty with your hearing limits or hampers your personal or social life?

   1) almost never (or   2) occasionally   3) about half of   4) frequently   5) practically
      never)              (about ¼ of the      the time         (about ¾ of      always (or
                          time)                                 the time)        always)

8. Does any problem or difficulty with your hearing upset you?

   1) almost never (or   2) occasionally   3) about half of   4) frequently   5) practically
      never)              (about ¼ of the      the time         (about ¾ of      always (or
                          time)                                 the time)        always)

Other people

9. Do others suggest that you have a hearing problem?

   1) almost never (or   2) occasionally   3) about half of   4) frequently   5) practically
      never)              (about ¼ of the      the time         (about ¾ of      always (or
                          time)                                 the time)        always)

10. Do others leave you out of conversations or become annoyed because of your hearing?

   1) almost never (or   2) occasionally   3) about half of   4) frequently   5) practically
      never)              (about ¼ of the      the time         (about ¾ of      always (or
                          time)                                 the time)        always)

---

*Reprinted by permission from Schow, R. L., and Nerbonne, M. A., Communication screening profile; use with elderly clients. *Ear Hear.*, 3, 135–147 (1982).

---

## Appendix 14.5  Significant Other Assessment of Communication (SOAC)

### SIGNIFICANT OTHER ASSESSMENT OF COMMUNICATION (SOAC)*

Name _____

Form filled out with reference to _____(client/patient)

Relationship to client/patient_____(for example, wife, son, friend)

Date _____ Raw Score _____ × 2 = _____ − 20 = _____ × 1.25 _____%

Please select the appropriate number ranging from 1 to 5 for the following questions. Circle only one number for each question. If the client/patient has a hearing aid, please fill out the form according to how he/she communicates when the hearing aid is not in use.

Various Communication Situations

1. Does he/she experience communication difficulties in situations when speaking with one other person? (for example, at home, at work, in a social situation, with a waitress, a store clerk, with a spouse, boss, etc.)

   1) almost never (or   2) occasionally   3) about half of   4) frequently   5) practically
      never)              (about ¼ of the      the time         (about ¾ of      always (or
                          time)                                 the time)        always)

2. Does he/she experience communication difficulties in situations when conversing with a small group of several persons? (for example, with friends or family, co-workers, in meetings or casual conversations, over dinner or while playing cards, etc.)

   1) almost never (or     2) occasionally        3) about half of      4) frequently        5) practically
      never)                   (about ¼ of the        the time              (about ¾ of          always (or
                               time)                                        the time)            always)

3. Does he/she experience communication difficulties while listening to someone speak to a large group? (for example, at church or in a civic meeting, in a fraternal or women's club, at an educational lecture, etc.)

   1) almost never (or     2) occasionally        3) about half of      4) frequently        5) practically
      never)                   (about ¼ of the        the time              (about ¾ of          always (or
                               time)                                        the time)            always)

4. Does he/she experience communication difficulties while participating in various types of entertainment? (for example, movies, TV, radio, plays, night clubs, musical entertainment, etc.)

   1) almost never (or     2) occasionally        3) about half of      4) frequently        5) practically
      never)                   (about ¼ of the        the time              (about ¾ of          always (or
                               time)                                        the time)            always)

5. Does he/she experience communication difficulties when in an unfavorable listening environment? (for example, at a noisy party, where there is background music, when riding in an auto or bus, when someone whispers or talks from across the room, etc.)

   1) almost never (or     2) occasionally        3) about half of      4) frequently        5) practically
      never)                   (about ¼ of the        the time              (about ¾ of          always (or
                               time)                                        the time)            always)

6. Does he/she experience communication difficulties when using or listening to various communication devices? (for example, telephone, telephone ring, doorbell, public address system, warning signals, alarms, etc.)

   1) almost never (or     2) occasionally        3) about half of      4) frequently        5) practically
      never)                   (about ¼ of the        the time              (about ¾ of          always (or
                               time)                                        the time)            always)

Feelings About Communication

7. Do you feel that any difficulty with his/her hearing limits or hampers his/her personal or social life?

   1) almost never (or     2) occasionally        3) about half of      4) frequently        5) practically
      never)                   (about ¼ of the        the time              (about ¾ of          always (or
                               time)                                        the time)            always)

8. Does any problem or difficulty with his/her hearing visibly upset them?

   1) almost never (or     2) occasionally        3) about half of      4) frequently        5) practically
      never)                   (about ¼ of the        the time              (about ¾ of          always (or
                               time)                                        the time)            always)

Other People

9. Do you or others suggest he/she has a hearing problem?

   1) almost never (or     2) occasionally        3) about half of      4) frequently        5) practically
      never)                   (about ¼ of the        the time              (about ¾ of          always (or
                               time)                                        the time)            always)

10. Do you or others leave him/her out of conversations or become annoyed because of his/her hearing?

    1) almost never (or     2) occasionally        3) about half of      4) frequently        5) practically
       never)                   (about ¼ of the        the time              (about ¾ of          always (or
                                time)                                        the time)            always)

---

*Reprinted by permission from Schow, R. L., and Nerbonne, M. A. Communication screening profile: use with elderly clients, *Ear Hear.*, 3, 135–147 (1982).

# Appendix 14.6  Alpiner-Meline Aural Rehabilitation Screening Scale (AMAR)

## ALPINER-MELINE AURAL REHABILITATION (AMAR) SCREENING SCALE

### ADMINISTRATION INSTRUCTIONS

#### INTRODUCTION

The Alpiner-Meline Aural Rehabilitation Screening Scale (AMAR) is designed to identify adults who may need aural rehabilitation. The AMAR allows identification of problems related to hearing loss in three categories: (a) self assessment, (b) visual aptitude, and (c) auditory aptitude.

#### APTITUDE

1. The scale should be administered in a quiet room. Items are presented in an interview format.
2. Each subtest is scored independently. Part I, Self Assessment has nine items rated in terms of five possible responses: ALWAYS, USUALLY, SOMETIMES, RARELY, and NEVER. For all of the items, (except number five), ALWAYS refers to maximum negative response possible, that is, a problem exists. For item five, NEVER REFERS TO THE MAXIMUM NEGATIVE RESPONSE.

   A problem is indicated when the response is either ALWAYS, USUALLY, or SOMETIMES. For number five, a problem is counted for either NEVER, RARELY, or SOMETIMES. The possible number of problems for Part I can range from 0 to 9. Problems are designated by a minus sign.
3. The five visual aptitude sentences are presented face to face at a distance of three to five feet, with a normal to slow articulatory rate and no voice. Client's oral responses are scored on the basis of whether or not the client identifies the thought or idea of the stimulus sentence. Minus signs are circled for sentences not identified.
4. For auditory aptitude, six CVC or CV items are presented. For each of the six items, the examiner asks the client to circle one of two words. The word is presented live voice in a quiet room at a distance of five feet. A perforated $5 \times 8$ card is held three inches from the examiner's mouth so that no visual cues can be received by the client. The minus sign is circled for each incorrect response.
5. AMAR scores are calculated as the total number of problems indicated on the test form.
6. Total time required for administration, scoring, and interpretation is approximately 15 minutes.
7. Scoring (according to present norms):
   00–10 PROBLEMS = NO NEED FOR AURAL REHABILITATION
   11–13 PROBLEMS = QUESTIONABLE NEED
   14–20 PROBLEMS = ABSOLUTE NEED

REFERENCE: Alpiner, J. G., Meline, N. C., and Cotton, A. D., An Aural Rehabilitation Screening Scale: Self Assessment, Auditory Aptitude, and Visual Aptitude. *J. Acad. Rehabilitative Audiology, 24, 1991.*

## Appendix 14.7  Abbreviated Profile of Hearing Aid Benefit (APHAB)

### ABBREVIATED PROFILE OF HEARING AID BENEFIT, FORM A.

INSTRUCTIONS: Please circle the answer that comes closest to your everyday experience. Notice that each choice includes a percentage. You can use this to help you decide on your answer. For example, if a statement is true about 75% of the time, circle "C" for that item. If you have not experienced the situation we describe, try to think of a similar situation that you have been in and respond for that situation. If you have no idea, leave that item blank.

A  Always (99%)

B  Almost Always (87%)

C  Generally (75%)

D  Half-the-time (50%)

E  Occasionally (25%)

F  Seldom     (12%)

G  Never (1%)

|  | Without My Hearing Aid | With My Hearing Aid |
|---|---|---|
| 1. When I am in a crowded grocery store, talking with the cashier, I can follow the conversation | A  B  C  D  E  F  G | A  B  C  D  E  F  G |
| 2. I miss a lot of information when I'm listening to a lecture | A  B  C  D  E  F  G | A  B  C  D  E  F  G |
| 3. Unexpected sounds, like a smoke detector or alarm bell are uncomfortable | A  B  C  D  E  F  G | A  B  C  D  E  F  G |
| 4. I have difficulty hearing a conversation when I'm with one of my family at home | A  B  C  D  E  F  G | A  B  C  D  E  F  G |
| 5. I have trouble understanding dialogue in a movie or at the theater | A  B  C  D  E  F  G | A  B  C  D  E  F  G |
| 6. When I am listening to the news on the car radio, and family members are talking, I have trouble hearing the news | A  B  C  D  E  F  G | A  B  C  D  E  F  G |
| 7. When I am at the dinner table with several people, and am trying to have a conversation with one person, understanding speech is difficult | A  B  C  D  E  F  G | A  B  C  D  E  F  G |

Reprinted by permission from Cox, R. M., and Alexander, G. C., The abbreviated profile of hearing aid benefit. *Ear & Hearing,* 16, 176–186 (1995).

## Appendix 14.8  Hearing Handicap Inventory for Adults (HHIA)

### HEARING HANDICAP INVENTORY FOR ADULTS (HHIA)

Instructions: The purpose of the scale is to identify the problems your hearing loss may be causing you. Check Yes, Sometimes, or No for each question. Do not skip a question if you avoid a situation because of a hearing problem.

|  | | Yes (4) | Sometimes (2) | No (0) |
|---|---|---|---|---|
| S-1. | Does a hearing problem cause you to use the phone less often than you would like? | _____ | _____ | _____ |
| E-2.* | Does a hearing problem cause you to feel embarrassed when meeting new people? | _____ | _____ | _____ |

*HHIA Items for Seniors.

| | Yes (4) | Sometimes (2) | No (0) |
|---|---|---|---|
| S-3.    Does a hearing problem cause you to avoid groups of people? | ____ | ____ | ____ |
| E-4.    Does a hearing problem make you irritable? | ____ | ____ | ____ |
| E-5.*   Does a hearing problem cause you to feel frustrated when talking to members of your family? | ____ | ____ | ____ |
| S-6.    Does a hearing problem cause you difficulty when attending a party? | ____ | ____ | ____ |
| S-7.*   Does a hearing problem cause you difficulty hearing/understanding coworkers, clients, or customers? | ____ | ____ | ____ |
| E-8.*   Do you feel handicapped by a hearing problem? | ____ | ____ | ____ |
| S-9.*   Does a hearing problem cause you difficulty when visiting friends, relatives, or neighbors? | ____ | ____ | ____ |
| E-10.   Does a hearing problem cause you to feel frustrated when talking to coworkers, clients, or customers? | ____ | ____ | ____ |
| S-11.*  Does a hearing problem cause you difficulty in the movies or theater? | ____ | ____ | ____ |
| E-12.   Does a hearing problem cause you to be nervous? | ____ | ____ | ____ |
| S-13.   Does a hearing problem cause you to visit friends, relatives, or neighbors less often than you would like? | ____ | ____ | ____ |
| E-14.*  Does a hearing problem cause you to have arguments with family members? | ____ | ____ | ____ |
| S-15.*  Does a hearing problem cause you difficulty when listening to TV or radio? | ____ | ____ | ____ |
| S-16.   Does a hearing problem cause you to go shopping less often than you would like? | ____ | ____ | ____ |
| E-17.   Does any problem or difficulty with your hearing upset you at all? | ____ | ____ | ____ |
| E-18.   Does a hearing problem cause you to want to be by yourself? | ____ | ____ | ____ |
| S-19.   Does a hearing problem cause you to talk to family members less often than you would like? | ____ | ____ | ____ |
| E-20.*  Do you feel that any difficulty with your hearing limits or hampers your personal or social life? | ____ | ____ | ____ |
| S-21.*  Does a hearing problem cause you difficulty when in a restaurant with relatives or friends? | ____ | ____ | ____ |

---

*HHIA Items for Seniors.

Reprinted by permission from Newman, C. W., Weinstein, B. E., Jacobson, G. P., and Hug, G. A. Test-retest reliability of the Hearing Handicap Inventory for Adults. *Ear Hear,* 12(5), 355–357 (1991).

## Appendix 14.9  The Denver Scale of Communication Function for Senior Citizens Living in Retirement Centers

### THE DENVER SCALE OF COMMUNICATION FUNCTION FOR SENIOR CITIZENS LIVING IN RETIREMENT CENTERS

by
Janet M. Zarnoch, M.A. and Jerome G. Alpiner, Ph.D.

_____ Initial Evaluation
_____ Final Evaluation

NAME: _____

ADDRESS: _____

AGE: _____ SEX:_____

DATE OF PRE-TEST: _____

DATE OF POST-TEST: _____

EXAMINER: _____

| CATEGORY | MAIN QUESTION | PROBE EFFECTS | EXPLORATION EFFECTS | PROBLEM | NO PROBLEM |
|---|---|---|---|---|---|
| Family | 1 [+] [−] | a b c □ □ □ | a. _____ b. _____ c. _____ d. _____ | | |
| Emotional | 2 [+] [−] | I a b c □ □ □  II a b c □ □ □ | a. _____ _____ | | |
| Other Persons | 3 [+] [−] | a b c □ □ □ | a. _____ _____ b. _____ c. _____ | | |
| General Communication | 4 [+] [−] | a b c d □ □ □ □  e □ | a. _____ b. _____ c. _____ _____ | | |
| Self Concept | 5 [+] [−] | a b c □ □ □ | a. _____ _____ | | |
| Group Situations | 6 [+] [−] | a b c □ □ □ | a. _____ b. _____ c. _____ d. _____ e. _____ | | |
| Rehabilitation | 7 [+] [−] | a b □ □ | Ia. _____ b. _____ IIa. _____ b. _____ | | |

Key  + = person responded yes to question

  − = person responded no to question

Additional Client Comments:

1. _____

2. _____

3. _____

4. _____

5. _____

6. _____

# 15. Augmentative and Alternative Communication

Mary Blake Huer

Augmentative and alternative communication (AAC) is a relatively new field of practice which *overlaps* with the field of speech-language pathology. During the past two decades, AAC has emerged from the disciplines of special education, physical therapy, occupational therapy, speech-language pathology, electrical engineering, rehabilitation fields within allied health, computer science, artificial intelligence, neurology, and medicine. The practice of AAC encompasses the use of several options and systems for communication, for example, the use of unaided techniques such as sign, or the use of aided strategies like communication boards or electronic devices. Although the scope of practice for AAC as defined by the American Speech-Language-Hearing Association (ASHA) is "an area of clinical practice that attempts to compensate (either temporarily or permanently) for the impairment and disability patterns of individuals with severe expressive communication disorders (i.e., the severely speech-language and writing impaired)" (ASHA, 1989, p. 107), AAC is, in reality, a *transdisciplinary field,* with practitioners uniting to serve the many needs of persons with severe physical and mental challenges. The typical AAC client may be nonverbal and in a wheelchair, referred for services pertaining to communication as well as mobility, access, literacy, and independence. Often a team treats the AAC consumer, family, and significant others in order to improve communication, increase involvement in everyday activities, and contribute to quality of life.

Since 1982, the profession of AAC has established an organizational structure, journal, series of conferences, and training programs. There are several excellent books that provide the novice practitioner with an overview of current practices for evaluation and intervention in AAC (Baumgart, Johnson, & Helmstetter, 1990; Beukelman & Mirenda, 1992; Beukelman, Yorkston, & Dowden, 1985; Blackstone, 1986; Church & Glennen, 1992; Fishman, 1987; Musselwhite & St. Louis, 1988; Reichle, York, & Sigafoos, 1991). It is beyond the scope of this chapter to discuss typical clinical practices in AAC; rather this chapter focuses on issues pertaining only to counseling in AAC. However, to assist interested readers, several appendices have been included at the end of the chapter, with fact sheets pertaining to the topics of evaluation (Appendix 15.1), selection of technology (Appendix 15.2), addresses and phone numbers of manufacturers (Appendix 15.3), and professional organizations (Appendix 15.4). Persons wishing to complete self-study in AAC should refer to those materials, as well as to citations listed in the reference section. In addition, as will be discussed, the fact sheets will become useful when counseling AAC consumers.

A review of the AAC literature reveals very little, if any, information pertaining to counseling. The content within this chapter in part is based on the author's personal clinical experiences over a 17-year time span across several work settings. The clinical guidelines proposed, areas for needed research, and other commentary within this chapter are based on the literatures in AAC, disability, and counseling, in general.

The organization of this chapter includes an identification of those persons who would typically be involved during counseling in AAC; a discussion of the variables and components of counseling which are regarded as critical to practices in AAC; suggestions for the acquisition of competence before counseling in AAC; a brief review of the classic approaches to counseling in the context of typical AAC practices; specific ideas for counseling different age groups and disability types; a commentary on the practice of AAC counseling across cultures; and general conclusions. As the target audience for this book is speech-language pathologists (SLPs) and audiologists, the counseling practices that are recommended within this chapter will be relevant to the scope of practice of speech-language pathology, in particular.

## WHO IS THE AAC CONSUMER?

The AAC consumer is identified, most accurately, as the family unit, or the members within a particular communication dyad. Individuals requiring AAC intervention may exhibit severe physical challenges (e.g., cerebral palsy) or persons may have no physical disabilities but they may be cognitively challenged. It is the "lack of" a communicative exchange between such individuals and their partners that is often the presenting problem in AAC. Without the presence of any speech, *both* the person who is severely physically challenged, as well as the person who is the primary caretaker, are at a loss during the *transmission* of spoken or written communication. Communication, spoken or written, always takes place between two or more persons. In AAC, it is not uncommon to see as much frustration in the eyes of the significant others as it is in those of the person who has the disability.

Disabling conditions that may require increased reliance on augmentative and alternative communication have been categorized into four types (Blackstone, 1986): congenital conditions, acquired disabilities, progressive neurologic diseases, and temporary conditions. Some examples of congenital conditions include cerebral palsy, mental retardation, deaf, blindness, and autism. The insult suffered during a closed head injury or cerebral vascular accident, and surgeries mandating a laryngectomy or glossectomy are examples of acquired disabilities that warrant AAC intervention. In addition, numerous progressive diseases impact an individual's communication: amyotrophic lateral sclerosis, multiple sclerosis, muscular dystrophy, Parkinson's disease, and acquired immune deficiency syndrome. Finally, many persons are unfortunate enough to experience accidents, which result in shock or trauma for which intubation may be required minimally, or maximally which may result in chronic conditions (e.g., severe facial burns).

An individual experiencing any one or a combination of the above-described disabling conditions may need AAC services. Communication partners will also need AAC services just as badly, if not more so, sometimes, because they too suffer a severe communication disability when interacting. That is, they must learn to be the receiver of alternative messages.

In addition to classifying AAC consumers and their families or significant others by disabling condition, it is typical to group consumers with reference to skill areas (or lack of skill areas). For example, AAC consumers may be referred to speech-language pathologists and other professionals because of the lack of skills in any one or a combination of the areas of: speech, gestures, nonverbal communication, paralinguistic communication, mobility, auditory perception and memory, cognition, gross and fine motor skills, hand use, finger dexterity, positioning, receptive and expressive language, visual memory and perception, access, control over their environments, and interpersonal relationships. Practitioners may note constraints in the consumer's environment, including the home, school, and community. The constraints may be in the form of fear, caution, or other attitudes that prohibit successful communicative exchanges. The following case studies illustrate three AAC consumers, as examples.

**Case Number One.**  A young boy, age two years and seven months, and his mother met with a speech-language pathologist for an initial consultation for an AAC system. The presenting diagnosis was severe Goldenhar syndrome/type III. On meeting the family, the speech-language pathologist noted the initial loss of, and function of, facial structures: a left facial cleft, no hard palate, no left facial bones, and no left eye or ear. After testing the child and meeting with the mother, it appeared that the young preschooler had a language age equivalent of 36 months receptively; 18 to 21 months expressively; apparently normal hearing; and appropriate motor skill and cognitive development. The child was undergoing a series of eleven surgeries to rebuild the facial structures. What were the critical issues for this AAC consumer?

It was apparent that an expressive and receptive language gap was emerging owing to the severe facial anomalies. An AAC system was introduced to this normally developing, active child who had a congenital condition which was expected to be temporary. An AAC system was designed to meet the child's communication needs during the course of the surgical repairs. As the child acquired more speech, the AAC system would be modified, and AAC techniques would be eliminated as speech production skills increased as a result of surgery. The plan was to facilitate the development of normal speech and language through AAC.

Because of the child's medical needs, it was particularly important to establish a close working relationship with the child's parents. It was especially important that the child was able to communicate with persons in the medical community because visits were so frequent and answers directly from the child to the doctors and nurses were so necessary. There was one critical issue, however: the parents did not allow anyone to see their child because of his facial features. This presented several problems in terms of programming speech and language goals. Counseling was warranted.

**Case Number Two.**  A 36-year-old business man who held two Master's degrees suffered a cerebral vascular accident that left him nonverbal and in a wheelchair. The director of the skilled nursing facility requested an AAC evaluation. During the initial meeting between the client, his personal care attendant, and AAC specialist, it was noted that the employer wanted to facilitate the client returning to work. During the course of several weeks of therapy, it was determined that the client was nonverbal, but able to use one hand for typing, and was capable of performing many of the duties of his job as an accountant. That is, he could complete tax forms, read and process financial data, and so forth. An AAC system was prescribed with special software in a lap top computer, configured for one-handed typing, with word prediction. The employer paid for the rehabilitation. There was one remaining problem, however: the client was angry. As a nonverbal individual, he had not yet developed appropriate communication skills to explain his daily frustrations. Through his anger he abused therapists, his girl friend, and his personal care attendant. He destroyed property. Therefore, it was difficult for him to find professional services and personal care, the very therapies he needed. His anger threatened the purchase of the expensive AAC system which had been custom designed and configured for him, and resulted in his placement in a nursing home rather than in the home of his girl friend. Counseling was warranted.

**Case Number Three.** A 65-year-old gentleman had been in an automobile accident several years previously. His wife faithfully sat near his bed side in their retirement community one afternoon when an AAC expert came for an initial evaluation. Although the gentleman had received years of speech therapy at different intervals, he had failed to develop meaningful communication with strangers, especially therapists. On meeting the family, the wife explained to the AAC counselor that her husband frequently liked to sleep during therapy and was usually uncooperative. As the AAC expert began the evaluation, it was noted that the gentleman was indeed sleeping and unresponsive. The therapist observed the gentleman closely, looked around the room at the television and stereo, and questioned his wife about hobbies, likes, dislikes, and their history together. After 30 minutes of conversation between the wife and therapist, which focused on his large video and audio tape collections (which were nicely catalogued and arranged meticulously); and after several attempts at requesting that he participate during the evaluation by following simple commands and moving his head and hands, the therapist spoke directly to the gentleman about his collections. Suddenly, the gentleman opened his eyes widely, looked deep into the AAC experts' eyes, smiled, gave a little wink and began participating. His employment history revealed that he had been an engineer. When the AAC expert discussed strategies through which he might select from his favorite videotape and audio tape collections, he listened and evidently decided that this therapist was "OK!" His behavior changed; he appeared to awaken; and he participated fully during the rest of the evaluation, moving his hands and head. He smiled broadly and appeared to trust the therapist. The critical element during that particular therapy session was the AAC intervention. It was novel from all the other therapies, which, to the gentleman, had appeared to waste his time. He knew the therapists' routines well and was choosing not to have to participate through faking a sleepy behavior. A plan for AAC intervention began.

These three case studies illustrate scenarios challenging practitioners serving the AAC consumer. AAC practices often necessitate the need for counseling the consumer. Who is the AAC consumer? The consumer is the individual with the disabling condition as well as the family members and significant others involved in communication exchanges. What are the challenges that warrant counseling in AAC? In the next section, those issues frequently identified by families and others are described.

## IDENTIFYING THE VARIABLES OR COMPONENTS CRITICAL TO COUNSELING IN AAC

The practice of AAC is multidimensional. No two clients are alike; rather each AAC user appears as a bundle of needs. The typical AAC user is best described as a corpus of ten individuals in one, all with differing problems to be dealt with during therapy, such as, communication, mobility, behavior, emotions, sensory, physical, health, environmental, financial, and educational crises. Practitioners serve consumers with needs across the life span, from birth to death. AAC specialists deal with death and dying issues frequently; speech-language pathologists deal with such to a lesser extent. The factors causing the need for AAC are diverse. The population of AAC users is growing (Huer, 1994). As a young discipline, AAC practices are still being identified and defined. Historically, the practice has emerged from a Euro-American perspective (Huer & Soto, 1996); that is, the vocabulary depicted in the symbol sets and the strategies for teaching interaction have been driven by practitioners who are Euro-American. The practice of AAC, however, is now expanding to include the provision of services to children and adults across cultures. Therefore, clinicians are learning new ways of practicing through multicultural studies of communication styles and patterns in order to serve all persons in need of AAC. Thus, the variables or components of counseling practices in AAC are multifaceted.

Mittler (1995) provided an excellent summary of the range of counseling needs experienced by families of persons with disabilities. Based on an international research project examining the perspectives of families' experiences of disability, Mittler (1995) articulates issues similar to those addressed by professionals who interact with AAC consumers, the process through which parents:

- find out about the disability
- first reactions
- wanting to know
- social attitudes
- the roles of individual family members
- effects on family life
- families' experiences with professionals
- additional costs
- families' ideas for improvement

Without a doubt, families will remember how they are initially told about their child's or parent's communication difficulty. It is critical that AAC practitioners become aware of their styles of message delivery, both positive and negative. During the initial discoveries of disabilities, it is important that practitioners facilitate communication between family members and between the family and the practitioner, as persons are seldom prepared with coping strategies during moments of shock and grief. The "sharing" of feelings and experiences is an important element during counseling.

Practitioners will want to take the opportunity to provide information about AAC practices to consumers and their families. Several fact sheets are included within the Appendices at the end of this chapter, to provide information. Parents often ask for explanations and advice as to how they can help the consumer make progress (Mittler, 1995). Families also may express concerns about others' attitudes toward the family. They may seek assistance in responding to members of their communities regarding: what to tell others'; whose fault is it?; what happens to "social life?" Practitioners should be prepared to hear stories of discrimination and abuse because of the disability. It is important to assist the families in developing responses to such comments or to discuss positive coping strategies when they feel hurt and angry. The financial burden of disability is another subject of concern. The practitioner should expect to become involved in securing sources of funding for the family for the technology and therapies that the AAC consumer will need.

On the more positive side, practitioners also hear stories of the joys the family experiences because of the disability. AAC consumers can make important contributions to everyday family life. Roles of individual family members and friends and neighbors do change when an AAC consumer enters their lives. As families get over the initial shock of discovery, they begin to plan for the future of the child or adult in their lives. The AAC practitioner will assist families in their planning for a quality of life for the AAC consumer. This is an extremely important role. In fact, it may be the AAC practitioner who establishes a positive role model for other professionals in the eyes of the consumers.

> Throughout the lifetime of a disabled person, the family are likely to come into contact with a variety of professionals. Many parents . . . tell of one professional or another who treated them and their disabled relative respectfully and humanely and who gave significant help and advice. (Mittler, 1995; p. 75)

Huer and Lloyd (1990) identified a similar issue to those shared by families, expressed directly by AAC consumers: frustration toward professionals, including speech-language pathologists and doctors. During a content analysis of publications pertaining to 165 different AAC users, Huer and Lloyd (1990) reported that the topic of frustration appeared more frequently than any other. With regard to speech-language pathologists in particular, the AAC users felt that some were not competent to provide treatment, were not qualified to conduct evaluations, and took a casual approach to making life-long decisions for communication for other individuals. The AAC consumers were frustrated that SLPs were not helpful. As AAC consumers, in particular, and families of persons with disabilities, in general, express these themes of concern, practitioners in AAC must pay attention to what consumers are saying. There are critical issues which need to be addressed. Such concerns impact not only counseling of families of persons with disabilities in general, but identify the salient components of counseling of the AAC consumer in particular. In essence, professionals ought to be listening to the perspectives of the families as well as the consumer, as historically we are in a period of "rediscovery of the family" (Dybwad, 1995).

When one listens to the family stories, especially the stories of those who have numerous experiences along the life cycle, it is remarkable to recognize the journeys from:

> "trauma to strength and achievement . . . the stresses and difficulties that they contend with but equally importantly the gains, benefits and joys that the experience of living with and caring for a family member with . . . disabilities can bring . . . the resourcefulness, creativity and fighting spirit of the families themselves." (Mittler, 1995; p. 3)

Almost universally, family members report that what they need from professionals is accurate information, practical advice, and contact with professionals. In addition, they need support during the experience of being told about the disability; support when persons react adversely to them and their family member; and conversations regarding the changing roles of and impact on family members. These are several of the components critical to counseling in AAC.

## PREREQUISITE KNOWLEDGE AND SKILLS FOR COUNSELING IN AAC

When counseling within the field of AAC, what one immediately notices is the lack of participation on the part of the person with the disability. That is, the *voice* of the disabled person will rarely be heard directly. Instead, the voice of the disabled is initially heard indirectly through another individual. Other persons may speak for the AAC user throughout the course of several sessions of therapy until an AAC system has been configured and put in place. Like working with an individual who is bilingual, AAC practices often require a translator. The information, the stories, the interpretations, will come through the parent, the spouse, the teacher, the caretaker, or written reports. In fact, in addition to the lack of *speech* during the counseling session, the therapist may also note in the client the absence of gesturing, body movement, independence during mobility, and the lack of the ability to reposition. The physical challenges which are sometimes present impact on the paralinguistic skills often noted during conversation; for example, nonverbal communication, spatial relationships between speakers, spontaneity in response, and signals of power, conversational control, and implied action.

It is interesting to contrast the communication styles and patterns of the typical AAC user with those of the typical voice-, language-, or hearing-impaired client. The communication patterns of persons who are physically challenged and nonverbal are not the same as their able-bodied, speaking peers. Speech-language pathologists and audiologists must deal with persons with such severe disabilities. Although historically, it has been rare for all speech-language practitioners to have such severe cases, it is now expected that they do provide services to persons with severe physical and communication challenges; that is, individuals who experience a total lack of speech as well as total lack of movement. Initially, SLPs may need some time to adjust to the severity of the presenting condition often found in the AAC user. The verbal as well as the nonverbal forms of communication familiar to most SLPs are not present in the AAC user; thus, there is a need for extensive involvement with the family or a familiar partner for interpretation of communicative intent.

Historically, professional training programs in speech-language pathology have incorporated very little information within their curriculum regarding counseling; they have incorporated even less information pertaining to the scope of AAC practice. The American Speech-Language-Hearing Association has published only eight papers since 1981 regarding the practice of AAC. In 1991, in the position statement on AAC, only seven roles and responsibilities were provided (ASHA, 1991). Two of those published have some relevance to this chapter to:

> utilize a service delivery approach that incorporates the goals, . . . and knowledge of various disciplines, as well as that of the individual and family members"; and to "facilitate the individual's integration of AAC use in daily life. (ASHA, 1991; p. 8)

Although the paper does not explicitly address the role of counseling, it does address the need to work with practitioners of various disciplines, the family, and to integrate AAC into daily life. Thus, one prerequisite for AAC counseling might be the capacity to work not only with the individual, but also with the family, and other professionals. A second skill that should be acquired by SLPs is the ability to assist a family to integrate AAC therapy goals into everyday life activities.

George and Cristiani (1986) describe the variety of roles that counselors may take: trainer/educator; expert/prescriptive; negotiator; and collaborator. These roles are often observed in the field of AAC. It is not uncommon for a SLP to be hired to teach staff particular skills with regard to evaluation, for example. Other times, an AAC expert will be under contract to diagnose the problem and prescribe the appropriate technology. It is common in AAC to find oneself in the position of mediator between the parents and a school district. Often there is conflict between professionals and family members because of limited funding, resources, staff time, area of expertise, and so forth. The AAC expert may be outside of the particular system in which there is conflict, and therefore may be able to provide objective feedback regarding the situation. Finally, the AAC expert may take the role of collaborator and assist all parties in problem-solving and in establishing relationships for joint decision-making. The collaborator role is particularly appropriate when making decisions regarding the purchase of technology. The manufacturer's representative, consumer, family, therapist, and AAC professional need to work together to select the components within the overall AAC system. This is a time-consuming and costly process, especially if not planned carefully. Thus, another prerequisite recommended for counseling in AAC is the acquisition of the necessary skill and competence in shifting between roles as counselor.

The counseling literature is filled with descriptions regarding the necessary traits, personalities, and qualities that characterize an effective counselor (Arbuck, 1962; George & Cristiani, 1986; Herr & Weakland, 1979; Jageman & Myers, 1986; Pedersen, Draguns, Lonner, & Trimble, 1976; Wolfgang, 1984). Such competencies must be developed through careful reading of the literature, coursework, workshops, and/or extensive clinical experience under the supervision of trained personnel. Persons wishing to develop their skills more fully as a counselor in the field of AAC should possess effective human relation skills. Recommended prerequisite skills, which should be acquired by SLPs wishing to counsel effectively with AAC consumers, include the development of a range of interpersonal skills that meets the consumer needs. For example, it is important that practitioners have the capacity for empathy and be able to understand others' experiences and feelings (Dinkmeyer & Carlson, 1973; p. 237). An understanding of human needs, "psychological dynamics, motivations, and purpose of human behavior" are necessary. The capability to establish relationships through mutual trust and respect are particularly important as the practitioner works with the family unit, across cultures. The ability to inspire confidence in others with the courage to be imperfect as a clinician are qualities which should be acquired. Many other personal traits include: the willingness to make mistakes, to be creative, spontaneous, and imaginative; the ability to be flexible, yet structured as the case demands; and the acquisition of leadership as well as collaborator skills. AAC, as a field, is a social science. As such, the practitioner needs to be able to deal with social problems and human needs as they arise.

Although it is beyond the scope of this chapter, the provision of services in AAC warrants careful training during the coursework and practicum sequence required for certification by the American Speech-Language-Hearing Association. Appropriate graduate instruction and advanced clinical experiences in diagnostics and intervention should incorporate the prerequisites discussed within this section of the chapter. It is mandatory that clinicians prepare themselves to provide quality services that serve the welfare of the public. Through coursework, clinical supervision, and internships, it is possible to acquire the skill to work with the AAC consumer (refer to Appendix 15.5 for a sample list of competencies).

## APPROACHES TO COUNSELING

Historically, many different theories have been developed to explain the underlying rationale for the various approaches to counseling (Barnes, 1977; Bootzin, Bower, Zajonc, & Hall, 1986; Corey, 1991; George & Cristiani, 1986; Glasser, 1965; King & Neal, 1968; Pedersen, Draguns, Lonner, & Trimble, 1989). Some of these are summarized within chapters 4 and 5 of this book. It is interesting to note that, with few exceptions, the advocates of such theories developed their thinking and established their hypotheses when counseling human beings who could speak, walk, and move through their life with increasing independence from birth to death. The field of AAC would have presented several special problems to the "fathers" of counseling practices. For example, how would Adler have expected individuals to "take control over their lives" if they are in wheelchairs and totally dependent on others for their very survival? In the next section, commentary is provided regarding the applicability of several of the classic approaches to counseling in the context of typical AAC practices. At the end of the chapter, several guiding principles are drawn from the literature on counseling, which will be proposed for counseling practice in the context of AAC.

### Classic Approaches to Counseling: Relevance to AAC

Consider the consequences of many of the disabling conditions found within the practice of AAC. Typically, the AAC client is unable to speak, gesture, walk, be spontaneous, make independent decisions, and move about the room freely. During conversation, the AAC user is not an equal partner. The most basic conversation skills require years and years of training and extensive technology. Persons with disabilities, in general, are powerless. In contrast, the typical clients needing counseling are able to speak, gesture, walk, and exert control over their own lives. Therefore, the historical approaches to counseling need some modification before application to AAC. Let's look at a few examples that pertain to the therapeutic relationship (Corey, 1991) from the classic, cognitive-behavioral, and experiential approaches.

Adlerian therapy (classic) focuses on examining the lifestyles of individuals, with the concept that people have control over their own lives (George, & Cristiani, 1986). There is attention to the presence of feelings of inferiority, and to striving for security, perfection, and an awareness of self-defeating behaviors. The therapist, through mutual trust and respect, assists the client in understanding and interpreting positive changes in behavior. The client is encouraged to make change because of motivational factors arising from social and interpersonal factors. From the perspective of AAC, this approach to counseling creates several problems. First, AAC clients, in reality, have very little control over their lives. Sometimes the self-defeating behaviors are the result of a physical disability and can not be changed. The families of AAC users also have less control over their lives because of the complexities of the disability. This approach appears to oversimplify complex human problems and is too dependent on common sense. Depending on how one views causation of the problem, the Adlerian and other approaches may be inappropriate. That is, if one views the needs for counseling (symptoms) as behavioral, then one will select a treatment based on that belief. However, if one views the need from a physiologic perspective, then the treatment becomes very different.

Gestalt therapy (experiential approaches) emphasizes self-integration (George & Cristiani, 1986). Believing that a person is a composite whole made up of interrelated parts and that a person is a part of his or her own environment and cannot be understood apart from it, gestalt therapists would assist a person in becoming fully aware of the moment-to-moment experiences. The focus is on the *now*. On the surface this might appear as an attractive approach to counseling in AAC. However, the therapy itself would prove difficult as there is much emphasis on role playing, dialogue about feelings, discussions of dreams, and interpretation by the client. As the AAC consumer is nonverbal, it would be difficult for the consumer, as well as the family, to participate.

Similar limitations appear when viewing other historical approaches to counseling (cognitive-behavioral) from the context of AAC. The cognitive processes of thinking, perceiving, remembering (ego counseling), and feeling require *expressive language* to respond and explain to the therapist. AAC users have problems with expressive language. The abstract descriptions of emotion and reason (rational-emotive therapy), thoughts and feelings, analyzing, and experiencing, are lost in the limited vocabulary available within most AAC systems (e.g., communication boards, gesture, or an electronic aid). Thus, at the present time, the specialty area of counseling within AAC is underdeveloped and limited by the lack of verbal skills. It is also influenced in terms of a reduced range of nonverbal expression because of the presence of severe physical challenges.

Because, by definition, counseling incorporates the ability to solve problems and find new solutions, the question is then asked, "How would counseling be approached in AAC?" There is no easy answer to this question. In AAC, counseling involves an interaction with the family unit or significant others in addition to the individual experiencing the physical and/or mental disabling condition. The types of counseling used are strained by nature of client, clinician, and family interaction. The physical location (e.g., at home versus in a residential facility) in which the consumer lives impacts the nature of counseling. There will be time constraints and significant monetary concerns. It will not be uncommon to find a large number of participants involved directly in the counseling; for example, parents, consumer, teachers, therapists, personal care attendant, friends, and siblings. The viewpoints and expectations of each member of the team will influence the therapeutic relationships. Sometimes the projected goals for school, home, and social will not match real life expectations. Finally, each cultural group will demonstrate differing viewpoints and expectations. Each of these factors impacts on the success of the therapy. There are no wrong or right ways as yet. Thus, this chapter provides a few guiding principles based on the author's clinical experiences.

In the following sections some general approaches to counseling are provided by age group. It is not the author's intent to develop a theory or to utilize one of the more historical approaches to counseling. Rather, as the field of AAC is still young, it seems more appropriate to provide general commentary for the reader.

Probably one critical element that will be immediately noted in counseling in AAC is the presence of technology. Individuals using AAC tend to rely heavily on communication through technology that is sophisticated and more speedy than communication through a simple spelling or picture board, for example. Moore (1994) reminds us that in this age of telecommunications, we are suffering from "distant connections." Counseling in AAC may be best described as a series of distant connections. To reach the inner thoughts of the consumer, all persons must go through mechanical, electronic, and outer means. Although communication is becoming more efficient, at the same time it is less intimate when transmitted through a device rather than through speech. The physical limitations of the body add an additional layer that must be uncovered through counseling.

## Families of Children Using AAC

Children spend more time at home with their families than anywhere else. One critical aspect of counseling the young school-age child, therefore, must be to develop a plan to involve the parent(s). McFarlane, Fujiki, and Brinton's (1984) statement, "let's pool our resources and see what we can come up with" (p. 11), is an appropriate philosophy from which to begin to develop a comprehensive program of parent involvement. Several researchers (Angelo, Jones, & Kokoska, 1995 are suggesting that:

> professionals adopt a social systems perspective of families . . . as a social unit . . . viewed as interdependent . . . events in any one unit can . . . influence other social units . . . the child is seen as a member of a family system . . . events both within and outside the family unit affect the success of intervention. (p. 199)

From a counseling perspective, then, the practitioner's role is to monitor those events within the AAC clinical process which are apparently stressing the *system*, that is, the family unit. It is easy to identify some aspects of the typical AAC interventions that might cause stress on the family.

Parents are often given many responsibilities by practitioners (Beukelman, 1991; Huer & Lloyd, 1990): they serve as the informants during the selection of vocabulary (Fried-Oken & More, 1992; Yorkston, Dowden, Honsinger, Marriner, & Smith, 1988; Yorkston, Fried-Oken, & Beukelman, 1988); promote the social and linguistic experiences of children who are AAC users; provide practice opportunities; become facilitators for communication; contribute to literacy learning (Koppenhaver, Evans, & Yoder, 1991); and play an essential role in the operational competence and transfer of information about technology (Angelo et al., 1995; Berry, 1987). Angelo et al. (1995) noted that "professionals should recognize the need to address family issues" (p. 199). Practitioners should also prepare families for these newly added commitments.

Angelo et al. (1995) provided a list of concerns expressed by the mothers and fathers in 59 families. In brief, the parents shared the needs for increased:

> knowledge of assistive devices . . . integrating assistive devices in the community, developing community awareness and support for . . . AAC users, getting computer access, finding professionals . . . advocacy groups . . . volunteers to work with their child, getting funding for devices or services, knowing how to teach their child, and integrating assistive devices at home. (p. 193)

It would appear reasonable to use this list as a beginning from which to counsel the family, providing appropriate information and access to the necessary resources.

Parent programs are successful when there is a focus on the development of mutual respect between parents and professionals. An important ground rule is the establishment of true appreciation of all persons in an AAC user's life; an appreciation of the knowledge, competence, and experience which each person may contribute. A second rule is to encourage reciprocal interaction between all of the AAC user's communication partners when selecting goals. This is time consuming for the SLP, given the size of some caseloads and paperwork requirements. However, the time will be well spent as a future working plan will grow out of a team effort. If the SLP takes careful notes and listens to the stories that parents may tell during conferencing, the SLP will collect data regarding previous approaches to treatment, the outcomes of previous treatments, and information regarding parent motivation, knowledge, and attitudes. Such information is useful to collect before selecting final goals and it is mandatory for understanding and meeting the needs of the family.

It is also important to involve parents because it is mandated by the law; that is, a team must be used to evaluate a child who receives services from a federally funded program. Parents, therefore, are to be included in the planning and placement of their child before treatment may begin. The extent of parental involvement will be determined by the type of program in which the young AAC user is placed. Salisbury and Evans (1988) noted an important difference between parental involvement in regular versus special education. Typically, in regular education programs, the role of parents has been one of support. Parents have historically been involved through participation in the social functions of the schools and have usually been receivers of information regarding their child's educational progress. It has been rare for parents to contribute to the development of curriculum, to plan for their child's education, or to establish educational policy.

Unlike the parents of children in regular education, however, parents of children receiving special education have been legally mandated to enter into the planning process and to be involved in establishing a plan for their child's education. Because parents of children receiving special education have been more involved, they have had opportunities to influence the educational policy and the development of curricula for their child. Opportunities for increased parent involvement have become a challenge to SLPs working with children in special education. SLPs are not used to as much parental involvement as one finds in the AAC population. It is important, therefore, to plan for parental involvement. A careful plan for parental involvement will facilitate the establishment of an improved, comprehensive program. SLPs need to develop plans to assist parents in becoming active participants and eventually partners in the process of decision-making. How does one develop such a plan?

The literature in parent counseling, education, and training offers assistance for the SLP wishing to involve parents in management of the young AAC user. Moses (1985) notes that parents sometimes bring emotions of frustration, grief, a sense of failure or disappointment, anxiety, hope, sadness, anger, and anticipation to meetings with professional service providers. The SLP should identify each parent's feelings during parent conferences. Sometimes parents need to "vent" feelings and just need someone to listen for a moment. Although it is the role of the SLP to provide information and resources for the young AAC user, SLPs will achieve greater success if they acknowledge parent feelings, as necessary, before moving into discussions of goals and objectives, and expectations for parent assistance. It is a challenge for SLPs to learn to identify the parent expectations at conferences, particularly as services are provided across various ethnic groups. SLPs have to develop competence in recognizing parents' needs, across cultures. It is important to make careful observations, and to practice *active listening* to identify at which point in time, if any, the parents may need to have counseling versus specific training regarding AAC treatment strategies. Often the practitioner can take advantage of the opportunity, when actively listening, to attempt to mirror the parents' feelings, to check the perceptions of each individual, and to wait for opportunities to redirect and guide the parents in order to integrate appropriate objectives for the child. An SLP's skill at switching strategies during conferencing in response to parent expectations does take time to develop, but it is a worthwhile objective.

When SLPs meet during parent conferences, they should be careful to avoid "professional jargon" and to pace the demands placed on parents. Goals and objectives must be slowly identified as the SLP and parents establish a good working relationship. During conferences, the SLP should outline the strategies through which specified goals will be attained. An example of a program that includes home activities may be taken from the work of Fey (1986).

Fey (1986) lists eight steps that might be "taken to enhance the likelihood that trained intervention procedures will be applied correctly and routinely in the home" (p. 316). Within the eight steps, responsibilities are assigned to either the SLP or the parent. Examples of assigned responsibilities include: (a) deciding who will be involved in achieving which goal; (b) setting beginning and ending dates; establishing schedules for record keeping, phone calls, and face-to-face meetings; (c) writing contracts for rental or loan of equipment, if required; and (d) determining a plan for securing funding. If parents are actively involved in the management program, Fey's model offers useful suggestions for the SLP.

Berry (1987), describes "strategies for involving parents in programs for young children using augmentative and alternative communication" (p. 90). She suggests the following strategies: (a) provide information to parents; (b) utilize a family systems approach, viewing the family as an individual system; (c) create support networks that offer day camps, counseling services, recreational activities, and baby-sitting; and (d) advocate teamwork between parents and professionals serving together on the team. These strategies offer novice SLPs several good ideas how to proceed when involving parents in programs. Several other suggestions have been compiled by Blackstone (1989).

Blackstone (1989) offers nine suggestions to SLPs to help families add AAC approaches to already existing intervention programs:

1. Discuss and demonstrate the reason for an individual's speech problem. Explain what is involved in producing speech and how the speech system develops.
2. Introduce the concept of parallel programming. Talk about sound stimulation, articulation, language and communication training using AAC techniques . . . . Ask caregivers (as primary team members) to help set priorities, assign tasks, and measure effectiveness.
3. Set up an activity to demonstrate what the individual with AAC needs can do using a particular AAC technique.
4. Offer family members written information about AAC. Follow up with discussion.
5. Arrange to have family members talk with others whose child has been successful using recommended aids or techniques.
6. Show videotapes of individuals with similar problems communicating successfully using AAC.
7. If possible, make a videotape of case examples illustrating improvement in speech, language, and communication skills over time.
8. If the family does not want to use AAC aids and techniques at home, begin at school or in some other context.
9. Be patient and honest. If caregivers refuse to allow the team to implement special AAC techniques, recommend working on speech and standard augmentative techniques (gestures, vocalizations, drawing). Teach conversational repair strategies, letter cueing, and so forth. Periodically, reintroduce the idea of special AAC approaches.

Musselwhite and St. Louis (1988) discuss the "responsibilities of professionals in relation to parents" (p. 60) in their chapter on supportive services. Their discussion focuses on sharing information with parents, providing emotional support to parents, and the approaches to training parent(s) to assume greater responsibility. A "sample priority rating form for communication-related services" (p. 61) is offered as a form that is extremely useful during initial parent/professional contacts. The form, adapted from Canseler, Martin, and Valand (1975), offers a framework within which initial questions can be posed during the meeting between the SLP and parent(s).

Although it is often assumed that clinicians know what the parents' preferences are, clinicians should exercise caution in making such assumptions. Some parents might want to be included in their child's program through weekly meetings to discuss current issues in AAC, to provide updates on available techniques for communication, and to share problems, successes, and follow-up; others may not wish to get as involved. A notebook may be utilized, as an appropriate strategy to communicate between the home and school. The notebook serves as a diary for parents to record the progress, or lack thereof, in communicating. Frustrations of the parents, and child may be communicated immediately in the notebook, facilitating a check within the system when needed. Practitioners should always ask the parents about their wishes whether or not to become involved in the therapy and to respect such wishes as expressed by the parents. It is important that clinicians take the time to expand their understanding of parents.

Training the siblings of AAC users is useful. Brothers and sisters serve an invaluable role vital to the development of communication. Throughout each day, siblings provide opportunities for communication. Children who have received training may assist in identifying communication breakdowns during the day. They may offer the SLP critical insight regarding family issues and needs. Given a role, siblings have a positive impact on family dynamics.

SLPs may want to form support groups for parents. There are many excellent models from which to learn: the Association for Retarded Citizens, United Cerebral Palsy Foundation, the National Special Education Alliance, and the National Association for Retarded Citizens. Kirstein, Peters, Cottier, & Blau (1988) describe strategies for establishing a parent support group. They list six questions that may facilitate conversation during meetings. In addition, they provide a bibliography of reading materials made available to communication enhancement center parents. Appendices 15.1 and 15.2 of Kirstein et al., (1988) offer excellent resources to the SLP wishing to establish a support group.

Parents expect education, training, and support from the SLP. Therefore, it is extremely important that the SLP is equipped to meet the parents' expectations, be it on an intellectual or an emotional level. Often, parents do not want the theoretic training requested by service providers (Behrmann, 1995, p. 214). Rather, parents need information regarding awareness and attitude training and support in using the specific AAC devices. Beukelman and Mirenda (1992) note that

> AAC interventions never end! Once an AAC user has mastered a device for today . . . begin to prepare for one that is . . . more accurate, efficient, and non-fatiguing for tomorrow. Once these new skills are acquired, today becomes yesterday, tomorrow becomes today, and planning can begin for a new 'tomorrow'!" (p. 156)

If the AAC user is a child, this cycle is likely to require repetition at each transition from preschool to kindergarten, from elementary school to junior high, from junior high to senior high, and from senior high to either employment or postsecondary school. Thus, when working with families of children using AAC, it is reasonable to expect that there will be a cycle of need. That is, during each transition to a new school, or device, or social situation, parents will become more dependent on the AAC practitioner for support and guidance, as well as for continual information about the cause of the disabling condition and future prospects for such.

## Adults Using AAC

There are several different populations of adults using AAC (Beukelman & Mirenda, 1992; Garrett, 1992): adults with acquired physical disabilities (e.g., amyotrophic lateral sclerosis, multiple sclerosis, Parkinson's disease, and spinal cord injury); adults with severe aphasia as a result of a cerebral vascular accident; adults with traumatic brain injury (e.g., caused by vehicle accidents and recreational- and sports-related injuries); and adults who are unable to communicate either temporarily or permanently as a result of a medical condition (e.g., a traumatic brain injury, intubation, and tracheostomy). Typically, the adult using AAC as well as their family members, spouses, friends, and significant others will seek counseling during the course of the intervention, especially during the time periods where there is a change in the AAC system. For some individuals, changes are frequent; for others, change occurs more slowly. Generally, adults using AAC may be divided into two groups: "adults with congenital (e.g., cerebral palsy) or acquired, non-degenerative impairments (e.g., spinal cord injury)"; and "adults with degenerative illnesses (e.g., ALS, multiple sclerosis)" (Beukelman & Mirenda, 1992, pp. 156–157). The former group requires less frequent change to their AAC system whereas the latter may require "frequent system changes as their abilities deteriorate and living situations change." Both groups as well as their families or personal care attendants will require counseling.

The age of onset differs across the various populations of adult AAC users. The course of the loss of language, speech, communication, and physical abilities is not the same for each adult AAC user. In general, it appears that there is more frustration, grief, and shock observed by clinicians working with adults with acquired disabilities than with those working with adults with congenital disabilities. That is, there tends to be stronger feelings exhibited, the closer to the discovery of disability. Over time, reactions settle and the course of intervention may begin. This section focuses on counseling tips for practitioners serving adults with acquired disabling conditions that warrant AAC intervention.

Initially, it is important to meet with the individual who has suffered the loss as well as with the significant others in that individual's life. The purposes of the first meetings are to establish the extent of loss in the areas of communication and the changes taking place during participation in daily life activities. Beukelman and Mirenda (1992) describe a *participation model* which is an effective framework for organizing an approach to AAC intervention. From the participation model we know that it is important to ask questions pertaining to dramatic changes in the individual's life. For example, adults may now center their new lives around their home, rather than around their community. They may have been forced to retire early owing to the disability or they may be encouraged by their employer to return to the workplace. However, the workplace, including the computer, telephone, office furniture, and so forth, have to be made accessible for persons with disabilities. Some AAC users may no longer feel like or have the physical stamina to participate in social activities with their friends. Their communication partners may be limited. Their message needs may be more basic than before. It is the AAC practitioner's responsibility to make accurate observations of all the changes that have occurred since the acquisition of the disability. Careful note taking is mandatory; listening to the family, the user, and caregivers is necessary. The accurate perceptions of all of the changes will form the basis from which intervention may begin.

The clinician should also assess constraints which are affecting the person with the acquired communication disorder. Often family members do not agree on the course of treatment for an individual. Some family members are more optimistic, whereas others are pessimistic. The person's age, young or elderly, will have an impact on decision-making and discussion regarding the desired course of action. Family members will need someone to talk to, to seek advice from, to provide information regarding the disability, and to provide training pertaining to the technology involved in AAC programming. Adult AAC users will need the same services, with and separate from their significant others.

SLPs providing AAC services to adults have to work as a member of a team. SLPs need to become knowledgeable regarding access to services that provide electronically controlled beds, powered mobility, portable respiratory ventilation systems, modified public and private transportation, and computer technology, as adults may want to attend colleges and hold regular jobs (Beukelman & Mirenda, 1992). As a member of the AAC team, SLPs will advocate for the needs of the consumer to ensure the full return to and participation in everyday life activities.

Although the AAC intervention focuses on restoring the communication skills of the individual, the counseling for AAC must focus on issues such as the need for independence and social closeness. Adults who become disabled often lose their independence. Events in their lives become rather automatic. They experience a sense of loss and they may not wish to become dependent on their loved ones. Adults in skilled nursing facilities or those at home alone may reach out to the SLP because of their need for social closeness. Often persons with disabilities feel alienated and lonely. It is necessary to facilitate opportunities for persons with disabilities to socialize and communicate with others. Be prepared to answer questions regarding issues related to dating, employment, education, and the future as persons experiencing a major change in their lifestyles have questions and need answers to remain motivated for their futures.

### The Significant Others: What to Do?

In AAC, one not only works with families and consumers, one works closely with many of the significant others in the lives of AAC consumers. Typically, during the course of daily practice in speech-language pathology, a practitioner meets a parent or spouse who drives the child or adult to and from therapy. Also, the SLP consults with persons in the educational system, teachers, administrators, therapists, and nurses. However, SLPs rarely see large groups of persons attending a therapy session or participating in the intervention strategy. In the practice of AAC, it seems that the clinician meets many more people in the life of each AAC consumer.

It is often the case that the AAC expert is found much later during the course of treatment than are other health care providers and educators. Historically, there are probably several good reasons for this timeline: the physician makes the initial diagnosis; issues of life and death are dealt with before communication and access; the field of AAC is relatively new as a professional discipline; because AAC is a new field, educators and health care professionals have not had many referrals, or it has been difficult to know how to make appropriate referrals; there are very few professionals practicing AAC so they simply are not available nor are they on the staff of medical facilities or employed within educational systems; funding was not available; or it did not appear necessary as other professionals could take care of the presenting problems. Nevertheless, eventually families find the AAC expert if they keep looking and expecting that appropriate services will become available. Usually, at the end of a long search, there is a rich history of treatment practices and practitioners who find the AAC expert. These individuals have many questions and need answers. If the AAC intervention is successful, then the AAC practitioner finds another client for life! There is a saying in the field of AAC: "How many persons can one adopt in a professional lifetime?" AAC practitioners find their case loads continually increasing!

The approach to counseling the significant others is best defined as that of advocate and resource. The significant others of AAC users are often highly resourceful persons, full of energy and stamina, with determined spirits to seek the full range of services available to their loved ones. Because of years and years of meeting the needs of their loved ones (the consumers), significant others may appear as confrontational, angry, tired, religious, optimistic, helpful, or any combination of these traits. Most significant others are extremely helpful individuals who continually meet the needs of the AAC user. The significant others have often developed coping strategies to deal with the problems presented by the disability. Sometimes the coping strategies that are already in place may appear to be functional; sometimes they may appear as dysfunctional in best meeting the needs of the consumer. What these individuals need from the AAC expert is continual access to information pertaining to the latest technology, to best practices, the dates and places of conferences, including exhibits, and time for re-evaluation and intervention whenever the AAC user is moving to a new school, teacher, or employer, or has exhibited a physical or cognitive change. They also need support groups, information about funding sources, and encouragement as they think about the future. The approach to counseling the significant others may take any one of the forms: trainer/educator; expert/prescriptive; negotiator; and collaborator.

## ACQUIRED VERSUS CONGENITAL DISORDERS: DOES IT MAKE A DIFFERENCE?

It is never easy to accept the news that one's child, spouse, family member, or friend has a disabling condition. It is also not easy for the professional to discuss the realities of a loss of speech, language, communication, and physical ability. The impact of the announcement of disability is rarely forgotten by the consumer or professional for the rest of their lives. Does it make a difference if the disabling condition is congenital or acquired? Probably not—during the initial moment of discovery. All disabling conditions stir strong feelings at deep levels within human beings. On the surface, however, the reactions to such knowledge probably differ. In addition, the time span between the original discovery and any given moment in the present, probably makes a difference in the ability to take action and plan for the intervention.

Family members who experience a loved one's disability have lost a known relationship. Moore (1994) writes eloquently regarding the loss of relationships. His writings are applicable to AAC. When any relationship ends, strong feelings and anger stirs. The hopes for the future, the experience of grief and mourning are essential elements within lives shaken. A father or mother may never be the same. The family roles may need to shift. Parents, anticipating the birth of a newborn, may not have visualized a child with a disability. The shock and tragedy of an automobile accident leaves scars on the lives of all family members. Financial concerns, access to new information, and lack of preparation for a life changed have a great impact on the AAC consumer.

After the initial announcement and shock of discovery, a few subtle differences are noted in counseling persons with congenital versus acquired disabilities. In general, a congenital problem (e.g., cerebral palsy) creates little change throughout the course of treatment so the need for counseling is fairly steady. On the other hand, acquired, progressive degenerative diseases (e.g., amyotrophic lateral sclerosis) cause gradual to rapid change over time. "Sound clinical management dictates early preparedness" (Yorkston, Smith, Miller, & Hillel, 1991; p. 10). The counselor needs to prepare facilitators for such changes.

Recovery from spinal cord injury progresses through several stages (Beukelman & Mirenda, 1992): "paralysis, sensory loss, and loss of the reflexes below the level of the injury" (p. 324). Depending on the location of the spinal cord lesion, there may be interference with handwriting and keyboard control. Persons may be ventilator dependent and "learn to speak by venting air past their tracheostomy tube and through the larynx as the ventilator forces air into the lungs" (Beukelman & Mirenda, 1992; p. 325). The communication abilities of persons with traumatic brain injury (TBI) can change dramatically during the course of treatment. An individual suffering from TBI may initially be totally dependent on an AAC system, but later re-establish natural speech for communication (Yorkston, et al. 1992). Thus, the role of the counselor would be to answer questions and to prepare individuals to cope with change, as necessary; change can result in improvement as well as in further loss of function.

In summary, if there is a difference in counseling approaches for persons with acquired versus congenital conditions, the difference focuses on the extent of change in disabling condition. Any time there is a change in a person's condition, there will probably be a need for counseling. Persons with acquired disabilities tend to exhibit greater change more frequently than persons with congenital disabilities. More importantly, as a rule of thumb, the shorter the time interval between the discovery of disability or change in condition, the greater the need for counseling. Practitioners should expect the counseling to focus on issues pertaining to: emotional reactions of AAC consumer, changing view of self, attitudes expressed by others, memories of lost relationships, responsibilities, abandonment, and loss of expressions of intimacy.

## COUNSELING ACROSS CULTURES: AAC CONSUMERS—THE FUTURE

Communication styles and patterns vary across cultures (Dillard, 1988; Lynch & Hanson, 1992; Schaffer; 1993). Historically, most of the health care practices, including those in speech-language pathology, as well as AAC in the United States have evolved from a model based on Euro-American perspectives (Kreps & Kunimoto, 1994). In Chapter 5 of this book, there is an extensive discussion focusing on multicultural considerations in counseling persons with communication disorders and their families. However, it is appropriate to insert a brief discussion of culturally bound communication issues that pertain to counseling in AAC as there is some interesting research emerging in this area (Huer, 1995; Ponterotto, Casas, Suzuki, & Alexander, 1995), which will have direct impact on all counseling practices in AAC.

Future projections of the populations of AAC consumers indicate that although the population of Euro-American AAC users (approximately 0.8 % of the total population) will continue to grow, the populations of Asian/Pacific Islanders, Hispanic/Latino, American Indian, and African American AAC users will expand at an accelerated rate in comparison. Rough estimates indicate that by the year 2020 there may be 2.3 million consumers in need of AAC services in the United States. Of that group, approximately 1.3 million will be Euro-American (0.8%); 366,000 African American (0.1%); 343,000 Hispanic/Latino (0.07%); 229,000 Asian/Pacific Islanders (0.03%); and 34,000 Native American (0.01%) (Huer, 1994). These estimates are probably low. Nevertheless, an examination of the current delivery of AAC services reveals a severe shortage of AAC practitioners trained to provide AAC across cultures (Huer, 1993). Persons with disabilities come from a variety of ethnic groups and socioeconomic classes. At the present time, very few AAC services are found among the various ethnic groups. Little knowledge is available to prepare practitioners for meeting the needs of AAC users across cultures.

What are some of the critical issues AAC practitioners should understand as they begin to provide counseling services to AAC consumers from various ethnic groups? First, it is necessary for the professional to learn as much about *culture*, their own as well as that of other's, as possible. A few authors are beginning to identify issues pertaining to AAC across cultures (Harrison-Harris & Soto; 1994; Huer, 1993; Huer, 1995; Soto, Huer, &

Taylor, in press). Specifically, researchers in the subspecialty of AAC across cultures are examining:

- the definition of culture
- the importance of designing culturally valid AAC assessment and intervention processes
- varying attitudes toward the use of technology for communication
- mixed attitudes toward AAC systems as a strategy for communicating
- extent of knowledge regarding health and disorder
- home language proficiencies; second language acquisition
- learning environments
- educational demands
- models of service delivery
- severity of disorders
- communication styles and patterns across cultures
- discourse styles
- acceptance of disabling conditions

Knowledge about such issues will become mandatory as professionals expand their practices. In becoming culturally competent, it has been useful to use the literature from the related fields of speech communication, interpersonal communication, intercultural communication, sociologic prediction, psychology, ethnolinguistics, language, nonverbal communication, psycholinguistics, and bilingual education (see the reading list in Appendix 15.6 for a list of recommended readings).

An extensive awareness of one's own culture as well as that of other's is the best preparation for a counselor beginning to practice across cultures in AAC. An understanding of culture is the foundation of good counseling practices. Why? Because counseling deals with solving problems and finding solutions within given systems, in this case "family systems." For practitioners to work effectively with families, they must understand the culture (system) of each family. Consider one definition of culture (Huer, 1995): "Culture is the totality of those shared, learned, owned 'X' by members of the particular cultural grouping. What is the composite 'X'? 'X' equals all those beliefs, values, traditions, behaviors, communication patterns, laws, myths, religions, perceptions, assumptions, attitudes, identities, socialization practices, and views of health and education." Thus, in order for a counselor to be effective in solving problems and finding solutions for any given family, that counselor must acquire an understanding of that family's systems. How might one accomplish such?

There are several explicit strategies for learning about culture that can be taught. First, one begins by reading the history of various ethnic groups, including the literatures describing their histories, immigration patterns, language and linguistic origins, sociocultural patterns, and socialization practices of particular groups. During such reading, general patterns of communication styles and patterns begin to emerge. One may attempt to develop profiles of various cultures, being careful not to stereotype and realizing that there is much variability across cultures. The counselor might ask a series of questions or make observations to identify cultural groups. Collectible information might pertain to the structure of the group; roles of various members; rules for decorum; rules for discipline; standards for health and hygiene; attitude toward disability; education; rules for interpersonal interactions; communication style; language use, chants; religious beliefs, prayers, spiritual songs; family rituals; celebrations; ceremonies; important events in life; rituals to honor persons, events; holidays; food preferences; dress and personal appearance; perceptions of time and space; explanations of natural and supernatural phenomena; jokes; morals; attitude toward pets and animals; artistic tastes; colors; famous people; and life expectations and aspirations (Taylor, 1994; Soto, et al., in press). As therapists begin to collect this type of information about the AAC consumer, they will find effective ways to discover solutions and solve problems within the context of the family system and with respect for the culture of the particular family. Let us look at some examples.

## Culturally Bound Communication Issues

Consider the question, "Who is the decision maker in a particular culture?"

Decision makers change across cultures. The counselor, seeking to establish an AAC program, may approach the parents of a child from a Euro-American culture. The counselor, with the parents, agree on a course of therapy. In working with parents from other cultures, it is necessary to understand the decision-making process within that particular culture. For example, it might be that the grandparents are the decision makers, not the parents, in some cultures. The counselor may need to invite other family members of Asian or African-American consumers, for example, to the evaluation. If a counselor does not include or invite the decision maker (in this case the grandmother) to the meetings, the counselor may be failing to understand how decisions are made within that particular family system. It is the responsibility of counselors, working across cultures, to become familiar with the *rules* and communication styles and patterns of the individuals with whom they are working. Communication styles and patterns are culturally bound. Not all communication styles and patterns are universal. If the counselor takes the time to acquire competence and understanding regarding the relationship between communication style and culture, then that counselor will begin to design more effective culturally valid AAC assessment and intervention processes.

Several competencies for the provision of AAC and multicultural services are provided in the appendices (Appendices 15.5 and 15.7). Several of these proposed competencies are universal across cultures; others are culture dependent. The practitioner in AAC needs to acquire skill across cultures during coursework and practicum experiences in graduate school. One example of a culture-dependent competency is the ability to evaluate AAC candidacy (see Appendix 15.5; trainee competency 2). For the practitioner to interpret effectively the evaluation information, that practitioner must identify those parameters within the assessment that are culturally sensitive (see Appendix 15.1). Three examples of cultural issues that might be manifested during an evaluation are: (a) observation of paralinguistic aspects of language; (b) interactive language skills across partners; and (c) environmental constraints and attitudes/support services. Of the 15 areas proposed for evaluation (see Appendix 15.1), these three parameters are more sensitive to the culture of the consumer.

Collectivistic cultures demonstrate different interactive language styles than do individualistic cultures. The paralinguistic aspects of language, for example, the use of nonverbals, eye gaze, and facial expressions signal different communicative intent across cultures. Some families may have very positive attitudes toward disabilities; other families may exhibit judgmental behaviors, have different opinions, or challenging attitudes. Clinicians practicing AAC must be competent in correctly interpreting their observations during evaluation. Without appropriate training in AAC across cultures, counselors may misread the communication patterns and styles of those with whom they are interacting.

An awareness of the various attitudes toward learning, disability, and education is needed when prescribing technology for the AAC user across cultures. In a Euro-American culture, for example, parents may advocate for and fully support the decision to purchase technology. With reference to those 25 or so critical parameters for fit and selection of AAC systems and components (see Appendix 15.2), it would appear that most families would appreciate the *independence* and *assertability* factors offered through technology. Not so! In some cultures, *dependence* and *silence* are valued. An AAC expert prescribing technology must understand the culture of the family in which the device will be placed to be an effective trainer of such a system.

*Color* is culturally bound. The colors depicted in some of the symbols and device overlays, which are commercially available, may be offensive or may signal different meanings to persons in different cultures. Thus, the "cosmesis" of a system (see Appendix 15.2) is an important consideration for many cultures.

There are cross-cultural differences in learning and conversational styles. For example, careful attention should be paid to polychronic versus monochronic communication styles during the initial meetings with families as well as when teaching the skills of interaction. Cultures with communication styles that are low context (e.g., Euro-American) differ from those with high context (e.g., Asian and Hispanic-Latino) styles. Thus, the content extent conveyed by the counselor must be modified during counseling of persons from different cultures. Although beyond the scope of this chapter, there are numerous readings recommended for the interested practitioner wishing to pursue the study of multiculturalism and its relevance to AAC practices. A multicultural reading list is included in Appendix 15.6 for that purpose.

There are cross-cultural differences in attitudes toward health and disorders. In some cultures, disorders are accepted and viewed as blessings from God. In other cultures, AAC users may be viewed as a curse. These differing beliefs directly impact the perceived treatability of the disorders (Wyatt, 1995). The extent to which families may seek health care services may be directly related to their perceptions of disability. The willingness, or lack thereof, for some families to accept AAC intervention may be impacted by cross-cultural differences in attitudes.

In summary, it is becoming increasingly apparent that the age-old practices of counseling have emerged from practitioners who are of Euro ancestry (Ponterotto et al., 1995). AAC practices still reflect a single point of view, but this is slowly changing. Expect to see future research in AAC counseling that reflects a shift from a monolithic to a pluralistic perspective; research that questions the validity of current theories, techniques, and strategies used in the profession. This is a time of change. Why? Because clinicians are becoming aware that there is a need to acquire a broad range of multicultural competencies if they are to remain responsible as counselors. An understanding of the threat the perpetuation of ethno-centrism represents in AAC exposes biases which impair good and fair practices. Counselors in AAC need to understand these critical cultural issues in order to recognize the impact of such on the success of their practices, and before they can develop new strategies to minimize cultural dissonance when practicing.

## GENERAL GUIDELINES FOR COUNSELING IN AAC

Within this chapter, there has been a discussion of the variables and components of counseling practices that are relevant to counseling the AAC consumer. Numerous strategies have been discussed that are relevant for counseling persons requiring AAC across cultures and across the life span. Of all those qualities and traits that counselors might acquire and given the vastly different roles counselors play when meeting the specific needs of the array of individuals, this section of the chapter concludes with a list of general guidelines for counseling the AAC consumer. This simple list is profoundly important:

1. AAC is a transdisciplinary field. Therefore, it is a common practice for SLPs to consult with other professionals to seek guidance and instruction regarding appropriate services for persons with severe physical and/or mental challenges.
2. When counseling the AAC consumer, the SLP provides services to the family unit, however that unit may be configured or defined. Counseling involves treatment of the communication partners as well as the individual who is communicatively different.
3. The practice of AAC is multidimensional. No two clients are alike.
4. The SLP should be prepared to assume a variety of roles to meet individual needs. For example, at times the SLP will be providing education and training to the family. On other occasions, the SLP may become the negotiator between members of the family and professional team members.
5. SLPs wishing to counsel AAC consumers effectively should possess human relation skills, understand human needs, and have the capability to influence the therapy process through mutual trust and respect.
6. Do not make assumptions about the preferences of families. Although some families may wish to become very involved in the clinical process, others may not, or may be unable to become active participants. Clarify the expectations within the family unit and respect the boundaries expressed.
7. Always remember that the counseling process involves working with "human beings," whose lives have been shaken because of a lost relationship, shifting roles, unmet expectations, or gradual change.
8. Communication styles and patterns vary across cultures. Therefore, different practices, processes, and procedures should be implemented, as appropriate.
9. Expect to see continued change in counseling practices in AAC during the next decade.
10. SLPs may assume vastly different responsibilities when counseling individual AAC consumers.

REFERENCES

Angelo, D., Jones, S., & Kokoska, S. (1995). Family perspective on augmentative and alternative communication: Families of young children. *Augmentative and Alternative Communication, 11,* 193–201.
Arbuck, D. (1962). *Counseling: An introduction.* Boston: Allyn and Bacon.
American Speech-Language-Hearing Association. (1989). Competencies for speech-language pathologists providing services in augmentative communication. *ASHA, 31,* 107–110.
American Speech-Language-Hearing Association. (1991). Report: Augmentative and alternative communication. *ASHA, 33* (Suppl. 5), 9–12.
Barnes, G. (Ed.), (1977). *Transactional analysis after Eric Berne.* New York: Harper's College Press.
Baumgart, D., Johnson, J., & Helmstetter, E. (1990). *Augmentative and alternative communication systems for persons with moderate and severe disabilities.* Baltimore: Paul H. Brookes.
Behrmann, M. (1995). Assistive technology training. In K. Flippo, K. Inge, & M. Barcus (Eds.), *Assistive technology: A resource for school, work, and community* (pp. 211–222). Baltimore: Paul H. Brookes.
Berry, J. O. (1987). Strategies for involving parents in programs for young children using augmentative and alternative communication. *Augmentative and Alternative Communication, 3* (2), 90–93.
Beukelman, D. (1991). Magic and cost of communicative competence. *Augmentative and Alternative Communication, 7,* 2–10.
Beukelman, D., & Mirenda, P. (Eds.). (1992), *Augmentative and alternative communication: Management of severe communication disorders in children and adults.* Baltimore: Paul H. Brookes.
Beukelman, D. R., Yorkston, K. M., & Dowden, P. A. (1985). *Communication augmentation: A casebook of clinical management,* San Diego, California: College Hill Press.
Blackstone, S. W. (Ed.). (1986), *Augmentative communication: An introduction.* Rockville, MD: American Speech-Language-Hearing Association.
Blackstone, S. (1989). Future issues. *Augmentative Communication News, 2* (2), 2.
Bootzin, R., Bower, G., Zajonc, R., & Hall, E. (1986). *Psychology Today: An Introduction.* New York: Harper & Row.

Canseler, D., Martin, G., & Valand, M. (1975). *Working with families.* Winston-Salem, NC: Kaplan Press.

Church, G., & Glennen, S. (1992). *The handbook of assistive technology.* San Diego, CA: Singular Publishing.

Corey, G. (1991). *Theory and practice of counseling and psychotherapy* (4th ed.). Los Angeles, CA: Brooks/Cole.

Dillard, J. (1988). *Multicultural counseling, toward ethnic and cultural relevance in human encounters.* Chicago: Nelson-Hall.

Dinkmeyer, D., & Carlson, J. (1973). *Consulting: Facilitating human potential and change processes.* Columbus, Ohio: Charles E. Merrill.

Dybwad, G. (1995). Foreword (pp. i–ii). In H. Mittler (Ed.), *Families speak out: International perspectives on families' experiences of disability.* Cambridge, MA: Brookline Books.

Fey, M. E. (1986). *Language intervention with young children.* Boston: College Hill Press.

Fishman, I. (1987). *Electronic communication aids selection and use.* Boston: College Hill Press.

Fried-Oken, M., & More, L. (1992). An initial vocabulary for nonspeaking preschool children based on developmental and environmental language sources. *Augmentative and Alternative Communication, 8,* 41–56.

Garrett, K. (1992). Adults with severe aphasia. In D. Beukelman, and P. Mirenda (Eds.), (1992). *Augmentative and alternative communication: Management of severe communication disorders in children and adults* (pp. 331–343). Baltimore: Paul H. Brookes.

George, R., & Cristiani, T. (1986). *Counseling: Theory and practice.* Englewood Cliffs, NJ: Prentice-Hall.

Glasser, W. (1965). *Reality therapy.* New York: Harper & Row.

Harrison-Harris, O., & Soto, G. (1994). *Assistive technology: ASHA's building bridges: Mulitcultural preschool project.* Rockville, MD: American Speech-Language-Hearing Association.

Herr, J., & Weakland, J. (1979). *Counseling elders and their families: Practical techniques for applied gerontology.* New York: Springer-Verlag.

Huer, M. (1993). *A master's program in speech-language pathology with special emphasis in augmentative and alternative communication and multiculturalism* (1994–1999) Funded through the U.S. Department of Education, Preparation of Personnel/Careers in Special Education, CFDA 84.029B (Grant Award Number:H029B40232).

Huer, M. (1994). *Diversity now: Multicultural issues in AAC.* A miniseminar presented at the National Annual Meeting for the American Speech-Language-Hearing Association, New Orleans, LA.

Huer, M. (1995). *A multicultural perspective of AAC Needs of school children and their families.* A Teleseminar at the Visions Conference for the American Speech-Language-Hearing Association, Atlanta, GA.

Huer, M., & Lloyd, L. (1990). AAC users' perspectives on augmentative and alternative communication. *Augmentative and Alternative Communication, 6,* 242–249.

Huer, M., & Soto, G. (1996). *Critical and emerging issues in AAC across cultures.* A miniseminar proposal submitted for the Meeting of the International Society for Augmentative and Alternative Communication (ISAAC), Vancouver, BC.

Jageman, L., & Myers, J. (1986). *Counseling mentally retarded adults: A procedures and training manual.* University of Wisconsin-Stout, WI: School of Education and Human Services.

King, P., & Neal, R. (1968). *Ego psychology in counseling.* Boston: Houghton Mifflin.

Kirstein, I. J., Peters, N. A., Cottier, C., & Blau, R. (1988). Establishing a parent support group (pp. 6–1–6–2). In *Augmentative communication: Implementation strategies.* Rockville, MD: American Speech-Language-Hearing Association.

Koppenhaver, D., Evans, D., & Yoder, D. (1991). Childhood reading and writing experiences of literate adults with severe speech and motor impairments. *Augmentative and Alternative Communication, 7,* 20–33.

Kreps, G., & Kunimoto, E. (1994). *Effective communication in multicultural health care settings.* Beverly Hills, CA: Sage Publications.

Lynch, E., & Hanson, M. (1992). *Developing cross-cultural competence: A guide for working with young children and their families.* Baltimore: Paul H. Brookes.

McFarlane, S. C., Fujiki, M., & Brinton, B. (1984). *Coping with communicative handicaps: Resources for the practicing clinician.* San Diego, CA: College Hill Press.

Mittler, H. (1995). *Families speak out: International perspectives on families' experiences of disability.* Cambridge, MA: Brookline Books.

Moore, T. (1985). *Soul mates: Honoring the mysteries of love and relationship.* New York: Harper Collins.

Moses, K. L. (1985). Dynamic intervention with families (pp. 82–98). *In hearing-impaired children and youth with developmental disabilities: An interdisciplinary foundation for service.* Washington, DC: Gallaudet College Press.

Musselwhite, C. R., & St. Louis, K. W. (1988). *Communication programming for persons with severe handicaps: Vocal and augmentative strategies.* Boston: College Hill Press.

Pedersen, P., Draguns, J., Lonner, W., & Trimble, J. (1976). *Counseling across cultures.* Honolulu, HI : The University Press of Hawaii.

Pedersen, P., Draguns, J., Lonner, W., & Trimble, J. (1989). *Counseling across cultures.* Honolulu: University of Hawaii Press.

Ponterotto, J. , Casas, J., Suzuki, L., & Alexander, C. (1995). *Handbook of multicultural counseling.* Beverly Hills, CA: Sage Publications.

Reichle, J., York, J., & Sigafoos, J. (1991). *Implementing Augmentative and Alternative Communication: Strategies for Learners with Severe Disabilities.* Baltimore, MD: Paul H. Brookes.

Salisbury, C., & Evans, I. M. (1988). Comparison of parental involvement in regular and special education. *The Journal of the Association for Persons with Severe Handicaps, 13*(4), 268–272.

Schaffer, R. (1993). *Racial and ethnic groups.* New York: Harper Collins.

Soto, G., Huer, M., & Taylor, O. (in press). Multicultural issues in augmentative and alternative communication, In L. Lloyd, D. Fuller, & H. Arvidson (Eds.), *Augmentative and alternative communication.* Newton, MA: Allyn and Bacon.

Taylor, O. (1994). Communication and communication disorders in a multicultural society (pp. 43–76). In F. Minifie, (Ed.) *Introduction to communication sciences and disorders.* San Diego, CA: Singular Publishing.

Wolfgang, A. (Ed.). (1984). *Nonverbal Behavior: Perspectives, Applications, Intercultural Insights.* New York: C. J. Hogrefe, Inc.

Wyatt, T.(1995). *Cross-cultural communication and learning style differences in culturally diverse child populations.* Unpublished paper, California State University-Fullerton, Fullerton, CA.

Yorkston, K. (1992). *Augmentative communication in the medical setting.* Tucson, AZ: Communication Skill Builders, Inc.

Yorkston, K., Dowden, P., Honsinger, M., Marriner, N., & Smith, K. (1988). A comparison of standard and user vocabulary lists. *Augmentative and Alternative Communication, 4,* 189–210.

Yorkston, K., Fried-Oken, M., & Beukelman, D. (1988). Single word vocabulary needs: Studies from various non-speaking populations. *Augmentative and Alternative Communication, 4,* 149.

Yorkston, K., Smith, K., Miller, R., & Hillel, A. (1991). *Augmentative and alternative communication in amyotrophic lateral sclerosis.* Unpublished manuscript, University of Washington, Seattle, WA.

## Appendix 15.1. Initial Assessment Consideration in AAC

### FACT SHEET 1: EVALUATION

Augmentative and alternative communication evaluations are multi-dimensional. Frequently, an AAC evaluation is transdisciplinary and may incorporate information from different professional practitioners. Consumers using AAC for communication typically have special needs. It is important for the clinician to compile as much information as possible, regarding all the skills of the client, during a first meeting. Experience as a clinician has suggested that there are 15 areas in which the initial information should be collected before determination of the need for AAC or not. A practitioner need not personally assess each of the 15 areas, rather he or she may compile descriptive information from a variety of team members to summarize the skills of the consumer.

*15 Areas for Assessment in AAC (initial Assessment, not in any order)*

Auditory perception and memory
Visual memory and perception
Cognitive skills including the ability to handle codes
Environmental constraints and attitudes/experiences within the home, school, and community, including support services/persons
Suitability of graphic systems, including traditional orthography, pictures, symbols, etc.
Gross and fine motor skills
Hand use skill, including finger dexterity
Interactive language skills across partners and situations
Method(s) of access to system/technique
Mobility
Paralinguistic aspects of language, such as facial expression and natural gesture
Positioning/seating needs for the potential AAC users as well as for the technique or system
Receptive and Expressive language

Speech (phonetic inventory)
Efficiency of Present Communication, Across Partners

REFERENCE

Huer, M. B. (1987). 1986 ISAAC Round Table Discussion—Formal assessment tools: What we have, what we
    need. *The ISAAC Bulletin, 10,* 14

## Appendix 15.2. Evaluation for Fit and Selection of AAC Systems and Components: A Process for Decision Making

The selection of components within AAC systems is a process. Technology is expensive and should not be purchased without careful consideration of multiple parameters. A review of the literature suggests that there are approximately 25 to 30 different issues which should be considered before the clinician determines the type and nature of the components of a consumer's AAC system.

Critical Parameters for Fit and Selection of AAC Systems and Components mutually exclusive, but not in any order:
Openness
Environmental Control Functions
Speed, Rate
Ease of Learning for User
Assertability
Reliability
Display Permanence
Privacy
Projection
Ease of Setup
Correctability
Ease of Learning for Receiver
Expandability
Physical Construction
Portability
Vocabulary Manipulation
Independence
Output Format
Intelligibility
Cognitive Selection Method
Appropriateness
Response Set, Physical Array
Durability
Representational System, Set
Cost
Reflective of Cultural Diversity
Cosmesis
Vocabulary Size
Training
Mirrors Communication Patterns, Styles of Consumer using the system and their family
Adaptability
Interdevice Compatibility

REFERENCES

Blackstone, S. W. (1986). *Augmentative communication: An introduction.* ASHA. [See Chapter 3 by Vanderheiden and Lloyd]. ASHA: Rockville, MD.

Cook, A. M., & Coleman, C. L. (1987). Selecting augmentative communication systems by matching client skills and needs to system characteristics. *Seminar in Speech and Language, 8* (2), 153–167.

Fishman, I. (1987). *Electronic communication aids selection and use.* Boston: College Hill Press.

Rosen, M. J., & Goodenough-Trepagnier, C. (1989). The Tufts-MIT prescription guide: Assessment of users to predict the suitability of augmentative communication devices. *Assistive Technology, 1,* 51–61.

## Appendix 15.3. Selected Publishers/Manufacturers of Augmentative and Alternative Communication Equipment/Materials for the Child Using AAC

Ablenet Inc., 1081 Tenth Avenue S. E., Minneapolis, MN 55414–1312, 800–322-0956

Crestwood Company, 6625 N. Sidney Place, Milwaukee, WI 53209–3259, 414–352-5678

Don Johnston Developmental Equipment, Inc., P. O. Box 639, 1000 N. Rand Road 115, Wauconda, IL 60084–0639, 708–526-2682 or 800–999-4660

Imaginart Communication Products, 307 Arizona Street, Bisbee, AZ 85603, 800–828-1376

IntelliTools, Inc., 55 Leveroni Court, Suite 9, Novato, CA 94949, 800–899-6687

Mayer-Johnson Company, P. O. Box 1579, Solana Beach, CA 920751579, 619–550-0084

Prentke Romich Company, 1022 Heyl Road, Wooster, Ohio 44691, 216–262-1984 or 800–262-1984

Sentient Systems Inc., 2100 Wharton, Suite 630, Pittsburgh, PA 15203, 412–381-4883 or 800–344-778

Southeast Augmentative Communication Publications, 2430 11th Avenue North, Birmingham, AL 35234, 205–251-0165

TASH, Inc. (Technical Aids & Systems for the Handicapped), Unit 1–91 Station Street, Ajax, Ontario, Canada L1S 3H2, 905–686-4129 or 800–463-5685

Words+, Inc., 40015 Sierra Highway, Building B-145, Palmdale, CA 93550, 800–869-8521

Zygo Industries, Inc., P. O. Box 1008, Portland, OR 97207–1008, 800–234-6006

## Appendix 15.4. Organizational Alliances for AAC in the USA

United States Society for Augmentative and Alternative Communication (USSAAC)
P. O. Box 5271
Evanston, IL 60204–5271
Phone: 847–869-2122; FAX: 847–869-2161;
America On-Line: USSAAC; Internet: USSAAC@aol.com

ASHA Special Interest Division, SID #12 for AAC
American Speech Language Hearing Association
10801 Rockville Pike
Rockville, Maryland 20852
Phone: 301–897-5700

RESNA, SIG-03, Special Interest Group on AAC
Suite 1540
1700 N. Moore Street
Arlington, VA 22209–1903
Phone: 703–524-6686

## Appendix 15.5.  Competencies for the Practice of AAC

1. Knowledgeable of Academic Content
    a. Knows history and development of AAC
    b. Knows AAC components, techniques, and strategies
    c. Knows characteristics of disabling conditions and implications for evaluation/intervention
    d. Knows principles of assessment
    e. Knows variety of evaluation instruments
    f. Knows available and effective materials and devices for effecting AAC
    g. Knows roles of interdisciplinary team members
    h. Knows funding sources and how to access
    i. Knows child development and AAC procedures for very young children
2. Demonstrates ability to evaluate AAC candidacy
    a. Uses screening procedures
    b. Uses comprehensive evaluation instruments
    c. Interprets evaluation information
3. Demonstrates ability to plan and implement AAC
    a. Selects and uses AAC components (e.g., symbols, communication devices, and so forth
    b. Uses techniques for developing interaction
4. Works effectively as part of interdisciplinary team
    a. Plans and participates as SLP in AAC evaluation, according to feedback of planning, and intervention professionals of other disciplines
    b. Communicates with other members of interdisciplinary team
5. Serves as advocate for AAC
    a. Knows updated information on laws impacting on AAC
    b. Utilizes community and professional resources on behalf of AAC client
6. Demonstrates professionalization in interactions with clients
    a. Participates in consultation and counseling AAC user
    b. Presents inservice training

Note: This form was developed with the assistance of Carole Zangari and Raymond Quist while Mary Blake Huer was a Postdoctoral Fellow at Purdue University.

## Appendix 15.6.  Multicultural Bibliography

Adler, S. (1993). *Multicultural communication skills in the classroom.* Boston: Allyn and Bacon.
Battle, D. E. (1993). *Communication disorders in multicultural populations.* Boston: Andover Medical Publishers.
Clark, L. W. (1993). *Faculty and student challenges in facing cultural and linguistic diversity.* Springfield, Illinois: Charles C Thomas.

Conklin, N. F., & Lourie, M. A. (1983). *A host of tongues: Language communities in the United States.* New York: The Free Press.

Damico, J. S., & Hamayan, E. V. (1992). *Multicultural language intervention.* Buffalo, NY: EDUCOM Associates, Inc.

Gudykunst, W. B. (1994). *Bridging differences: Effective intergroup communication* (2nd ed.). Beverly Hills, CA: Sage Publications.

Gudykunst, W. B., & Kim, Y. Y. (1992). *Communicating with strangers: An approach to intercultural communication* (2nd ed.). New York: McGraw-Hill.

Gudykunst, W. B., & Nishida, T. (1994). *Bridging Japanese/North American differences.* Beverly Hills, CA: Sage Publications.

Gudykunst, W. B., Ting-Toomey, S., Sudweeks, S., & Stewart, L. P. (1995). *Building bridges: Interpersonal skills for a changing world.* Boston: Houghton Mifflin.

Hamayan, E. V., & Damico, J. S. (1991). *Limiting bias in the assessment of bilingual students.* Austin, TX: Pro-Ed.

Harry, B. (1995). *Cultural diversity, families, and the special education system.* New York: Teachers College Press, Columbia University.

Kayser, H. (1995). *Bilingual speech-Language pathology: An Hispanic focus.* San Diego, CA: Singular Publishing.

Kelly, M. M., & DeVito, J. A. (1990). *Experiences activities manual to accompany messages: Building interpersonal communication skills.* New York: Harper & Row.

Kreps, G. L., & Kunimoto, E. N. (1994). *Effective communication in multicultural health care settings.* Beverly Hills, CA: Sage Publications.

Langdon, H. W., & Cheng, L. (1992). *Hispanic children and adults with communication disorders.* Rockville, MD: Aspen Systems.

Lynch, E. W., & Hanson, M. J. (1992). *Developing cross-cultural competence: A guide for working with young children and their families.* Baltimore: Paul H. Brookes.

Ponterotto, J., Casas, J., Suzuki, L., & Alexander, C. (1995). *Handbook of Multicultural Counseling.* Thousand Oaks, CA: Sage Publications.

Roseberry-McKibbin, C. (1995). *Multicultural students with special language needs: Practical strategies for assessment and intervention.* Oceanside, CA: Academic Communication Associates (1995).

Screen, R. M., & Anderson, N. B. (1994). *Multicultural perspectives in communication disorders.* San Diego, CA: Singular Publishing.

Taylor, O. L. (Ed.) (1986). *Nature of communication disorders in culturally and linguistically diverse populations.* Austin: Pro-Ed.

Taylor, O. L. (Ed.) (1986). *Treatment of communication disorders in culturally and linguistically diverse populations.* Boston: College Hill Press.

Valletutti, P. J., McKnight-Taylor, M., & Hoffnung, A. S. (1989). *Facilitating communications in young children with handicapping conditions: A guide for special educators.* Boston: College-Hill Press.

## Appendix 15.7. Necessary Competencies for Practice Across Cultures

1. Knowledgeable of academic content
   a. knows history, development, attitudes, policy of multiculturalism
   b. knows grammatical/phonological features of non-English languages such as Spanish, and nonstandard English dialects such as African-American English
   c. awareness of the cross-cultural differences in communicative behavior among culturally/linguistically diverse populations

    d. understanding of normal speech/language acquisition in the second language/ dialect of bilingual/bidialectal child speakers

2. Demonstrates ability to evaluate linguistically diverse persons:
    a. uses screening procedures
    b. uses comprehensive evaluation instruments
    c. interprets evaluation information
    d. competence in assessment, diagnosis and intervention when providing services to bilingual/bicultural clients

3. Demonstrates ability to plan and implement therapy
    a. identify the characteristics associated with disorders in culturally diverse populations
    b. accurately differentiate between difference and disorder in bilingual and non-standard English speaking populations
    c. evaluate strengths and weaknesses of current assessment and treatment approaches for culturally/linguistically diverse clients
    d. design an appropriate intervention for culturally/linguistically diverse clients
    e. design an appropriate intervention and/or English as a Second Language (ESL) instruction program for culturally/linguistically diverse students/clients

4. Works effectively as part of interdisciplinary team
    a. uses culturally sensitive interview and counseling techniques
    b. conducts a nonbiased assessment
    c. evaluates non-native English and ESL or Standard English as a Second Dialect (SESD) instruction
    d. communicates with other members of interdisciplinary team

5. Serves as advocate for multicultural persons (MC)
    a. knows updated policy and laws impacting on MC
    b. utilizes community & professional resources on behalf of client

6. Demonstrates professionalization in interactions with clients

# Index

Page numbers in *italics* denote figures; those followed by "t" denote tables.